EXERCISE IN PREGNANCY

EXERCISE IN PREGNANCY

Editors

Raul Artal (Mittelmark), M.D.

Associate Professor
Obstetrics, Gynecology, Physical Education
and Exercise Sciences
Department of Obstetrics and Gynecology
Division of Maternal-Fetal Medicine
and the Department of Physical Education
and Exercise Sciences
University of Southern California School of Medicine,
Los Angeles, California

Robert A. Wiswell, Ph.D.

Associate Professor and Chairman
Department of Physical Education and
Exercise Sciences
Research Associate
Andrus Gerontology Center
University of Southern California
Los Angeles, California

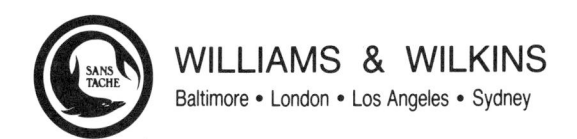

WILLIAMS & WILKINS
Baltimore • London • Los Angeles • Sydney

Editor: Carol-Lynn Brown
Associate Editor: Victoria M. Vaughn
Copy Editor: William Vinck
Design: Bob Och
Illustration Planning: Reginald R. Stanley
Production: Raymond E. Reter

Copyright ©, 1986
Williams & Wilkins
428 East Preston Street
Baltimore, MD 21202, U.S.A.

All rights reserved. This book is protected by copyright. No part of this book may be reproduced in any form or by any means, including photocopying, or utilized by any information storage and retrieval system without written permission from the copyright owner.

Accurate indications, adverse reactions, and dosage schedules for drugs are provided in this book, but it is possible that they may change. The reader is urged to review the package information data of the manufacturers of the medications mentioned.

Printed in the United States of America

Library of Congress Cataloging in Publication Data

Main entry under title:

Artal, Raul.
   Exercise in pregnancy.

   Includes bibliographies and index.
   1. Pregnancy. 2. Exercise for women—Physiological aspects. I. Wiswell, Robert A. II. Title. [DNLM: 1. Exertion—in pregnancy. 2. Pregnancy. WQ 200 A784e]
RG558.7.A77 1986   618.2′4   85-9270
ISBN 0-683-00257-0

Composed and printed at the   85 86 87 88 89
Waverly Press, Inc.   10 9 8 7 6 5 4 3 2 1

This book is dedicated to our children:
Roy, Dalia, Orna, Grant and Gavin

Foreword

Exercise has become a way of life for a significant portion of our population. Whether it prolongs life is still a hotly debated question, with the most recent evidence seeming to favor a longer life for the individual who continues to exercise. However, there is little question that the person who exercises regularly feels better both physically and psychologically.

The amount of exercise performed by an individual varies widely from the runner who covers 60–100 miles per week to the walker who spends one-half hour every evening doing a brisk walk.

The question facing a woman when she becomes pregnant is not whether she should exercise; obstetricians have recommended exercise in normally pregnant women for years. The major question is how much exercise will benefit both mother and fetus? A supplemental question relates to the amount of exercise tolerated in an abnormal pregnancy (i.e., preterm labor, hypertension or diabetes in pregnancy, etc.). Before one can answer these questions it is necessary to understand the normal physiologic changes which occur during pregnancy and how they are altered by exercise. Drs. Artal and Wiswell have approached the problem in a very methodical way by delineating the principles of exercise physiology, examining the work done in animals, examining the physiologic changes of normal pregnancy, looking at how these responses are altered by exercise during pregnancy, and examining the fetal response to maternal exercise.

I think this is an important book which should be read by all physicians who attempt to advise pregnant women with regard to an exercise program.

E. J. Quilligan, M.D.
Professor and Chairman
Department of Obstetrics and Gynecology
University of California at Davis
Davis, California
January 22, 1985

Preface

The impetus for writing a book on exercise in pregnancy stemmed from a common interest we shared for the past 5 years. The fascination with and the contemporary attitudes toward physical fitness are frequently carried into pregnancy. Unfortunately, no standards for exercise in pregnancy are available. Pursuing a common interest has allowed invaluable interactions between exercise physiologists and obstetricians. We set out to compile existing information and yet no authoritative source could be identified. The information that we have initially reviewed was rather scarce, anectodal, and largely related to animal studies.

We see our attempt as a first step toward creating a reference source for exercise prescription in pregnancy. We have included much of our own data; many of the opinions expressed in the book are our own. Some of the opinions may be biased and are based upon long hours of study and observation of pregnant women exercising under laboratory conditions.

We hope this book will generate a stimulus for new research that will help solve the question posed throughout the text: Is exercise beneficial and safe for the mother and her fetus?

Much of the data presented in this text have been the product of collaboration. We would like to express our gratitude to all the contributors who have joined us in this endeavor. We are also very indebted to our research associates whose contribution and input was invaluable: Rao Kammula, Lydia Puglisi, Nazareth Khodiguian, and Fred Dorey. Also, many thanks to the hundreds of volunteers who were willing to accept our curiosity as researchers. Thanks also to our editors Carol-Lynn Brown and Victoria Vaughn for their dedication and for sharing our enthusiasm.

It is our hope that this book will provide a useful resource for all those interested in this topic.

Raul Artal, M.D.
Robert A. Wiswell, Ph.D.

Contributors

Raul Artal (Mittelmark), M.D.
Associate Professor
Obstetrics, Gynecology and Physical Education and Exercise Sciences
Department of Obstetrics and Gynecology
Division of Maternal-Fetal Medicine and Department of Physical Education and Exercise Sciences
University of Southern California School of Medicine
Los Angeles, California

Samuel P. Bessman, M.D.
Professor and Chairman
Department of Pharmacology and Nutrition
University of Southern California School of Medicine
Los Angeles, California

Gail Butterfield, Ph.D., R.D.
Assistant Professor of Nutrition
Department of Nutritional Sciences
University of California
Berkeley, California

Denys J. Court, M.B., Ch.B.
Senior Lecturer
Department of Obstetrics and Gynecology
National Women's Hospital
Auckland, New Zealand

Val Davajan, M.D.
Professor Department of Obstetrics and Gynecology
Division of Endocrinology and Infertility
University of Southern California School of Medicine
Los Angeles, California

Marc J. Friedman, M.D.
Co-Director, Diagnostic Knee Clinic, UCLA
Los Angeles, California
Consultant, New York Jet Football Team and
New York Knicks Basketball Team

Susan Kelemen Gardin, M.S., R.P.T., M.P.H.
Doctoral Candidate
School of Public Health
Division of Population, Family and International Health
University of California
Los Angeles, California

Raymond D. Gilbert, Ph.D.
Professor of Physiology, Obstetrics and Gynecology
Division of Perinatal Biology
Department of Physiology
Loma Linda University School of Medicine
Loma Linda, California

Jeffrey Greenspoon, M.D.
Instructor, Maternal-Fetal Medicine
Department of Obstetrics and Gynecology
Division of Maternal-Fetal Medicine
University of Southern California School of Medicine
Los Angeles, California

Janet C. King, Ph.D.
Professor of Nutrition
Department of Nutritional Sciences
University of California
Berkeley, California

Brian J. Koos, M.D., D.Phil.
Assistant Professor of Physiology, Obstetrics and Gynecology
Division of Perinatal Biology
Loma Linda University School of Medicine
Loma Linda, California

Lawrence D. Longo, M.D.
Professor of Physiology, Obstetrics and Gynecology
Division of Perinatal Biology
Department of Physiology
Loma Linda University School of Medicine
Loma Linda, California

Frederick K. Lotgering, M.D., Ph.D.
Department of Obstetrics and Gynecology
Erasmus University
Rotterdam, The Netherlands

James Metcalfe, M.D.
Professor of Medicine
Oregon Heart Association
Chairman of Cardiovascular Research
Oregon Health Sciences University
Portland, Oregon

Mark J. Morton, M.D.
Assistant Professor of Medicine
Oregon Health Sciences University
Portland, Oregon

Julian T. Parer, M.D., Ph.D.
Professor and Director of Obstetrics
Associate Staff
Cardiovascular Research Institute
University of California, San Francisco, California

Gordon G. Power, M.D.
Professor of Physiology and Obstetrics and Gynecology
Division of Perinatal Biology
Department of Physiology
Loma Linda University School of Medicine
Loma Linda, California

Edward J. Quilligan, M.D.
Professor and Chairman
Department of Obstetrics and Gynecology
University of California at Davis
Davis, California
Editor, *American Journal of Obstetrics and Gynecology*

Yitzhak Romem, M.D.
Instructor, Maternal-Fetal Medicine
Department of Obstetrics and Gynecology
Division of Maternal/Fetal Medicine
University of Southern California
School of Medicine
Los Angeles, California

Wendy E. St. John Repovich
Doctoral Candidate
Department of Physical Education and Exercise Sciences
University of Southern California
Los Angeles, California

Janet P. Wallace, Ph.D.
Assistant Professor of Physical Education
Director, Adult Fitness
San Diego State University
San Diego, California

Robert A. Wiswell, Ph.D.
Associate Professor and Chairman
Department of Physical Education and Exercise Sciences
Research Associate
Andrus Gerontology Center
University of Southern California
Los Angeles, California

Itzhak Zaidise, M.D., Ph.D.
Department of Pharmacology and Nutrition
University of Southern California
School of Medicine
Los Angeles, California

Contents

Foreword		vii
Preface		ix
Contributors		xi

Chapter 1	Historical Perspectives Raul Artal and Susan Kelemen Gardin		1
Chapter 2	Exercise Physiology Robert A. Wiswell		7
Chapter 3	Exercise in Pregnancy in the Experimental Animal Frederick K. Lotgering, Raymond D. Gilbert, and Lawrence D. Longo		21
Chapter 4	The Effect of Exercise on the Menstrual Cycle Val Davajan		51
Chapter 5	Physiological and Endocrine Adjustments to Pregnancy Yitzhak Romem and Raul Artal		59
Chapter 6	Fuel Metabolism in Pregnancy Itzhak Zaidise, Raul Artal, and Samuel P. Bessman		83
Chapter 7	Nutritional Needs of Physically Active Pregnant Women Janet C. King and Gail Butterfield		99
Chapter 8	Changes in Maternal Hemodynamics during Pregnancy Mark J. Morton and James Metcalfe		113
Chapter 9	Maternal Cardiovascular Response to Exercise during Pregnancy Janet P. Wallace, Robert A. Wiswell, and Raul Artal		127
Chapter 10	Hormonal Responses to Exercise in Pregnancy Raul Artal		139
Chapter 11	Pulmonary Responses to Exercise in Pregnancy Raul Artal, Robert A. Wiswell, Jeffrey Greenspoon, and Yitzhak Romem		147
Chapter 12	Placental Oxygen Transfer with Considerations for Maternal Exercise Brian J. Koos, Gordon G. Power, and Lawrence D. Longo		155
Chapter 13	Altered States of Fetal Circulation Julian T. Parer and Denys J. Court		181
Chapter 14	Fetal Responses to Maternal Exercise Raul Artal and Yitzhak Romem		195
Chapter 15	Sports Activities and Aerobic Exercise during Pregnancy Wendy E. St. John Repovich, Robert A. Wiswell, and Raul Artal		205

Chapter 16 Orthopaedic Problems in Pregnancy
            Marc J. Friedman 215
Chapter 17 Exercise Prescription in Pregnancy
            Raul Artal and Robert A. Wiswell 225

Index 229

1
Historical Perspectives

In recent years there has been a dramatic increase in the number of women engaging in physical fitness activities. The exercise spirit has enraptured women of all ages, including women in their childbearing years. Confronted suddenly with this revolution, health care providers, obstetricians in particular, are faced with many questions: What are the effects of exercise on the mother and her fetus? What types of exercise? How much exercise is safe? Who may exercise in pregnancy? What are the legal and ethical issues involved in recommending prenatal exercise? And, finally, is exercise necessary or desirable in pregnancy? Answers to the above questions remain indefinite as there is no convincing evidence that exercise in pregnancy is either beneficial or harmful vis-à-vis labor, delivery, and birth outcomes.

Throughout history, recommendations for exercise were based on "commonsense" notions of the relationship between maternal physical activity and birth outcomes. In biblical times it was recognized that Hebrew slave women had easier labors than their Egyptian masters: " . . . the Hebrew women are not as the Egyptian women; for they are lively, and are delivered ere the midwife come unto them" (Exodus 1:19). One may speculate that Hebrew slave women, while being physically prepared for the demands of childbirth, delivered relatively small infants. Another possible explanation is a higher incidence of premature precipitous deliveries. Conversely, the sedentary lifestyles of Egyptian women predisposed them to the delivery of large babies and associated dystocia.

In the third century B.C., Aristotle also attributed difficult childbirth to a sedentary maternal life-style (1). Two thousand years later, James Lucas (1788), surgeon at the Leeds General Infirmary in England, strongly advocated maternal exercise in a paper presented to the Medical Society of London. Lucas suggested that maternal exercise could decrease the size of the infant and allow easier passage through the maternal pelvis (2).

The philosophy of the 18th century was to encourage exercise, albeit with strong limitations. In 1781 Alexander Hamilton (1781) published his *Treatise of Midwifery*. In the chapter entitled, "Rules and Cautions for the Conduct of Pregnant Women," he cautioned pregnant women to exercise only in moderation, avoiding "agitation of the body from violent or improper exercise, as jolting in a carriage, riding on horseback, dancing and whatever disturbs the body or mind" (2).

Although the concept of "moderation" was not based on scientific research, it was consistently maintained up to and including much of the 20th century. Further, it was enforced by moral exhortations regarding the responsibilities of the pregnant woman. In an 1892 book entitled *Advice to Women in the Care of their Health before, during and after Confinement*, the author writes: "When you neglect, risk or injure your own health during pregnancy, you do a direct injustice to, and commit a real crime against your unborn baby" (3).

The 19th century also brought forth the first serious attempts at scientific examination of the relationship between maternal activity and birth outcomes. In 1895, A. Pinard published a study of 1000 births demonstrating a relationship between social class and birth weight. He explained this by differential physical activity in women of heterogenous social classes (4). Letourneur published a similar study in 1896, based on 627 deliveries in Paris, and concluded that physical work at the end of pregnancy was a stronger determinant of birth weight than maternal morphology. He commented that "robust" women engaged in strenuous work (e.g., housemaids) delivered infants of lower birth weight than thinner women involved in less demanding work (e.g., florists) (4). In 1917, Peller published data in Vienna demonstrating that maternal rest resulted in higher birth weights and lower perinatal mortality (5). Naeye and Peters (5) have more recently analyzed the outcome of 7722 pregnancies in four different groups of working women defined by: (*a*) presence or absence of children at home, and (*b*) home or outside employment. Their results suggest that women who have standing jobs and children at home deliver infants who have significantly lower birth weights.

At the turn of the century, there was concern in several countries about the poor health of volunteer recruits for military service. In England, it was estimated that only two-fifths of volunteers were in acceptable health for military service (6). Many British politicians expressed dismay about the "declining quality" of the British population (6). The studies of Pinard, Letourneur, Peller, and others provided a logical plan for improving the quality of the progeny. Legislation was enacted in England, as well as Holland, Belgium, Portugal, Austria, and Switzerland, prohibiting the employment of pregnant women in factories during the 2–4 weeks preceding childbirth and the 4–6 weeks following childbirth (7). Despite the fact that analogous concerns were voiced in the United States, similar legislation was not adopted (8). Neither was such legislation adopted in Turkey, Russia, Spain, Italy, or France (7).

Moderation in exercise and the need for outdoor air were the two themes of the early 20th century. A handbook for "prospective mothers" published in 1913 contained the following recommendations:

The amount of exercise which the prospective mother should take cannot be stated precisely, but what can be definitely said is this — she should stop the moment she begins to feel tired . . . Women who have laborious household duties to perform do not require as much exercise as those who lead sedentary lives; but they do require just as much fresh air. . . .

Walking is the best kind of exercise . . . Most women who are pregnant find that a two to three mile walk daily is all they enjoy, and very few are inclined to indulge in six miles, which is generally accepted as the upper limit. . . .

Very few outdoor sports can be unconditionally recommended to a prospective mother. Because athletic exercise is either too violent or else jolts the body a great deal, it is especially dangerous in the early months of pregnancy. . . .

All kinds of violent exertion should be avoided—a rule which at once excludes sweeping, scrubbing, laundry work, lifting anyting that is heavy, and going up and down stairs hurriedly or frequently. The use of a sewing machine is also emphatically forbidden (7).

The expanding list of arbitrary restrictions on activity during pregnancy were derived more from the cultural and social biases of each era than from scientific investigations. A 1935 book entitled *Modern Motherhood* allowed pregnant women to bathe, swim, golf, and engage in ballroom dance, while warning against the danger of excessive walking:

The expectant mother must, of necessity, curtail her usual physical activities because of her extra burden . . . she cannot exercise more than she is accustomed to; she should exercise less. She should not be persuaded to walk a lot because walking is supposed to make birth easier—this superstition is hundreds of years old and still prevalent (9).

The author also prohibits horseback riding and tennis, but notes that some expectant mothers indulge in these and like activities "with impunity."

While it is difficult to analyze the impact of various life-styles on pregnancy outcomes, it is clear that this question preoccupies contemporary researchers much as it did ancient and medieval thinkers. One may speculate as to possible differences in the pregnancy impact of pleasurable versus stressful work-related physical activity.

In the 1930s, a novel, different, and avant-garde approach to prenatal exercise was initiated: the specialized and unique prenatal exercise program. In England, Kathleen Vaughan advocated improving joint flexibility during pregnancy. The squat position was encouraged with promises of a widened pelvic outlet. Women were urged to adopt tailor-sitting positions and perform pelvic floor exercises in an attempt to prevent tears of the perineum. Women were also encouraged to perform breathing and posture exercises to improve fetal oxygenation and maternal health (10). Margaret Morris promoted maternal exercise from an entirely new slant: She promised improved appearance "in both face and figure" following childbirth as a result of maternity exercises (9). Dick Read developed specific progressive breathing patterns and aphysical exercises for improving health, muscle-tone and "sense of well-being," as well as decreasing the pain of childbirth (11). The psychoprophylaxis method of childbirth was also being developed during this time in Russia, although it was not introduced to the West until the 1940s by Dr. Fernand Lamaze (11).

The advice of the new prenatal programs was clearly directed at achieving new goals: first, the programs attempted to provide the pregnant woman with a sense that she could develop skills for controlling her experience of childbirth; second, there was a new emphasis on the prospective mother's "non-maternal" interests, both psychological and physical; third, there was a strong emphasis on the positive and active, i.e., what the pregnant woman could accomplish rather than what she was prohibited from attempting.

In the 1940s, the avant-garde recommendations of the 1930s were quietly ignored in favor of more traditional advice regarding moderation and fresh air. In a 1942 book entitled *Getting Ready to Be a Mother*, the following instructions appeared:

Regular out-of-door exercise promotes digestion, stimulates the activity of the skin and lungs, steadies the nerves, quiets the mind, and promotes sleep. Walking, which is probably the most satisfactory form of exercise, also strengthens some of the muscles that are used during labor ... The woman who does her own housework may not need additional exercise, but may get her quota of fresh air by resting out of doors each day. Hard work, such as washing, heavy lifting or much running up and down stairs, should not be the lot of the expectant mother.

All violent exercise and sports are, of course, to be avoided, particularly swimming, horseback riding and tennis (12).

Similar guidance appeared in the *Manual for the Conduct of Classes for Expectant Parents* published by the Cleveland Child Health Association in 1942:

A woman who does her own housework gets plenty of exercise; but she will find she profits by being in the open air for an hour or so each day. Walking is the best exercise (13).

In 1949, the United States Childrens' Bureau issued a publication in which they made standard recommendations for moderation in physical activity:

A moderate amount of exercise is good for anyone, and this is particularly true for a pregnant woman. Unless you have been ill or unless there is some complication, you can continue your housework, gardening, daily walks and even swim occasionally (14).

Many books of this era permitted housework, while prohibiting sports, despite the fact that housework could be more exhausting than sports.

Exercise advice of the 1950s and 1960s differed little from earlier advice. Three versions of *Expectant Motherhood* published in 1951, 1957, and 1963, respectively, each contained the identical bland exercise prescription:

Regular exercise in the open air ... should form part of your daily routine. For everyone, probably walking is the best type of exercise; for the pregnant woman there can be no question of its superiority ... For the average woman, a mile or so a day is about the right amount, but it is advisable to divide this into several short walks ... Light housework ... is a helpful form of activity and may be stopped short of fatigue, however, in no event should it include lifting of heavy objects.

Violent activity is to be avoided, particularly anything which involves jolting, sudden motion or running. Although physicians vary widely in the forms of exercise they permit in pregnancy, they usually disapprove of horseback riding, tennis and skating ... Dancing is harmless, as a rule, if indulged in moderately (15–17).

Kathleen Vaughan, one of the innovators of the 1930s, published another innovative book in the 1950s entitled *Exercises before Childbirth*. The book contains a forceful attack on the sedentary life of English women:

The mother who has lived a natural life from her own birth, who was breastfed herself and who has lived on plain, good food, with plenty of free movement in the fresh air when growing, she is the woman who will have an easy confinement when her time comes; while the more luxurious, wrapped-up, bottle-fed infant, kept long hours in a perambulator or indoors, with no exercise, and later sitting for long hours in school, is very likely to have difficulty in childbearing later on because the natural growth, shape and mobility of the pelvis and its joints have been stunted (1).

In her book, Vaughan recommends a series of exercises based on the movements of Kashmiri boatwomen at work. A novel approach in Vaughan's book is her recommendation that exercise be performed in group classes for the psychological boost to the prospective mother:

The advantage of attending a class is that you are stimulated by others also engaged in training for motherhood, with whom you make friends and can compare your babies later on (1).

Such arguments, though valuable from the social and psychological perspective, have also dominated the current line of thought of those who engage in organizing and promoting exercise programs for pregnant women. By and large, such programs are based on motivational arguments that often push pregnant women into activities they are more prepared to engage in mentally than physically. The emphasis in these programs is on giving the pregnant woman a sense of control over her body, her pregnancy, and her life. There is no doubt that the contemporary society is extremely preoccupied with a slim female appearance.

In a 1977 book entitled *Exercises for Increased Awareness in Education and Counselling in Childbirth*, Sheila Kitzinger (18) writes that "exercises should aim at developing poise and a sense of well-being." In discussing pelvic floor exercises she writes:

There is, therefore, room for exercises, always and flowing, which increases in women a happy consciousness of this part of their body as both good, clean and right, and as under their control (18).

In the *Exercise Plus Pregnancy Program* (1980), the authors write that:

Successfully completing an exercise program will give you a greater sense of control over your body. Being in control, while at the same time being relaxed, will give you the confidence and trust you'll need to "let go" for a smoother labor and delivery (19).

It is unfortunate that no standards for exercise have ever been developed for pregnant women. While the medical community has failed to systematically research and establish prenatal exercise programs based on scientific rationale, social reformers and sports advocates have promoted highly specific programs lacking a scientific basis of clinical trials, medical supervision, and follow-up. Typical programs of the 1970s and 1980s ignore basic physiologic changes of pregnancy such as the aortocaval compression syndrome, the increased laxity of joints and ligaments, and exaggerated lumbar lordosis. These programs promote the belief that physical fitness will ease labor and delivery; unfortunately there is no strong scientific evidence to support this view. The intensive birthing education of the 1980s provides women with a sense of command, but also leaves them with the fear that some minor dietary error or failure to engage in "prenatal exercises" will result in damage to their unborn children.

A *Wall Street Journal* article appearing in the August 17, 1984, issue, comments on the enormous change in expectations and procedures of childbirth during the last generation. Several statements in the article clearly capture the quandry in which the modern pregnant woman finds herself:

> ... today's middle class mother-to-be is often older and more ambitious than her mother was ... she approaches childbirth as she does any activity: She studies and prepares and trains as though labor were the bar examination or a sales campaign.
>
> She's so programmed to be in control, however, that if something goes wrong and childbirth doesn't meet her high expectations, she faces a profound sense of guilt and failure. That's the downside risk of the new motherhood.
>
> The variables a mother-to-be can control include diet and exercise. So the conscientious career women ... plunges into prenatal exercise classes that strengthen her back, abdomen and pelvic muscles. She also keeps going as long as she can (20).

It is difficult to determine what proportion of American women exercise regularly throughout their pregnancies. It is estimated that 85 million Americans are involved in some type of fitness programs and 25 million Americans jog regularly (21). Women of reproductive age constitute a significant proportion of this active American public (22). In a 1982 survey published in *MMWR*, only 10.8% of California women ages 18–34 years admitted to leading sedentary lives (23). In a recent article published in *Newsweek* magazine (July 23, 1984), the authors note that " ... as an outgrowth of the general fitness craze, women are flocking to exercise programs designed to get them in shape for labor and delivery" (24).

Our own experience is that many women, anxious to "get in shape" during their pregnancies, come to such programs mentally, but not physically, prepared. While the psychological benefits of exercise are unquestionable, such activities predispose unfit mother and infant to injury.

Between 1970 and 1973, 42% of all pregnant women worked for some portion of their pregnancy (25). Based on 1977 fertility rates, Kuntz (26) estimates that working American women will constitute over one million pregnancies each year. Seen in this light, injuries that could result from inappropriate prenatal exercise acquire national economic significance. Estimates of the direct and indirect costs of treating fitness related injuries in the general population are as high as 40 billion dollars annually.

In the case of pregnant women, one may speculate as to the source of payment for such injuries. According to Sheila Kamerman (25) of Columbia University,

> Unlike seventy-five other countries, including all other advanced industrialized societies and many among the less developed countries, the United States has no statutory provision that guarantees a woman the right to a leave from employment for a specified period, protects her job while she is on leave, and provides a cash benefit equal to all or a significant portion of her wage while she is not working because of pregnancy and childbirth. Nor does the United States guarantee a working mother the right to health insurance to cover her own medical expenses at the time of pregnancy and childbirth as well as those of her child. Benefits such as these cover most employed women in other countries. . . .

In 1976 the United States Supreme Court ruled in *Gilbert* v. *General Electric Corporation* that the exclusion of pregnancy-related disabilities from a company's disability insurance program is not considered sex discrimination, and employers are under no obligation to provide disability insurance benefits to pregnant women (25). The effects of this ruling were essentially reversed with the passage of the 1978 Pregnancy Disability Amendment to Title VII which requires employers to treat pregnancy and childbirth like other causes of disability under employee benefit plans such as health insurance, disability insurance, or sick leave plans (25). Only five states (California, Hawaii, New Jersey, New York, and Rhode Island) and Puerto Rico have mandatory state disability laws (25).

Analysis of the judicial aspects of such decisions are beyond the scope of this book; however, recommendations for prenatal activities must be viewed against this background. We have to be aware that certain activities may expose individuals to unwarranted risks (e.g., premature labor) for which unemployment compensation funds may not be available. This may be especially true in cases where an individual requires prolonged periods of hospitalization or confinement at home bed rest.

One obligation that we have as health care providers is to reassure women that it is also acceptable to limit exercise in pregnancy if their life-styles do not allow or they do not desire to do so. Limiting women to normal daily activities would in no way compromise her or her unborn child's health.

In view of the current trend toward a more physically active society, the medical community has an obligation to investigate, design, and promote activities that will be safe and maintain the well-being of both mother and fetus.

REFERENCES

1. Vaughan K: *Exercises before Childbirth*. London, Faber & Faber, 1951, pp 11–29.
2. Kerr JMM, Johnstone RW, Phillips MH: *Historical Review of British Obstetrics and Gynecology*. London, E.S. Livingstone, 1954.
3. Stacpoole F: *Advice to Women on the Care of their Health before, during and after Confinement*. London, Cassel, 1892, p 16.
4. Briend A: Maternal physical activity: birth weight and perinatal mortality. *Med Hypotheses* 6:1157–1170, 1980.
5. Naeye RL, Peters EC: Working during pregnancy: effects on the fetus. *Pediatrics* 69:724–727, 1982.
6. Oakley A: The origins and development of antenatal care. In Enkin M, Chalmers I (eds): *Effectiveness and Satisfaction in Antenatal Care*. London, published for Spastics International Medical Publications by Heinemann Medical Books, 1982, pp 1–20.
7. Slemmons JM: *The Prospective Mother: A Handbook for Women during Pregnancy*. New York, D. Appleton, 1913, pp 125–135.
8. Enkin M, Chalmers I: Effectiveness and satisfaction in antenatal care. In Enkin M, Chalmers I (eds): *Effectiveness and Satisfaction in Antenatal Care*. London, published for Spastics International Medical Publications by Heinemann Medical Books, 1982, pp 266–290.
9. Heaton C: *Modern Motherhood*. New York, Farrar & Rinehart, 1935, pp 38–40.
10. Blankfield A: Is exercise necessary for the obstetric patient? *Med J Aust* 1:163–165, 1967.
11. Enkin M: Antenatal classes. In Enkin M, Chalmers I (eds): *Effectiveness and Satisfaction in Antenatal Care*. London, published for Spastics International Medical Publications by Heinemann Medical Books, 1982, pp 151–162.
12. Van Blarcom C: *Getting Ready to Be a Mother*. New York, Macmillan, 1942, pp 48–49.
13. *Manual for the Conduct of Classes for Expectant Parents*. Cleveland, Cleveland Child Health Association, 1942.
14. *Prenatal Care*. Federal Security Agency and Social Security Administration: Children's Bureau Publication No. 4, 1949, pp 25–26.
15. Eastman NJ: *Expectant Motherhood*. Boston, Little, Brown, 1951, pp 74–75.
16. Eastman NJ: *Expectant Motherhood*. Boston, Little, Brown, 1957, pp 73–75.
17. Eastman NJ: *Expectant Motherhood*. Boston, Little, Brown, 1963, pp 79–80.
18. Kitzinger S: *Exercises for Increased Body Awareness in Education and Counselling for Childbirth*. London, Bailliere-Tindall, 1977, pp 165–171.
19. Cedeno L, Cedeno O, Monroe C: *The Exercise Plus Pregnancy Program*. New York, William Morrow, 1980.
20. Cox M: Many professional women apply career lessons to job of childbirth. *Wall Street Journal*, Section 2, August 17, 1984.
21. *Medical World News* (Psychiatry Edition), July 26, 1984, p 25.
22. Jarrett JC, Spellacy WN: Jogging during pregnancy: an improved outcome? *Obstet Gynecol* 63:705–709, 1983.
23. *MMWR Weekly Report*: Annual Summary 1982. Vol 31:128, December 1983.
24. Keerdoja E: Now, the pregnancy workout. *Newsweek*, July 23, 1984, p 70.
25. Kamerman S: *Maternity Policies and Working Women*. New York, Columbia University Press, 1983.
26. Kuntz WD: Pregnant working women: what advice should you give them? *Contemp Ob/Gyn* 15:69–79, 1980.

2
Exercise Physiology

Exercise physiology is the study of the functional changes that occur, within an organism, as a result of acute or chronic exposure to exertion. Acute exercise is a physiological stressor; and, as such, requires a major homeostatic adjustment in all organ functions if the exercise is to be continued. Very heavy exercise may require the body to increase its energy output by 20-fold. It may require up to an 8-fold increase in cardiac output. The exercise may stimulate a major increase in endocrine activity and an increased neuromotor recruitment. As well, the body has to adjust to accelerated heat production by modifying its normal mechanisms of thermoregulation. Fluid and electrolyte balance will be disturbed, and fuel sources may become depleted. Fortunately, the body adjusts quite well to this stress and, in fact, over time is able to perform at much higher levels without similar fatigue.

The magnitude of the adjustment to chronic stress (or exercise) is dependent on several factors, such as: (*a*) the age, sex, and body size of the individual; (*b*) the type of exercise (intensity of training, duration of the activity, the muscles involved and the body position); (*c*) the environment in which the exercise is performed (high altitude, heat, cold under water, in a polluted environment, etc.); as well as (*d*) the health and nutritional status of the individual.

In general, it is believed that the chronic adaptions in physiological function that accrue as a result of physical training are beneficial to the individual and may even affect mortality and morbity. As a result, exercise patterns in the United States over the past years have changed dramatically, showing a renewed interest in vigorous physical activity. Consequently, more and more people are participating in long-distance running and marathons. Millions are enrolling in organized aerobic and anaerobic exercise programs. New weight-training devices are available, and emphasis is being placed on strength training and power lifting. Academically, there has been an interest in studying special groups such as elite athletes, children, older people, and women.

With the interest in encouraging the participation of women in sport came several questions about performance capability, influence of menstrual cycling during participation, and possible risks involved while exercising. New and greater opportunites became available for females to compete. As a result, several studies have been conducted to assess their fitness potential (1–7).

Several authors have provided information as to the possible role of exercise on the maturation process of young girls (8–10) and on menstrual dysfunction in women that engage in rigorous physical training (11–16). As a result, a growing amount of literature is now available to assist the physician, therapist and exercise physiologist in understanding the effects and importance of exercise for their female patients.

Pregnant women are joining this fitness revolution, as well, and are beginning to participate in vigorous exercise throughout the duration of their pregnancy and are in need of relevant information to direct their exercise programs. Statements have been made about the exercise potential for childbearing women, but the scientific literature is not adequate. Several physicians recommend bed rest for some of their patients with complicated pregnancies. On the other extreme, we have examples of pregnant women running a marathon the day prior to delivery.

An attempt has been made to modify exercise programs for pregnant women from research studies conducted on normal nonpregnant females. The recommendations are conservative but, even so, do not have any kind of scientific basis. Fox (17) provides some very specific statements about exercise in pregnancy to support the concept that exercise is not harmful. He reports that complications of pregnancy are fewer in athletes, that performance returns to prepregnancy levels within 2 years, that pregnancy does not adversely affect athletic participation, and that serious injury to the breasts or the external and internal reproductive organs is very rare in female athletes. While these statement may have some documented support, the academic community is not willing to accept them without considerably more research.

Exercise during pregnancy is probably beneficial to most women. On the other hand, exercise in some may actually be detrimental to both mother and fetus; therefore, recommendation for exercise, as such, should be individualized.

In this chapter, information will be presented about basic physiological responses to exercise with special reference to pregnant women. As well, a brief introduction to the nomenclature of the field will be presented. More detailed information on exercise physiology is beyond the scope of this book; ample literature is available for the interested reader (17–19).

MEASUREMENT OF AEROBIC FITNESS

Exercise Metabolism

Prior to the application of science to physical fitness assessment, work capacity was measured in terms of running times, pounds lifted, distance covered, etc. With more sophisticated methodologies these performance measurements were replaced with laboratory measures. Fitness is now assessed using parameters such as oxygen-pulse, ventilatory equivalents, respiratory exchange ratios, lactic acid production, and maximal oxygen consumption. These terms will be elucidated later in this chapter; suffice it to say this time that with the new sophistication in fitness evaluation a more in-depth understanding of exercise physiology is required to interpret this new information.

It has been suggested that an individual's capacity for work is limited by the combined ability of the respiratory and cardiovascular systems to meet the increased oxygen demand of the muscles. Assessment of cardiorespiratory function can be made at rest but, by and large, is more definitive when appraised under exertional stress. Higher levels of stress up to maximal exertion seemingly allows a more reliable, valid measure of the adaptive capacities of an individual.

Of the noninvasive measures, maximal oxygen consumption is regarded by exercise physiologists as the best single measurement of physical working capacity (20–22). Maximal oxygen consumption is highly related to maximal cardiac output and is an excellent discriminatory measure of an individual's prior exercise history (23). In some instances, however, it is not advisable for the subject to perform at maximal exercise. For these individuals, submaximal tests may give some indication of exercise tolerance, but the interpretation of submaximal tests is difficult and often misleading.

Maximal Oxygen Uptake

Maximal oxygen consumption ($\dot{V}_{O_2max}$) is defined as the maximal rate at which oxygen can be utilized by the body. It relates to the power or capacity of the aerobic system (17). There are two very important equations that help describe the significant systems that influence and/or regulate the uptake of O_2. The first, the Fick equation, suggests that the two most important parameters in determining $\dot{V}_{O_2}$ is cardiac output and the arteriovenous oxygen difference.

$$\dot{V}_{O_2} = \text{cardiac output (Q)} \times \text{A-V } O_2 \text{ difference.}$$

Thus, there is a circulatory component to oxygen uptake (oxygen delivery) and an extraction component (oxygen utilization). The circulatory component is influenced by myocardial contractility, venous return, blood volume, oxygen carrying capacity, and peripheral resistance. It can also be influenced by intrinsic factors as well as neurogenic factors that may influence heart rate. Oxygen extraction, on the other hand, is related to cellular metabolic function and is regulated by enzyme activity and production as well as fuel availability.

Pregnancy is known to have a major impact on the circulatory system. The blood volume is increased, blood pressure may either increase or decrease, and there are significant changes in both resting and exercise heart rate. The literature related to the oxygen extraction side of the equation suggests that during pregnancy there is a significant decrease in A-V O_2 difference which has been attributed to the increase in blood volume and cardiac output rather than to any specific changes occurring at the cellular level (24).

It would be simple to calculate $\dot{V}_{O_2}$ if the inspired ventilatory volume were equal to the expiratory volume. However, this is only the case when the respiratory exchange ratio equals one, and this event occurs only during relatively moderate exercise, when the primary fuel for cellular metabolism is carbohydrate. To account for this problem of substrate utilization, adjustments have to be made to the expired oxygen concentration (25).

$$\dot{V}_{O_2} = \dot{V}_{E(STPD)} \times \frac{\%N_2 exp}{79.04} \times \frac{20.93}{100}$$
$$- \dot{V}_{E(STPD)} \times \frac{\%O_2 exp}{100}$$

$\dot{V}_{E(STPD)}$ = expired ventilatory volume corrected to standard temperature and pressure dry

$\%N_2 exp$ = the percentage expired nitrogen concentration

20.93 = the assumed inspired oxygen concentration

79.04 = the assumed inspired nitrogen concentration

$\%O_2 exp$ = the percentage of expired oxygen

This equation reveals that, in addition to those already mentioned parameters of circulation and extraction, one must consider ventilatory function as an important contributor to exercise tolerance and capacity.

For most individuals, oxygen uptake increases linearly with increasing work loads until a plateau is reached, at this point more work can be applied without further increases in $\dot{V}_{O_2}$ (Fig. 2.1). The usual criteria employed to ascertain whether or not max-

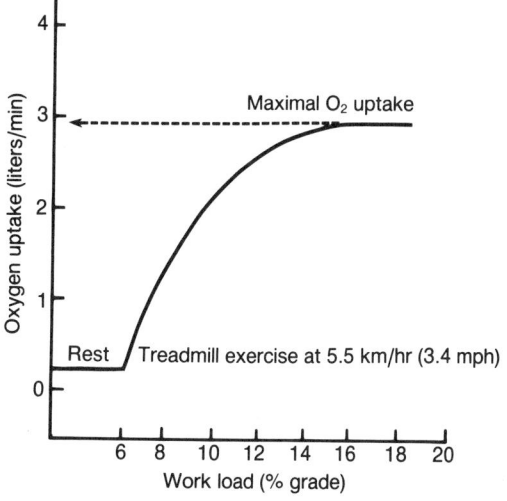

Figure 2.1. The plateau in oxygen uptake with increasing work load at maximal oxygen consumption. (From Lamb (19).)

imal oxygen uptake has been achieved are:
1. The subjects' having reached a plateau of decrease in $\dot{V}_{O_2}$ with increasing workload (26).
2. The respiratory exchange ratio having reached a level greater than 1.1.
3. The pulse rate reaching the age-adjusted maximal level. Maximal heart rate (HR) can be estimated by subtracting ones age from 220; this figure may slightly underestimate the actual HR_{max}; or by subtracting one-half age from 210 which gives a less conservative estimate (27).
4. The subject's inability to maintain the work load.

Unfortunately, during clinical practice, most of the subjects are not of sufficient physical condition to achieve a "true" $\dot{V}_{O_2max}$ and stop exercise prior to a plateauing of $\dot{V}_{O_2}$ due to a variety of symptoms which generally include shortness of breath and/or leg fatigue. In these subjects, the test is defined as a "symptom limited $\dot{V}_{O_2max}$ test" and only approximates the subject's actual aerobic capacity. Table 2.1 presents standards for $\dot{V}_{O_2max}$ ml/kg × min^{-1}.

If one uses these standards, it becomes obvious that pregnancy is affecting fitness or aerobic capacity because of the increase in body weight. The increase in weight may serve as a stimulus to improve oxygen uptake (29). In effect, the system adjusts to the increase in weight by improving its aerobic capacity.

However, when taking into consideration all parameters it may be more useful to describe aerobic capacity in terms of oxygen consumption in liters rather than the weight adjusted ml × kg^{-1} × min^{-1}. The method of expressing aerobic fitness, or the oxygen cost of an activity, has led to some major confusion within the field. Next we will present information related to the methods utilized to expressing energy expenditure.

Relative versus Absolute Work

It is common practice to report the cardiorespiratory responses to exercise as a function of absolute work intensity or as a function of relative work intensity, expressed as a percentage of the individual's maximal oxygen uptake. Clausen (30) suggests that heart rate and arterial pressure responses are closely related to the relative workload while cardiac output is more a function of absolute workload (31). Figure 2.2 illustrates the importance of utilizing either absolute or relative work in interpreting the physiological response. Thus, as one improves physical fitness, the metabolic and circulatory response to the same (absolute) work load may be reduced (e.g., lower ventilation) while when expressed relative to the $\dot{V}_{O_2max}$ the fit and unfit may have a similar response. There are several metabolic parameters that change significantly during exercise in pregnancy; yet if these changes are not viewed in light of the reduced fitness, the results could be misleading.

Energy Expenditure

Energy expenditure refers to the total calories required to complete a given task, and it is estimated from the amount of oxygen consumed during that activity (17). Measuring oxygen consumption can be utilized as an index of energy liberation and thus fuel catabolism. The specific use of oxygen during exercise is that of a hydrogen acceptor. The source of the excessive hydrogen pool is derived from substrate catabolism (ATP, creatine phosphate (CP), carbohydrate, fats, and proteins). For every liter of oxygen utilized by the body, approximately 5 kcal of energy could have been liberated from the substrate pool. During the high energy demands of exercise, oxygen uptake

Table 2.1. Aerobic Capacity Standards for Women[a]

Age	Maximal Oxygen Consumption (ml × kg^{-1} × min^{-1})				
	Low	Fair	Average	Good	High
20–29	28	29–34	35–40	41–46	47
30–39	27	28–33	34–38	39–45	46
40–49	25	26–31	32–37	38–43	44
50–65	21	22–28	29–34	35–40	41

[a] Adapted from Katch and McArdle (28), p. 291.

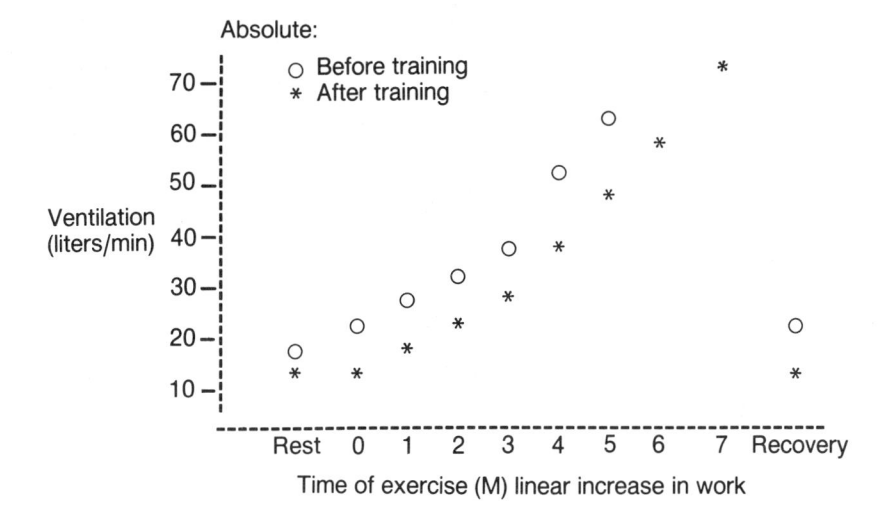

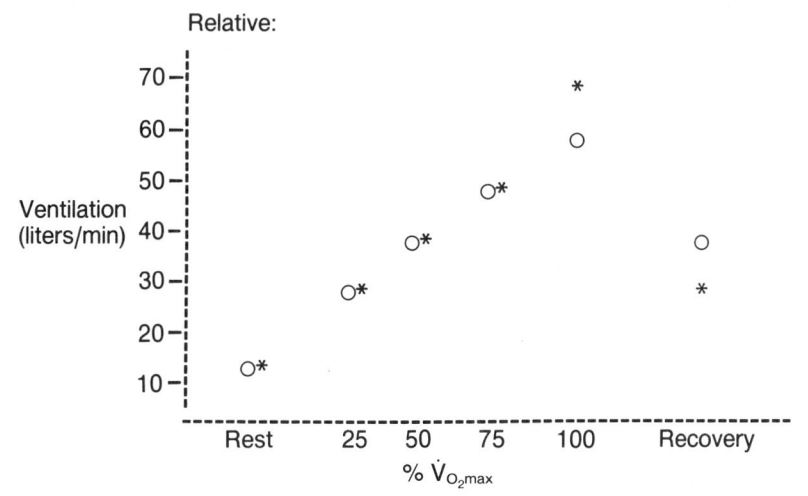

Figure 2.2. Hypothetical effect of training on a given metabolic parameter in absolute and relative terms.

goes up as much as 20 times, increasing the resting caloric expenditure from 1 kcal per minute at rest to as much as 20–25 kcal per minute during high intensity exercise. To obtain the approximate caloric expenditure of an activity, oxygen uptake in liters is multiplied by 5 kcal/liter.

Oxygen uptake can be expressed in liters per minute or as a function of one's body weight or body surface area. Expressing metabolic cost in liters gives an indication of the energy requirement of the task, while expressing the metabolic cost in ml $\times$ kg^{-1} $\times$ min^{-1} gives an indication of one's efficiency in utilizing oxygen based upon their own body weight. A normal exercise task, such as casual walking, may require 1 liter of oxygen per minute in absolute terms. In a 50-kg woman, the oxygen uptake per body weight would be 20 ml $\times$ kg^{-1} $\times$ min^{-1}, and in a 60-kg woman it would represent 16.67 ml $\times$ kg^{-1} $\times$ min^{-1}.

Another means of expressing energy cost of activity rather than the absolute oxygen cost is to express energy requirements in METs. One MET is equivalent to 3.5 ml $\times$ kg^{-1} $\times$ min^{-1}, which in most subjects it approximates metabolic rate at rest. A 3-MET activity would be an activity that raises the resting metabolic rate 3 times. The 1-

liter oxygen consumption during a 1-mile walk could be expressed as a 3–4-MET activity. The use of MET facilitates describing a relative scale of work intensity and is used for exercise prescription.

The advantage or disadvantage of one system over another in defining energy expenditure is solely based upon the preference and background of the investigator. It is unfortunate that there is no agreed upon uniform method of expressing energy requirements of work (Table 2.2).

It is a common trend in exercise prescription to suggest that individuals should be involved in an exercise program which elevates energy expenditure 150–300 kcal per day. The caloric cost of walking a mile is estimated to be approximately 80–120 kcal (depending on weight). Therefore, the exercise program of choice seems to be one that would be equivalent in energy expenditure terms to 1.5–3 miles of walking or running per day. It must be noted that these values have not been standardized for pregnant women. The oxygen cost of any weight-bearing exercise is greater during pregnancy due to the increase in body weight and reduced efficiency of oxygen utilization. It is interesting to note that speed is relatively unimportant in terms of energy expenditure, although it is believed that faster work rates lead to slightly (6–10%) greater caloric expenditures. This caloric difference is not, however, of major physiological significance. An excellent review of the caloric cost of various activities was reported by Passmore and Durnin (32).

Mechanical Efficiency

Based upon the published literature it is assumed that the oxygen cost of performing a given amount of work is the similar in all

Table 2.2. Methods of Classifying Energy Requirements of a Task

Activity			Weight (kg)			
			50	65	80	95
Caloric cost (kcal $\times$ min^{-1}):						
Sitting quietly			1.1	1.4	1.7	2.0
Walking			4.0	5.2	6.4	7.4
Running—5 mph			6.8	8.8	10.5	12.9
Running—6.6 mph			9.7	12.5	15.4	18.3
O$_2$ cost (liters $\times$ min^{-1}):						
Sitting quietly			0.22	0.28	0.34	0.40
Walking			0.80	1.04	1.28	1.48
Running—5 mph			1.36	1.76	2.10	2.58
Running—6.6 mph			1.94	2.50	3.08	3.66
O$_2$ cost (ml $\times$ kg^{-1} $\times$ min^{-1}):						
Sitting quietly			4.4	4.3	4.2	4.2
Walking			16.0	16.0	16.0	15.6
Running—5 mph			27.2	27.1	26.2	27.2
Running—6.6 mph			38.8	38.5	38.5	38.5
Metabolic equivalent (MET: O$_2$ cost = 1 $\times$ min^{-1}/caloric cost = kcal $\times$ min^{-1}):						
Sitting quietly	1	MET	0.18/0.9	0.23/ 1.2	0.28/ 1.4	0.33/ 1.6
Walking	3–4	MET	0.70/3.5	0.91/ 4.5	1.12/ 5.6	1.33/ 6.6
Running—5 mph	6–7	MET	1.20/6.2	1.59/ 7.9	1.96/ 9.8	2.33/11.6
Running—6.6	10–11	MET	1.92/9.6	2.50/12.5	3.08/15.4	3.65/18.3

Interpretation:
Caloric cost: A 65-kg person would expend approximately 5.2 kcal/min while walking
O$_2$ cost: An 80-kg person would have an oxygen uptake of approximately 0.34 liter per minute while sitting quietly. In relationship to his body weight, this would represent 4.2 ml/kg $\times$ min^{-1}
MET: Running at 5 mph is a 6–7-MET activity. It requires approximately 1.2 liters of oxygen per minute in a 50-kg person and represents a caloric expenditure of 6.2 kcal/min

individuals. However, while the oxygen cost of an activity is work load dependent, there are several factors which may influence the absolute amount of oxygen consumed. The economical use of oxygen by an individual is termed metabolic efficiency. Biomechanical factors can affect efficiency as well as type of activity and type or size of the muscles involved. Several different mathematical equations of mechanical efficiency have been applied to address the question of differences in O_2 cost between activities. With regard to these models, efficiency is defined as the ratio of useful work output to energy expended (33). In most machines efficiency is lost to friction between parts; extra energy required to overcome frictional factors serves to reduce efficiency of the machine. The human, even though not affected by friction, is less efficient than most machines in the use of energy sources. As a result, the human uses a disproportionate amount of fuel and generates an excessive amount of heat when performing physical work. Table 2.3 is an example of how mechanical efficiency is determined in individuals performing bicycle exercise.

The determination of work efficiency during treadmill testing is considerably more difficult due to problems related to calculating the amount of distance (both horizontal and vertical) transversed during the exercise task. An excellent review of the methods and mathematical procedures is provided by Fox and Mathews (33).

Donovan and Brooks (34) reported efficiencies for horizontal walking of 19.6–35.2%. Gaesser and Brooks (35) reported 20.6–43.0% efficiency for cycling. Pendergast et al. (36) found much lower efficiencies in swimming freestyle (2.9–7.4% in male subjects; 2.7–9.4% in female subjects). In general, tasks requiring larger muscle groups result in greater efficiency than those using smaller muscles. However, one must be cautious when comparing the efficiencies reported because of the different equations used and the fact that some authors report gross rather than net efficiencies.

Girandola et al. (9) reported efficiency difference between pre- and postpubescent girls. The younger girls were less efficient having higher $\dot{V}_{O_2}$ for similar work loads. The differences were attributed to shorter limb length causing more strides for the same running pace or a possible deficiency in motor development that may have resulted in more extraneous movement during the run. Another explanation could be that the taller, older girls may have been able to walk at the speed used for comparison; whereas, the younger girls may have been running.

Running has been reported to be less efficient (37). The literature with regard to running is not conclusive, and further research required.

The literature relating to efficiency difference during pregnancy is contradictory. Knuttgen and Emerson (38) reported a lower O_2 cost of treadmill walking at 14 weeks postpartum compared to prepartum values. This difference was attributed to maternal weight gain and was consistent with several

Table 2.3. An Example of Mechanical Efficiency Determinations Using a Bicycle Ergometer[a]

Work Output	Energy Expenditure
Work = Force × distance	
Bicycle resistance = 4 kg	Steady-level $\dot{V}_{O_2}$ = 1.2 liters
Wheel circumference = 2 meters	Caloric cost = 1.2 × 4.83[b]
	= 5.79 kcal
Revolutions per min = 60 rpm	(caloric cost × 426.8 converts to work units − kg)
Work = 4 kg × (60 × 2) = 480 kg	Work = 5.79 × 426.8 = 2474 kg
Efficiency = $\dfrac{\text{work output}}{\text{energy expenditure}} = \dfrac{480 \text{ kg}}{2474 \text{ kg}} = 19.4\%$	

[a] Adapted from Fox and Mathews (33).
[b] Assume an R = 0.83.

earlier studies (39, 40). Knuttgen and Emerson also reported that the O_2 cost of cycling was not significantly different in their study, implying no effect of pregnancy on efficiency. Seitchik (41) studied the oxygen requirement of a submaximal bicycle task in 195 pregnant women and concluded that pregnancy did not significantly increase oxygen cost of exercise. Edwards et al. (42) reported a significant increase in resting metabolism but no difference in submaximal oxygen uptake. Conversely, Pernoll et al. (29) reported that significantly greater exercise $\dot{V}_{O_2}$ occurs during mild, non-weight-bearing, steady-state exercise in pregnancy with a significant reduction in efficiency.

Ueland et al. (43) also support the finding that oxygen cost of exercise is greater in pregnancy. An explanation of the decreased efficiency is related to the increase in ventilation induced by pregnancy. The hyperventilation of pregnancy both at rest and at various levels of submaximal exercise increases the O_2 cost of breathing and therefore would reduce the efficiency of O_2 delivery to the working muscles. However, this ventilatory inefficiency accounts for less than 20% of the observed changes (43).

Cardiac output is greater in pregnancy, indicating a slightly greater myocardial oxygen consumption; but, again, the impact on total efficiency is slight. The actual mechanism for the decrease in efficiency during pregnancy is not fully understood, and further research is needed.

Exercise Protocol

Another area of confusion within the field of exercise assessment and prescription relates to the standardization of testing modality and protocol. The modalities that have been used to assesss fitness include step tests, bicycle ergometers, treadmills, swimming flumes, laddermills and several others. Even within the literature related to pregnancy, several different testing devices have been employed (Table 2.4).

The most commonly used device is the bicycle ergometer. However, it is obvious that the protocols used vary greatly. Pollack (53) compared four major treadmill protocols and found that for the most part the protocols yielded similar results (Fig. 2.3) (54). The use of the treadmill protocol during pregnancy is questionable. In determining $\dot{V}_{O_2max}$ in pregnant subjects, Artal et al. (52) used a modified Balke treadmill protocol in which the speed was held constant at 2.5 mph while the elevation was increased by 2% each minute until the subject reached her maximum capacity. As in any weight-bearing exercise, the metabolic cost is dependent upon the weight of the subject.

Table 2.4. Different Protocols Used in Evaluation Effect of Exercise on Pregnant Women

Protocol	Test	Evaluation
Widlund (40)	Step test	22-, 40-, 52-step frequency
Bader et al. (44)	Recumbant bicycle	10-min duration
Genzell et al. (45)	Bicycle ergometer	33, 66, 99 watts, 6-min duration
Ueland et al. (46)	Bicycle ergometer	100,200 kpm
Guzman and Caplan (47)	Bicycle ergometer	150, 250, 350 kg; 4 min/10 min rest
Knuttgen and Emerson (38)	Treadmill and bike	4% grade 4.5 km $\times$ hr^{-1}; 60 watts
Pomerance et al. (48)	Bicycle ergometer	450 kpm ($N = 49$) 600 (4), 300 (1)
Pernoll et al. (49)	Bicycle ergometer	Submaximal test 6 min
Erkkola and Makela (50)	Bicycle ergometer	3-stage 150, 300, 450 kpm/min each lasting 4 min on the day after a voluntarily maximal test
Edwards et al. (42)	Bicycle ergometer	10 min at 50 watts
Collings et al. (51)	Bicycle ergometer	150 kpm at 85 rpm for 4 min followed by 2-min rest; increments until subject reached heart rate = 150–160
Artal et al. (52)	Treadmill	2.5 mph, increased 2% min until exhaustion

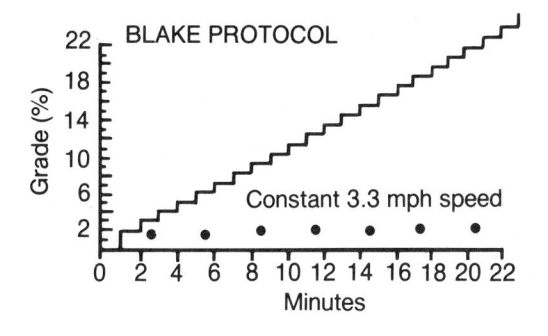

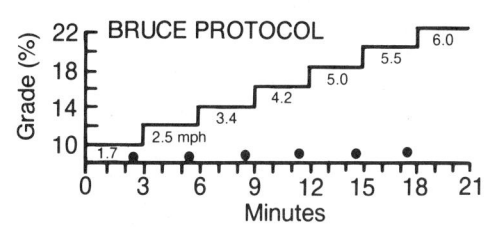

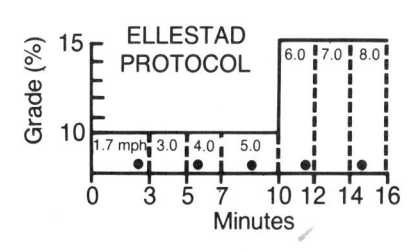

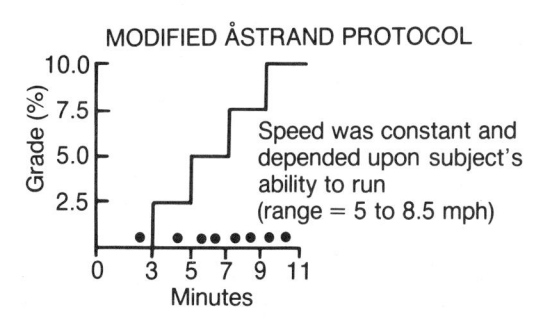

Figure 2.3. Commonly used exercise test protocols. ● = $\dot{V}_{O_2}$ determination. (From Pollock (53).)

During pregnancy, due to the disproportional increase in weight, the metabolic response to a similar increase in elevation or speed cannot be compared. For this reason, we recommend the use of a bicycle ergometer whenever attempting to evaluate the cardiovascular, respiratory, or metabolic response to submaximal exercise during pregnancy. If the purpose of study is to evaluate the effects of pregnancy on maximal aerobic power ($\dot{V}_{O_2max}$), the treadmill is the device of choice.

ACUTE METABOLIC RESPONSE TO EXERCISE

When an individual starts exercising there is a brief lag in the increase in oxygen uptake. After a short period, depending on the intensity of the exercise and the fitness of the individual, the $\dot{V}_{O_2}$ reaches a plateau or steady state. It is generally accepted that in a dynamic system, such as the body during exercise, there are always occurring homeostatic changes: to suggest that a steady state has been reached assumes some kind of static equilibrium within the system which, most likely, does not occur. The term steady-level exercise implies a more general adaption to a constant work load and does not attempt to imply a fixed physiological response.

For definitional purposes, any exercise intensity which results in a steady-level response in $\dot{V}_{O_2}$ is called submaximal exercise. If the work intensity is so great that $\dot{V}_{O_2}$ does not "level-off" but continues to increase without changes in work load, the exercise will not result in steady-level $\dot{V}_{O_2}$ and maximal oxygen consumption will be achieved. Any work load can lead to fatigue if performed long enough; but, by and large, the test of $\dot{V}_{O_2max}$ is of a reasonably short duration and is of sufficient intensity to involve recruitment of the greater tension-producing glycolytic, fast-twitch muscle fibers.

Oxygen Deficit/Debt

During the initial phase of exercise, the cardiorespiratory system is not capable of providing O_2 rapidly enough. As a result, the muscle uses high energy phosphates (ATP, CP) and cellular oxygen to meet this transitional need. This leads to the so called "oxygen deficit" (Fig. 2.4). At the end of exercise, during recovery, excess oxygen (above resting levels) is required to restore the muscles' energy pool back to equilibrium. This has been called the "oxygen debt." The rate of repayment or recovery is

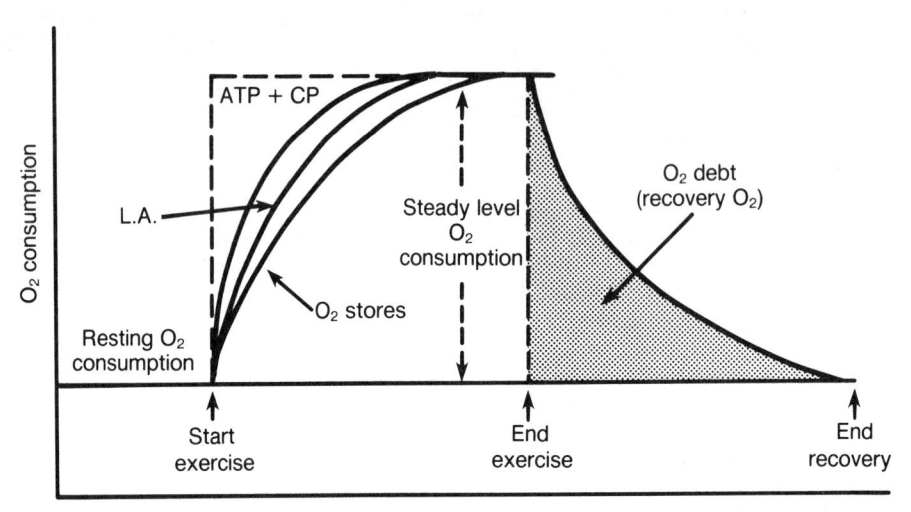

Figure 2.4. Oxygen deficit and debt. L.A. = lactic acid. (From H. A. DeVries: *Physiology of Exercise for Physical Education and Athletics*, Ed. 2. Dubuque, Iowa, William C. Brown Co., 1974.)

dependent on the work intensity and the fitness of the individual. The excess oxygen is used not just to replenish tissue O_2 stores and the high energy phosphates, but must also be used to supply the energy for lactate removal and glycogen and glucose resynthesis as well. The metabolic rate is elevated in recovery due, in part, to the increased body temperature (Q_{10} effect), and the very slow removal rate of several of the hormones that were released during the exercise.

Ready et al. (55) reported an increase in maximal O_2 debt of 19.8% during physical training of 6 weeks in young women. In other words, training has the effect of allowing one to tolerate greater levels of oxygen deficit and anaerobic metabolism. Pernoll et al. (49) reported a significant increase in exercise $\dot{V}_{O_2}$ in late pregnancy when compared to postpartum values. The oxygen debt incurred by standard non-weight-bearing exercise was greater in late pregnancy than early in pregnancy or 14 weeks postpartum. This may indicate a reduced tolerance for exercise or, perhaps, a change in fuel utilization patterns during exercise and/or recovery. Widlund (40) and Seitchik (41) also reported increased oxygen debt during pregnancy.

Oxygen Pulse

Oxygen pulse, or the quotient of oxygen consumed as a function of heart rate over the same period, is affected by and is an indirect measure of all of the aforementioned circulatory adjustments during exercise, a relationship that can be described by substitution as:

$$O_2 \text{ pulse} = \frac{\dot{V}_{O_2}}{\text{heart rate}}.$$

Therefore, any circulatory adjustment which improves A-V O_2 difference (e.g., redistribution of blood flow to the active muscle) or increases cardiac output (e.g., increased stroke volume due to greater venous return) will effect an improvement in oxygen pulse. Hence, oxygen pulse becomes elevated in muscular exercise due to increased stroke volume as well as increased oxygen extraction in the working muscle (56). The increase in oxygen pulse with work load (relative work load in percentage of $\dot{V}_{O_2max}$) is linear above 50% relative work loads (50). While no information is available in the literature with regard to oxygen pulse in pregnancy, several studies have reported higher heart rates during submaximal exercise, thus implying an elevated oxygen pulse during pregnancy. The work of Wiswell et al. (59) indicates a lowering of maximal heart rate during exercise, but the $\dot{V}_{O_2max}$ was also reduced, suggesting that maximal O_2-pulse may not change.

Ventilatory Equivalent for Oxygen

Ventilatory equivalent for oxygen, ($\dot{V}_E/\dot{V}_{O_2}$), or the quotient obtained by the ratio of ventilation to $\dot{V}_{O_2}$, is often used as a measure of respiratory efficiency. During the initial few moments of exercise the $\dot{V}_E/\dot{V}_{O_2}$ ratio rises rapidly, after which it gradually drops until reaching a lower stable value (Fig. 2.5). This is due to a rapid ventilatory acceleration (neural control) at the onset of exercise without a similar rise in $\dot{V}_{O_2}$. During steady level submaximal exercise the $\dot{V}_E/\dot{V}_{O_2}$ ratio reaches and maintains a plateau until certain anaerobic factors again begin to drive the ventilation up exponentially. It is assumed that the lower the plateau value, the more efficient the respiratory system is in delivering O_2 to the working muscles. In this case, it is efficient to have a higher $\dot{V}_{O_2}$ with a lower $\dot{V}_E$. Knuttgen and Emerson (38) reported an elevation in resting and submaximal exercise $\dot{V}_E/\dot{V}_{O_2}$ in prepartum versus postpartum subjects. The resting level decreased from 33.2 to 28.3, while the exercise value decreased from 33.7 to 29.3 after delivery. Submaximal $\dot{V}_E/\dot{V}_{O_2}$ has been used as a good predictor of $\dot{V}_{O_2max}$. However, due to the extremely high ventilation obtained by trained subjects, the maximal $\dot{V}_E/\dot{V}_{O_2}$ may not be a discriminator of fitness.

Respiratory Exchange Ratio

The respiratory exchange ratio (R) has been used to give an index of type of fuel being metabolized. R is calculated from a ratio of the $\dot{V}_{CO_2}$ to $\dot{V}_{O_2}$. By observing R during exercise one can estimate the foodstuff or substrate that is being utilized. Unfortunately, studies that have provided information about R and fuel metabolism do not always account for transient shifts in ventilation and the problems of interpreting the influence of protein metabolism on R (Table 2.5). This becomes relevant in the study of pregnancy due to the fact that there is a changing endocrine function, and some women become carbohydrate intolerant during late pregnancy. The relationship between R and fuel metabolism in pregnancy is not well established. However, Knuttgen and Emerson (38) have reported a decrease in R from 0.83 to 0.77 in prepartum versus postpartum women. They postulated that the elevated R of pregnancy is due in part to the increased expired CO_2 caused by the abnormally high ventilation at rest and during submaximal exercise. Blackburn et al. (57, 58) reported a reduced R when comparing prepartum to postpartum values on both bicycle ergometer and treadmill.

EXERCISE PRESCRIPTION

With the increased interest in exercise, particularly endurance type exercise, a need for exercise prescription evolved. Prescription was based upon the individual's age, sex, and physical fitness and/or health sta-

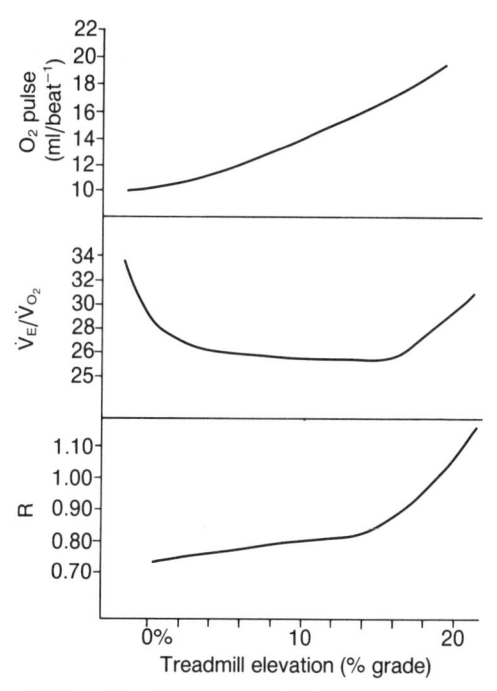

Figure 2.5. Time course of select metabolic parameters in pregnant women during maximal exercise. (From Wiswell et al. (59).)

Table 2.5. Expedience of Using R in Determining Type of Fuel Used Non-protein R[a]

Fuel	Respiratory Exchange Ratio	Example
Fats (palmitic acid)	R = 0.707 4.686 kcal/liter O$_2$	$C_{16}H_{32}O_2 + 23\,O_2 \rightarrow 16\,CO_2 + 16\,H_2O$
		$16\,CO_2/23\,O_2 = 0.707$
Carbohydrates (Glucose)	R = 1.0 5.047 kcal/liter O$_2$	$C_6H_{12}O_6 + 6\,O_2 \rightarrow 6\,CO_2 + 6\,O_2$
		$6\,CO_2/6\,O_2 = 1.0$

[a] Adapted from Fox and Mathews (33).

Table 2.6. Guidelines for Estimating Frequency, Intensity, Duration, and Distance of Aerobic and Anaerobic Training Programs of Running[a]

Training Aspect	Endurance (Aerobic) Training	Sprint (Anaerobic) Training
Frequency	4–5 days/wk	3 days/wk
Intensity	Heart rate = 85–95% of maximal heart rate	Heart rate = 180 beats or greater
Sessions/day	One	One
Duration	12–16 wk or longer	8–10 wk
Distance/workout	3–5 miles	1.5–2.0 miles

[a] From Fox (17), p. 219.

tus. As a prerequisite for exercise prescription, normal medical and physiological tests were required to ensure physical competence to perform exhaustive exercise. Prescriptions usually include information about what type of exercise modality should be employed, as well as the duration, frequency, and intensity of the activity. Table 2.6 shows an example of guidelines that have been used in developing an exercise plan.

The American College of Sports Medicine (27) recommends exercise that uses large muscle groups, is rhythmical and aerobic in nature, and can be maintained continuously. The intensity of training should be between 60 and 90% of maximum heart rate or 50–85% of $\dot{V}_{O_2max}$. The use of target heart rate has been a popular method of prescribing exercise. The target heart rate is determined by subtracting the individual resting heart rate from the maximal heart rate. The difference is then multiplied by the desired exercise intensity (60–90%, depending on age and fitness of the subject) and added to the resting heart rate to produce the exercise heart rate range.

Unfortunately, there are some major drawbacks in using heart rate as a means of prescribing exercise in pregnancy. Recent research in our laboratory causes us to question the usefulness of this equation in determining maximal heart rate during pregnancy. We have reported that maximal heart rate in pregnant females is considerably lower than that which has been estimated (59). Due to cardiovascular complications that may occur in pregnancy, unsupervised exercise prescription should be limited to a maximum of 140 beats/min.

REFERENCES

1. Brown CH, Harrower JR, Deeter MF: The effects of cross-country running on pre-adolescent girls. *Med Sci Sports* 4:1–5, 1972.
2. Brown CH, Wilmore JH: The effects of maximal resistance training on the strength and body composition of women athletes. *Med Sci Sports* 6:174–177, 1974.
3. Drinkwater BL: Physiological responses of women to exercise. *Exerc Sport Sci Rev* 1:125–153, 1973.
4. Drinkwater BL, Horvath SM, Wells CL: Aerobic power of females, ages 10–68. *J Gerontol* 30:385–394, 1975.
5. Plowman S: Physiological characteristics of female athletes. *Res Q* 45:349–362, 1974.

6. Sinning DW: Body composition, cardiorespiratory function, and rule changes in women's basketball. *Res Q* 44:313–321, 1973.
7. Spence DW, Disch JG, Fred HL, Coleman AE: Descriptive profiles of highly skilled women volleyball players. *Med Sci Sports Exerc* 12:299–302, 1980.
8. Wilmore JH, Brown CH: Physiological profiles of women distance runners. *Med Sci Sports* 6:178–181, 1974.
9. Girandola RN, Wiswell RA, Frisch F, Wood K: V_{O_2max} and anaerobic threshold in pre- and postpubescent girls. In Borms J, Hebbelinck M, Venerando A (eds): *Women and Sport: An Historical, Biological, Physiological and Sportsmedical Approach*. Basel, S. Karger, 1981, vol 14, pp 155–161.
10. Vaccaro P, Clarke DH: Cardiorespiratory alterations in 9- to 11-year-old children following a season of competitive swimming. *Med Sci Sports* 10:204–207, 1978.
11. Erdelyi GJ: Gynecological survey of female athletes. *J Sports Med Phys Fitness* 2:174–179, 1962.
12. Astrand PO, Engstrom L, Eriksson BO, et al: Girl swimmers: gynaecological aspects. *Acta Paediatr Scand* 147:33–38, 1963.
13. Rebar RW, Cumming DC: Reproductive function in women athletes. *JAMA* 246:1950, 1981.
14. Feicht CB, Johnson TS, Martin BJ, et al: Secondary amenorrhea in athletes. *Lancet* 2:1145–1146, 1978.
15. Dale E, Gerlach DH, Wilhite AL: Menstrual dysfunction in distance runners. *Obstet Gynecol* 54:47–53, 1979.
16. Speroff L, Redwine DB: Exercise and menstrual function. *Phys Sports Med* 8:42–52, 1980.
17. Fox E: *Sports Physiology*. New York, W. B. Saunders, 1984.
18. Brooks GA, Fahey TD: *Exercise Physiology: Human Bioenergetics and Its Applications*. New York, John Wiley & Sons, 1984.
19. Lamb DR: *Physiology of Exercise: Responses and Adaptations*. New York, Macmillan, 1978.
20. Åstrand PO: *Experimental Studies of Physical Working Capacity in Relation to Sex and Age*. Copenhagen, Munksgaard, 1952.
21. Mitchell JH, Sproule BJ, Chapman CB: The physiological meaning of the maximal oxygen consumption test. *J Clin Invest* 37:538–547, 1958.
22. Taylor HL, Wang Y, Rowell L, Blomqvist G: The standardization and interpretation of submaximal and maximal tests of working capacity. *Pediatrics* 32:703–722, 1963.
23. Åstrand PO, Rodahl K: *Textbook of Work Physiology: Physiological Bases of Exercise*. New York, McGraw-Hill, 1977.
24. Pritchard JA, MacDonald PC, Gant NF (eds): *Williams Obstetrics* ed 17. Norwalk, Conn., Appleton-Century-Crofts, 1985.
25. Consolazio CF, Johnson RE, Pecora LJ: *Physiological Measurements of Metabolic Functions in Man*. New York, McGraw-Hill, 1963.
26. Wyndham CH: Submaximal tests for estimating maximum oxygen intake. *Can Med Assoc J* 96:736–745, 1967.
27. American College of Sports Medicine: *Guidelines for Graded Exercise Testing and Exercise Prescription*. Philadelphia, Lea & Febiger, 1980.
28. Katch FI, McArdle WD: *Nutrition, Weight Control and Exercise*. Philadelphia, Lea & Febiger, 1983.
29. Pernoll ML, Metcalfe J, Sclhlenker TL, Welch JE, Matsumoto JA: Oxygen consumption at rest and during exercise in pregnancy. *Respir Physiol* 25:285–293, 1975.
30. Clausen JP: Circulatory adjustments to dynamic exercise and effects of physical training in normal subjects and in patients with coronary artery disease. *Prog Cradiovasc Dis* 18:459–495, 1976.
31. Lewis SF, Taylor WF, Graham RM, Pettinger WA, Schutte JE, Blomqvist CG: Cardiovascular responses to exercise as functions of absolute and relative workload. *J Appl Physiol* 54:1314–1323, 1983.
32. Passmore R, Durnin JVGA: Human energy expenditure. *Physiol Rev* 35:801, 1955.
33. Fox EL, Mathews DK: *The Physiological Basis of Physical Education and Athletics*. New York, W. B. Saunders, 1981.
34. Donovan CB, Brooks GA: Muscular efficiency during steady-rate exercise. *J Appl Physiol.* 43:431–439, 1977.
35. Gaesser GA, Brooks GA: Muscular efficiency during steady-rate exercise: effects of speed and work rate. *J Appl Physiol* 38:1132–1139, 1975.
36. Pendergast DR, diPrampero PE, Craig AB, Wilson DR, Rennie DW: Quantitative analysis of the front crawl in men and women. *J Appl Physiol* 43:475–479, 1977.
37. Howley ET, Glover ME: The caloric costs of running and walking one mile for men and women. *Med Sci Sports* 6:235–237, 1974.
38. Knuttgen HG, Emerson Jr K: Physiological response to pregnancy at rest and during exercise. *J Appl Physiol* 36:549–553, 1974.
39. Teruoka G: Labour physiological studies on pregnant women. *Arbeitsphysiol* 7:259–279, 1933.
40. Widlund G: The cardio-pulmonal function during pregnancy. *Acta Obstet Gynecol Scand* 25(Suppl 1):1–125, 1945.
41. Seitchik J: Body composition and energy expenditure during rest and work in pregnancy. *Am J Obstet Gynecol* 97:701–713, 1967.
42. Edwards MJ, Metcalfe J, Dunham MJ, Paul MS: Accelerated respiratory response to moderate exercise in late pregnancy. *Respir Physiol* 45:229–241, 1981.
43. Ueland KM, Novy J, Metcalfe J: Cardiorespiratory responses to pregnancy and exercise in normal women and patients with heart disease. *Am J Obstet Gynecol* 115:4–10, 1973.
44. Bader RA, Bader ME, Rose DJ, Braunwald E: Hemodynamics at rest and during exercise in normal

pregnancy as studied by cardiac catheterization. *J Clin Invest* 34:1524–1536, 1955.
45. Genzell D, Robbe H, Stron G: Total amount of hemoglobin and physical working capacity in normal pregnancy and puerperium (with iron medication). *Acta Obstet Gynecol Scand* 36:93–136, 1957.
46. Ueland KM, Novy MJ, Peterson EN, et al: Maternal cardiovascular dynamics; IV. The influence of gestational age on the maternal cardiovascular response to posture and exercise. *Am J Obstet Gynecol* 104:856, 1969.
47. Guzman CA, Caplan R: Cardiorespiratory response to exercise during pregnancy. *Am J Obstet Gynecol* 108:600–605, 1970.
48. Pomerance JJ, Gluck L, Lynch VA: Physical fitness in pregnancy: its effect on pregnancy outcome. *Am J Obstet Gynecol* 119:867–876, 1974.
49. Pernoll M, Metcalfe J, Kovach PA, Wachtel R, Dunham MJ: Ventilation during rest and exercise in pregnancy and postpartum. *Respir Physiol* 25:295–310, 1975.
50. Erkkola R, Makela M: Heart volumes and physical fitness of parturients. *Ann Clin Res* 8:15–21, 1976.
51. Collings CA, Curet LB, Mullin JP: Maternal and fetal responses to a maternal aerobic exercise program. *Am J Obstet Gynecol* 145:702–707, 1983.
52. Artal R, Wiswell RA, Romen Y: Hormonal responses to exercise in diabetic and non-diabetic pregnant subjects. *Diabetes* (in press).
53. Pollock ML: A comparative analysis of 4 protocols for maximal exercise testing. *Am Heart J* 93:39, 1976.
54. Ellestad MH: *Stress Testing: Principles and Practice.* Philadelphia, F. A. Davis, 1980.
55. Ready AE, Eynon RB, Cunningham DA: Effect of interval training and detraining on anaerobic fitness in women. *Can J Appl Sport Sci* 6:114–118, 1981.
56. Anderson KL, Seliger V, Rutenfranz J, Berndt I: Physical performance capacity of children in Norway; Part II: Heart rate and oxygen pulse in submaximal and maximal exercises—population parameters in a rural community. *Eur J Appl Physiol* 33:197–206, 1974.
57. Blackburn M, Calloway D: Basal metabolic rate and work energy expenditure of mature pregnant women. *J Am Diet Assoc* 69:24–28, 1973.
58. Blackburn M, Calloway D: Energy expenditure and consumption of mature pregnant and lactating women. *J Am Diet Assoc* 69:29–37, 1973.
59. Wiswell RA, Artal R, Romen Y, Kammula R: Hormonal and metabolic response to maximal exercise in pregnancy. *Med Sci Sports Exerc* 17:206, 1985.

3
Exercise in Pregnancy in the Experimental Animal

Energy demands of a living organism increase whenever its metabolism is stimulated. For example, during exercise the working muscles can increase their energy requirements drastically. Similarly, the pregnant uterus and its contents constitute a growing mass of tissue with increasing need for substrates. This places demands upon the cardiovascular system such as increases in blood volume and cardiac output which in these respects resemble those of ordinary physical training.

In this review we will explore what is known about physiologic adjustments when exercise stress is imposed upon that of pregnancy. Among the issues which we will consider are: (*a*) differences in metabolic, endocrinologic, respiratory, and circulatory responses between pregnant and nonpregnant animals; (*b*) temperature changes; (*c*) uteroplacental blood flow and the placental transport of respiratory gases and substrates; and (*d*) metabolic, respiratory, and circulatory adjustments in the nonhuman fetus.

MATERNAL RESPONSES

A fundamental question concerns the extent to which responses to exercise during pregnancy differ from those in the nonpregnant state. This problem can be investigated only in carefully controlled studies against a background of knowledge of the physiologic changes of both pregnancy and exercise.

Few well-controlled studies on the subject of exercise in pregnancy can be found in the literature, probably because of the many variables that affect the responses to both pregnancy and exercise. In addition, very few studies have been performed under the most extreme conditions, that is, during exhaustive exercise near term. Unfortunately it is therefore impossible in many instances to determine the exact extent to which exercise responses are different during pregnancy. Because of this, and the fact that fetal physiologic functions are difficult to determine in humans, laboratory animals are utilized for such studies. For the general reader, perhaps unacquainted with experimental methods in laboratory animals, an appendix is offered which details some of these techniques.

Oxygen Consumption

At rest all energy is generated by oxidative metabolism of nutrients (8). Resting O_2 consumption ($\dot{V}_{O_2}$) is influenced by several factors, including species, body size and composition, sex, age (see Chapter 12) (8, 35), position (53), and environmental factors (e.g., temperature). During pregnancy nutrients are also used for maternal weight increase and for the growth, metabolism, and muscular activity of the fetus. Strictly speaking, one cannot measure O_2 consumption or basal metabolic rate of the mother alone.

During pregnancy O_2 consumption measured at rest increases with advancing gestational age to a maximum near term (11, 139, 145, 173, 179). In humans this value is 16–32% above that of nonpregnant controls (49, 87, 92, 93, 95, 139, 173, 179), while in near-term pygmy goats it is increased 21% (51). Therefore the higher resting $\dot{V}_{O_2}$ during pregnancy could result from increased tissue mass, higher metabolic rate per gram of tissue, and/or more work for vital functions.

Maximal O_2 consumption during pregnancy has not been studied in great detail. In pregnant ewes Lotgering and co-workers (109) observed a 5.6-fold increase in O_2 consumption to 32 ml·min^{-1}·kg^{-1} during maximal exercise, but it is unknown whether or not this is higher than in nonpregnant sheep. If one could extrapolate from observations at submaximal work levels in humans, a given maximal task during pregnancy would require about a 10% higher absolute $\dot{V}_{O_2max}$. Physical training of a sedentary nonpregnant individual can increase $\dot{V}_{O_2max}$ up to 33% (153). Because during pregnancy every task requires a higher O_2 consumption than in the nonpregnant state, some training effect seems inevitable unless a more sedentary life-style is adopted. (See Chapter 11 for additional information.)

Physical Working Capacity

Physical working capacity, the highest external work output reached under a specific set of circumstances, is reflected by $\dot{V}_{O_2}$ peak, the highest O_2 consumption reached under such circumstances. In turn, this is affected by $\dot{V}_{O_2max}$ as well as by a variety of conditions, including somatic factors (sex, age, body dimensions, health), psychic factors (attitude, motivation), environmental factors (altitude, gas pressures, temperature, noise, air pollution), work characteristics (intensity, duration, rhythm, technique, position), training and adaptation (8, 149).

As $\dot{V}_{O_2max}$ probably increases during pregnancy working capacity will tend to increase. Brühl et al. (36) reported that fatigue was reached sooner in exercising pregnant rabbits than in controls; however, his methods were not reported.

Metabolism

During pregnancy the turnover rates of the different substrates must increase linearly with O_2 consumption, as pregnancy does not significantly affect the balance of carbohydrates and fats used for combustion. The observation that the glucose turnover rate increases in absolute terms but remains constant when normalized for body weight in humans (84) and horses (56) supports this suggestion. Turnover rates are important from a quantitative standpoint (77), whereas plasma concentrations merely reflect the balance between production (absorption and gluconeogenesis) and utilization of the different fuels. The maternal glucose concentration falls linearly with advancing gestational age in humans (86) and guinea pigs (167) but not significantly in sheep (169) and horses (56). The variations among these species seem to reflect their differences in blood volume increase with gestation.

In men (181) moderate exercise increases the rates of gluconeogenesis and glucose turnover, with glucose oxidation providing about 20% of the total energy requirements. However, whether glucose turnover rate changes similarly in exercising pregnant women has not been examined. In fed humans the blood glucose concentration decreases with the level and duration of exercise (143), but it increases in fasting man, both at rest (31, 58) and during exhaustive exercise (31). (For additional information, see Chapters 6 and 7.)

Above about 50% $\dot{V}_{O_2max}$, the blood lactate concentration increases with the level of exercise. Higher blood lactate concentrations are found in pregnant women than in controls during (92, 93) and following (20, 88, 92, 93) moderate hand crank or bicycle exercise, but elevated concentrations have not been observed during exercise of short duration and low intensity (173). Because pyruvate concentrations increase only slightly during (92, 93) and following exercise in both pregnant and nonpregnant women (20, 92, 93), the increase in lactate-to-pyruvate ratio is more pronounced in pregnant women than in controls, both during (92, 93) and following exercise (20, 92, 93). In sheep lactate concentrations increase with both the exercise level (43, 109) and duration (109), with incomplete recovery at 20 min following prolonged exercise at 70% $\dot{V}_{O_2max}$ (109). Although the lactate increase is larger than that of pyruvate, the increase in lactate-to-pyruvate ratio in this species was not significant (45, 109).

During exercise in sheep the free fatty acid concentrations increase (21). In dogs the contribution of free fatty acids to the energy expenditure increases with exercise duration (175), until at very high levels the free fatty acid turnover rate is reduced (76). Berg et al. (20) observed a slight decrease in the free fatty acid concentration during exercise in both pregnant and nonpregnant women, but it is unknown whether the turnover rate during exercise in pregnancy is different from that in the nonpregnant state. In sheep, in which acetate metabolism accounts for 20 (3) to 30% (137) of the total energy expenditure at rest, the free fatty acid concentration during exercise is increased (21). However, neither acetate metabolism (79, 83) or concentrations (43) change during exercise. The contribution of protein metabolism to the energy expenditure of exercise is small (47%) (8) and has not been studied during pregnancy.

Body Temperature

Immediately following ovulation, "basal" body temperature rises approximately 0.5°C in association with increased progesterone concentrations. During pregnancy this temperature increase persists until about midgestation, declining thereafter to normal levels (76). Although progesterone concentrations increase markedly toward term (171), the decline in basal body temperature has been attributed to the opposing effect of increased estrogen concentrations (76).

During exercise only 20–25% of the added energy expenditure is used for external work, the remaining 75–80% being transformed into heat, increasing total heat production by as much as 20 times resting values (5). The increased body temperature results in significant circulatory adjustments (33). Increased blood flow to the skin results in most of the heat being lost to the environment, but some is stored, primarily in the exercising muscles. As exercise proceeds, the body temperature gradually increases until it plateaus at a level which depends mainly upon the exercise intensity and to a lesser extent its duration (8). Following the termination of exercise, temperature initially decreases rapidly, then more gradually returns to normal over a period of an hour or so (126).

Figure 3.1 depicts maternal body temperature at several levels and durations of exercise in near-term pregnant ewes (109). Compared with that of humans, basal body temperature in sheep is approximately 2°C higher and heat loss across the skin is much lower. Within the first minutes of exercise, maternal body temperature increased rapidly, the rate of increase varying with the exercise level (Fig. 3.1). After the initial rapid rise it continued to increase further, and a plateau was not observed during even relatively prolonged (40 min) exercise at 70% $\dot{V}_{O_2max}$. At exhaustion, reached either by short-term maximal exercise or by prolonged exercise at 70% $\dot{V}_{O_2max}$, the ewe's body temperature averaged 40.7°C (Fig. 3.1). Following exercise maternal temperature initially declined sharply, then gradually returned to normal. The recovery time varied with the exercise intensity and duration, so that even one hour after 40 min of exercise at 70% $\dot{V}_{O_2max}$, recovery was not complete. As an aside, sheep employ panting to a greater extent than do humans, in whom sweating is a more important mechanism.

Physical training increases blood volume and enhances sweat production. This permits greater cutaneous perfusion at a given

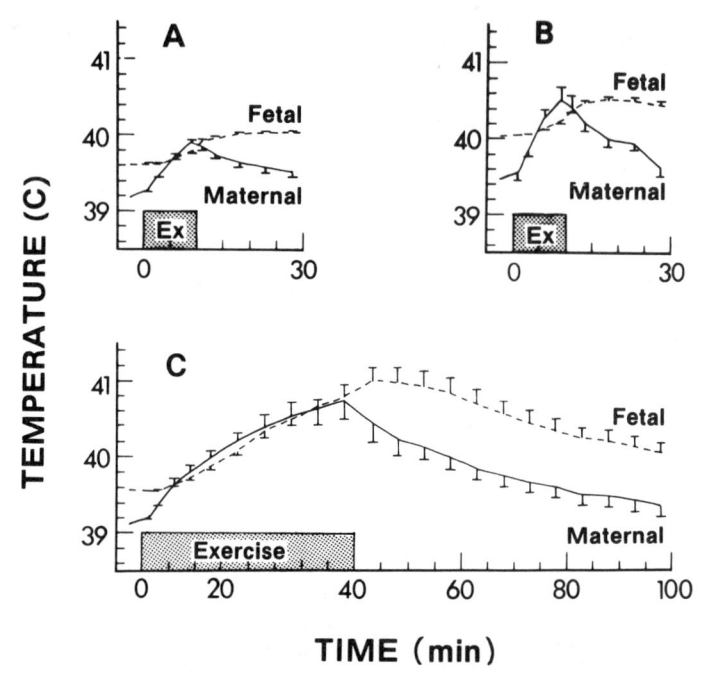

Figure 3.1. Maternal and fetal temperature changes in response to three different exercise regimens. (From Lotgering et al. (110).) (A) Ten-minute exercise at 70% $\dot{V}_{O_2max}$. (B) Ten-minute exercise at 100% $\dot{V}_{O_2max}$. (C) Forty-minute exercise at 70% $\dot{V}_{O_2max}$.

thermal load and results in increased capability of the organism to dissipate heat (8). The effect of training during pregnancy on body temperature control has not been studied.

Respiration and Blood Gases

The changes in resting respiratory function associated with pregnancy have been the subject of several reviews (29, 76, 127, 178).

Pregnant and postpartum pygmy goats which underwent only short-term moderate exercise showed a small decrease in arterial CO_2 tension, a small increase in O_2 content, and no change in pH (51). Larger decreases in CO_2 tension were observed during prolonged moderate exercise in sheep (43, 45, 54, 101), and these were associated with a marked increase in pH (43, 45, 54) and either a decrease or only slight increase in O_2 tension (43, 54).

In none of these studies were the blood gas values corrected for the exercise-induced temperature increase. Blood obtained anaerobically and analyzed for respiratory gases at a temperature below that of the body provides falsely low O_2 and CO_2 tensions and a falsely high pH (158). Therefore consideration of exercise-induced temperature changes is essential for a correct assessment of the blood gases in vivo. Lotgering and co-workers (109) observed that when the blood gas values were corrected for the temperature changes in vivo, no significant changes occurred during short-term (10 min) exercise at 70 and 100% $\dot{V}_{O_2max}$ in sheep. However, during prolonged (40 min) exercise in 70% $\dot{V}_{O_2max}$ the ewe's arterial O_2 tension increased 13% (to 117 Torr) and O_2 content 25% (to 13.3 ml·dl^{-1}), while CO_2 tension decreased 28% (to 28 Torr) and H$^+$ concentration decreased 22% (with a pH increase to 7.56). The increase in arterial O_2 content resulted largely from hemoconcentration. Recovery was virtually complete within 20 min.

In conclusion, the hyperventilation during pregnancy results in a decrease in CO_2 tension and buffering capacity not only at rest but also during and following exercise. These changes are more pronounced in ungulates, in which hyperventilation has a more important role in heat dissipation than it does in humans. In other aspects, respiration during exercise in pregnancy does not seem to differ from that in the nonpregnant state. (For additional information, see Chapter 11.)

Circulation

Since 1915, when Lindhard (95) first observed increased cardiac output during pregnancy, many investigators have further explored the maternal circulatory adjustments (116). Burwell et al. (39), using the acetylene method, reported a maximum increase of about 50% at about 30 weeks. Later studies have used the direct Fick method (11, 67, 130, 145), dye dilution (1, 91, 174), thermodilution (157), and echocardiography (150) to measure cardiac output. It is now generally agreed that by 12 weeks of gestation cardiac output is increased above nonpregnant levels, but opinions differ as to the subsequent changes. Cardiac output may further increase during the second trimester (67, 174), but not significantly according to some (9, 11, 91, 130, 145). Although earlier studies reported a decreased cardiac output during the third trimester to almost nonpregnant values near term, Lees et al. (91) suggested that the fall during the third trimester may be attributed to decreased venous return in the supine position. Nonetheless, other investigators (9, 10, 174) have observed in the lateral and sitting positions during the third trimester a decrease in cardiac output to about 10% above nonpregnant values. (For additional information, see Chapter 8.) In sheep (117) and goats (51) resting cardiac output during a third trimester remains 20–30% above nonpregnant or postpartum control values.

Hytten and Leitch (75) have reviewed the resting arterial blood pressure changes during pregnancy in humans. In early and midgestation diastolic pressure decreases about 10% below nonpregnant values, while systolic pressure decreases only slightly. During the third trimester both pressures return toward nonpregnant values if supine hypotension is prevented. Sheep (117) and goats (51) do not show a clear gestational age trend and have slightly lower mean arterial pressures near term than postpartum. Total peripheral resistance in midpregnancy decreases as much as 30% in humans (11, 145), sheep (117), and goats (51). The mechanisms of this decrease are only partially elucidated, but may include the formation of an effective arteriovenous shunt by the placenta (38), decreased uterine and systemic vascular wall tension mediated by hormones (e.g., the progesterone-to-estrogen ratio) (98), and lowered viscosity associated with a fall in hematocrit (68).

Upon the initiation of exercise total peripheral resistance decreases immediately and is inversely related to O_2 consumption. The lowered resistance in the exercising muscles results from local vasodilatation and is probably mainly of metabolic origin, whereas the increased resistance in nonexercising areas is mainly the result of sympathetic stimulation (149). The diastolic pressure remains virtually constant, whereas the systolic and thus the mean arterial pressures increase with work load intensity.

The arterial blood pressure response to exercise in pregnancy has been studied in humans (4, 11, 20, 53, 55, 89, 92, 93, 112, 138, 142, 145, 161, 165); sheep (45, 50, 54, 108); and goats (51, 72). These studies show an increase of up to 20% in mean arterial pressure during exercise, mainly because of increased systolic pressure (11, 20, 92, 93, 142, 145, 161, 165), with the systolic pressure increasing proportionately with the level of exercise at moderate work loads (20, 92, 93, 165). However, in sheep mean arterial pressure does not significantly increase any further when the exercise level is increased from 70 to 100% $\dot{V}_{O_2max}$, or when the duration of exercise is extended from 10 to 40 min (108). Increased pressure response to treadmill exercise reported in pregnant women (87) and goats (51), may have resulted from a higher work load due to pregnancy weight gain. However, with one exception (92, 93) a slightly higher pressure in pregnant women than in controls has also been reported in response to bicycle exercise (20, 53, 165). (For additional information, see Chapters 8 and 9.)

Because both the cardiac output increase and the arterial pressure response to submaximal exercise are only slightly altered by pregnancy, the exercise-induced decrease in total peripheral resistance during pregnancy must be of a magnitude similar to that in the nonpregnant state. The more marked decrease in total peripheral resistance calculated during weight-bearing exercise in pygmy goats (51) probably reflects a higher work load rather than a pregnancy effect.

With advancing gestation whole blood volume in humans increases gradually up to 50% near term, due to a 30–60% increase in plasma volume and a 20–30% increase in erythrocyte mass, but the increases are less pronounced in some other species such as sheep (99). This hypervolemia tends to increase mean systemic pressure, which combined with the decreased peripheral resistance mediates the increase in resting cardiac output and stroke volume during pregnancy.

During exercise plasma volume decreases as a function of exercise intensity, reaching a maximal reduction of 14% at about 60% $\dot{V}_{O_2max}$ in man (63). The decrease occurs rapidly, is virtually complete within 10 min, and does not change further with exercise duration. Some workers (63, 164) consider increased blood pressure the major force driving plasma filtrate across the capillary membrane in exercising muscles, while others (110) suggest a more important role for muscle tissue osmolality changes. This filtrate consists of water and electrolytes and, to a lesser extent, of plasma proteins (64). One could speculate that the rise in hematocrit during exercise could also be partially caused by catecholamine-induced red cell release by the spleen; however, this has not been studied in man.

The hematocrit increases during exercise in pregnant sheep (43, 108), probably as the result of a decrease in plasma volume without a change in red cell mass (108) (Fig. 3.2). The 20% decrease in plasma volume observed in exercising pregnant sheep (Fig. 3.2) (108) was slightly larger than the maximal change observed in nonpregnant humans (63, 110) and was associated with a smaller increase in plasma protein concentration. Inherent in the calculation of plasma and red cell volumes from hematocrit and whole blood volume is the assumption that the pool of circulating erythrocytes remains constant (108). However, the sheep spleen contains approximately 25% of the total red cell mass (175), and in dogs (12) and sheep (172) the erythrocytes sequestered in the spleen and other reservoirs can be released by catecholamine infusion. If labeled red cells were released from these reservoirs at the onset of exercise, the calculated whole blood and plasma volume decrease would be overestimated.

Cardiac Output Distribution

The most striking change in blood flow distribution during pregnancy is the increase in uterine blood flow with advancing gestational age. Indicator dilution methods (6, 26, 118) and electromagnetic flowprobes (7) have been used to study uterine blood flow acutely in pregnant women, but only under stressful conditions or under anesthesia, and with the subject supine. Therefore, the results from these studies showing a mean total uterine blood flow of 110–150 ml·min^{-1}·(kg total uterus)$^{-1}$ may well underestimate total uterine flow under more physiologic conditions. In chronically catheterized sheep the antipyrine technique (74) and radioactively labeled microspheres (146), give values of approximately 240 ml·min^{-1}·(kg total uterus)$^{-1}$, or absolute values near term of approximately 1300 ml·min^{-1}, a 50–60-fold increase above nonpregnant values. Blood flow to placental cotyledons increases with increasing fetal weight, whereas that to the myometrium and endometrium remains relatively constant (111), so that near term cotyledonary flow

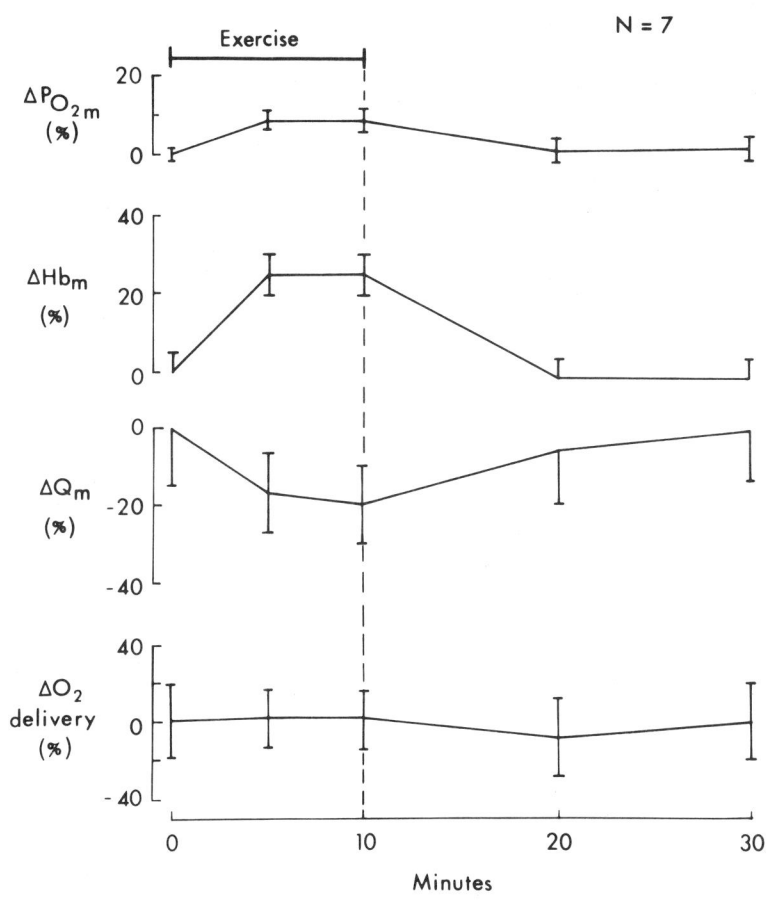

Figure 3.2. Changes in whole blood, plasma, and red cell volumes during exercise in pregnant sheep. (From Lotgering et al. (109).)

is approximately 85% of total uterine blood flow (140, 147). Because placental growth during the later part of gestation is small (113), the increase in cotyledonary flow during this period appears to reflect the increasing demands of the fetus. Acute studies (7, 115) showed a constant blood flow per kilogram of total uterine tissues during the course of gestation. However, in chronically instrumented animals the increase in uterine flow is less than the increase in total uterine or fetal weight, and blood flow per kilogram of total uterine contents or fetus decreases with advancing gestational age (74, 147).

Some factors affecting uterine blood flow have been reviewed (18, 19, 34, 144, 177). The large decrease in uterine vascular resistance during pregnancy probably results from vasodilation associated with increasing concentrations of estrogens produced by the fetoplacental unit and prostaglandins (PGE_2 and PGI_2) produced by the vessel wall. Estrogens may exert their action by the mediation of prostaglandins, but the intermediate steps in the vascular smooth muscle relaxation have not been clearly identified. Although the uterine vasculature during pregnancy is less sensitive to the effects of vasoactive agents, it responds to circulating prostaglandins and catecholamines. The response of myoendometrial flow to catecholamines is similar in the pregnant and nonpregnant state, whereas cotyledonary flow is less sensitive (65). Spontaneous decreases in uterine blood flow of as much as 20% have been reported (90, 176), and up to 50% in response to alkalosis (40, 128), hyperthermia (42, 128), and a variety of other stresses (120, 121, 160). Possibly these vasoconstrictive occurrences are catecholamine mediated (69).

The distribution of blood flow to other organs during gestation has been studied in sheep with the use of microspheres (146). Flow to the mammary glands increases and flow to the liver and adrenal glands decreases, while renal flow does not change significantly. In contrast, studies in humans show increases in both renal (96), and cutaneous (168) blood flow.

The effect of exercise of uterine blood flow during pregnancy has been studied in humans (123), sheep (43, 45, 50, 101, 108, 129), and pygmy goats (72, 73). Using the disappearance of ^{24}Na injected into the myometrium, Morris et al. (123) suggested a 25% decrease in perfusion of the human pregnant uterus during mild short-term bicycle exercise in the supine position. This probably represents an overestimate. In the supine position the presence of a large pregnant uterus may reduce venous return and cardiac output and consequently uterine blood flow. Furthermore, myometrial flow may not represent total uterine blood flow, because animal studies show that flow within the uterus is redistributed in response to exercise, favoring the cotyledons at the cost of the myometrium (50, 73).

Initial animal studies showed a variable change in uterine blood flow. In sheep Orr et al. (129), using a doppler flow probe around a distal branch of the uterine artery, and Curet et al. (50), using microspheres, concluded that uterine blood flow remains constant during treadmill exercise. However, their measurements were made shortly after, rather than during, the exercise, and uterine flow returns rapidly to control levels when exercise is discontinued (108). In preliminary studies Longo and co-workers (101) reported a decrease in uterine flow of up to 40% during prolonged exercise in sheep, while Hohimer and colleagues (72) reported only minimal changes in goats. Clapp (45) reported no change in total uterine blood flow during mild exercise in sheep, while flow decreased 28% near the point of exhaustion during prolonged exercise. Chandler and Bell (43) reported a mean decrease of 36% (range 17–47%) in blood flow to the pregnant horn during prolonged, moderately strenuous exercise in sheep. The exercise stress in these studies was expressed in work load rather than in physiologic terms. Hohimer and co-workers (73) reported a mean decrease in uterine blood flow of 32% during short-term exercise in 5 pygmy goats in which maternal heart rate increased from 129 to 195 beats/min (bpm). However, flow decreased only 18% in 4 other pygmy goats in which the mean heart rate increase was slightly greater, to 210 bpm.

Lotgering and co-workers (108) studied total uterine blood flow response to different levels (%$\dot{V}_{O_2max}$) and durations of exercise in sheep accustomed to the treadmill. The results are shown in Figure 3.3. Uterine blood flow decreased immediately at the onset of exercise, was significantly below control values throughout the exercise period, and returned to control values within 10 min of recovery. Mean uterine blood flow decreased 13% during a 10-min exercise period at 70% $\dot{V}_{O_2max}$, 17% during 10 min at 100% $\dot{V}_{O_2max}$, and 24% near the end of a 40-min period at 70% $\dot{V}_{O_2max}$ (Fig. 3.3). Although significantly different from the preexercise values, the flow values during the three regimens were not significantly different from each other, because of large spontaneous fluctuations in flow which persisted during exercise. However, regression analysis showed a significant decrease of flow with time, and flow varied linearly with heart rate (73, 108) (Fig. 3.4); thus, it seems likely that uterine blood flow decreases with both the level and the duration of exercise.

Although the exercise-induced increase in uterine vascular resistance probably results from active vasoconstriction caused by increased sympathetic activity, this has not been demonstrated. If it is true that the effects of increased sympathetic activity during exercise may be modified by local metabolic factors, one would expect my-

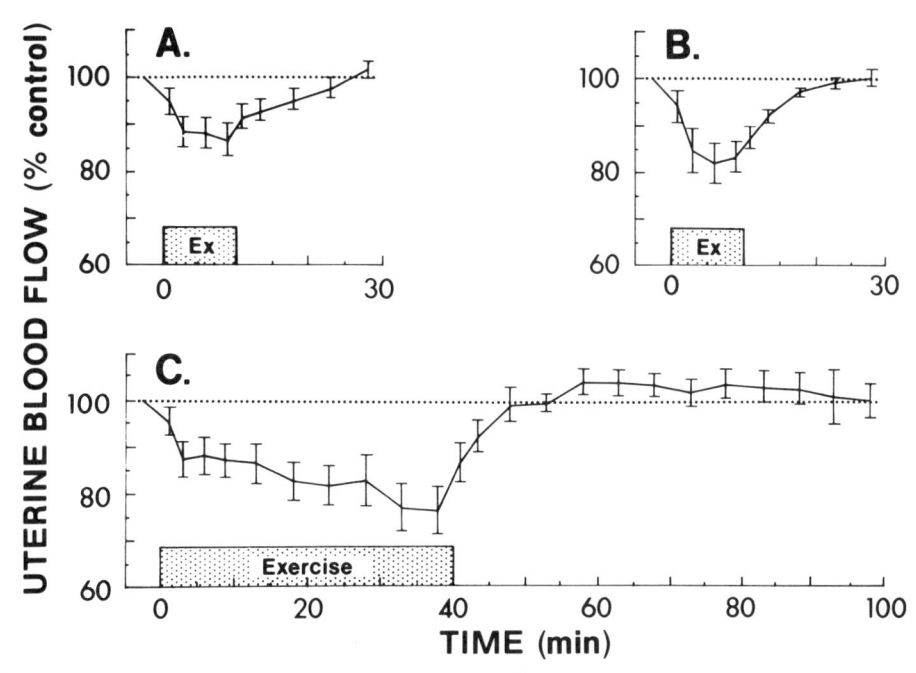

Figure 3.3. Uterine blood flow response to three different exercise regimens in pregnant sheep. (From Lotgering et al. (109).) (*A*) Ten-minute exercise at 70% $\dot{V}_{O_2max}$. (*B*) Ten-minute exercise at 100% $\dot{V}_{O_2max}$. (*C*) Forty-minute exercise at 70% $\dot{V}_{O_2max}$.

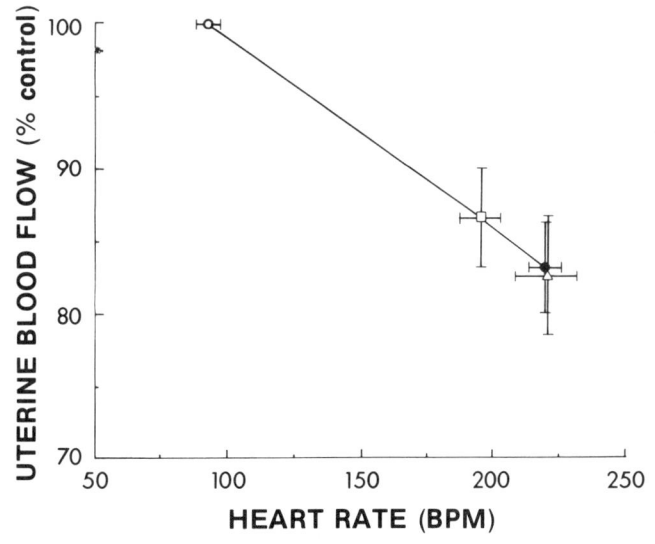

Figure 3.4. Relation between heart rate and total uterine blood flow in near term pregnant sheep. (From Lotgering et al. (109).). ○ = rest; □ = 10-min exercise at 70% $\dot{V}_{O_2max}$; ● = 10-min exercise at 100% $\dot{V}_{O_2max}$; △ = 40-min exercise at 70% $\dot{V}_{O_2max}$.

ometrial flow to behave like the flow to the splanchnic bed, whereas cotyledonary flow would decrease only to such an extent that the fetoplacental O_2 demands can still be met. There is some evidence that this is the case. Blood flow within the uterus is redistributed to the cotyledons at the expense of the myometrium, both during catecholamine infusion (44, 148), as well as during (73) and following (50) exercise. Hohimer and colleagues (73) reported only an 8% decrease in cotyledonary flow when total uterine blood flow decreased 18%, while myometrial flow decreased 52%.

From the observation that urinary 5-hydroxyindoleacetic acid following exercise is more reduced in pregnant women than in controls, it has been suggested that the decrease in visceral blood flow during exercise is more pronounced in pregnant women (52). However, more direct measurements are required to demonstrate this reduction. Bell and Hales (personal communicaion) observed no major effect of pregnancy on nonuterine regional blood flow distribution in sheep. Although Orr et al. (129) reported significant increases in carotid and iliac artery flow in pregnant ewes, they observed similar changes in nonpregnant sheep. Curet et al. (50) found no change in renal flow following exercise in pregnant sheep, but they made no comparison with nonpregnant ewes. Thus, with the exception of uterine flow, there is little evidence that regional blood flow distribution during exercise is altered by pregnancy.

Physical training increases maximal O_2 consumption and results in a lower physiologic level of exercise ($\%\dot{V}_{O_2max}$) of each work load. In turn, this results in reduced sympathetic activity in trained individuals in response to a given work load (46). One would expect a given work load in a trained individual to result in a smaller reduction in uterine blood flow during exercise, but this has not been investigated.

Curet et al. (50), studying the effect of physical training on postexercise uterine and renal blood flows in sheep observed no difference between trained and nontrained animals, but the numbers of animals were too small to allow a definite conclusion.

Uterine Oxygen Consumption

Uterine O_2 consumption increases during pregnancy in response to the increasing demands of the growing conceptus, as demonstrated in humans (6), sheep, and goats (74, 115, 124). With advancing gestational age the uterine arteriovenous O_2 difference rises 3- (124) to 10-fold (74). Thus, uterine O_2 consumption increases much more than would be expected on the basis of the blood flow increase alone. Acute studies have shown a constant uterine blood flow and O_2 consumption per kg of tissue with advancing gestational age in humans and sheep (7, 115), whereas studies in chronically catheterized sheep showed a decreasing uterine blood flow per kg uterine contents, but constant (124) or increasing (74) O_2 consumption per kg of tissue. In anesthetized sheep near term, the mean O_2 consumption of the uterus as a whole (myoendometrium, placenta, and fetus) was reported as 9.9 ml·min^{-1}·kg^{-1}, while that of the fetus, and of the placenta plus myoendometrium were 7.1, and 14.1 ml·min^{-1}·kg^{-1}, respectively (115). Moreover, recent studies in chronically catheterized sheep (114) show that about 45% of the O_2 used by the uterus is consumed by the placenta plus myoendometrium, so that the weight specific O_2 consumption of this compartment is about three times that of the fetus.

Uterine O_2 consumption during exercise has not been studied in pregnant humans, but it does not change significantly during prolonged submaximal treadmill exercise in sheep (43, 45, 109). Although total uterine blood flow reported by Lotgering and coworkers was markedly reduced, O_2 consumption was maintained as the result of hemoconcentration and increased O_2 extraction (109) (Fig. 3.2). During maternal exercise cotyledonary flow decreases less than myoendometrial flow (50, 73). Thus, in order to maintain the same metabolic rate during exercise, the myoendometrium must increase its O_2 extraction to a greater extent than do the cotyledons. However, myoendometrial O_2 consumption during exercise may decrease below resting values, while that of the fetus plus placenta increases. In addition, training may alter the distribution of flow and oxygen consumption within the uterus. The intriguing problem of autoregulation of blood flow and O_2 consumption within the pregnant uterus needs further study.

Table 3.1 summarizes some of the maternal responses to pregnancy, exercise, and the combination of the two.

FETAL RESPONSES

The fetus requires a continuous and increasing supply of oxygen and nutrients for its metabolism and growth. A prolonged severe reduction in this supply of substrates will result in fetal demise, but less severe reductions do not cause apparent damage. Our present understanding of the fetal adjustments and tolerance limits is limited for several reasons.

First, there is the absence of accurate and sensitive criteria for tolerance limits. Permanent structural or functional damage proves that tolerance was exceeded, but this criterion is relatively insensitive because small changes may be undetectable. Growth retardation demonstrates chronic adaptations within such limits, but this criterion lacks sensitivity because of the large normal variation. Physiologic variables such as heart rate, O_2 consumption, and oxygen, substrate, or hormone concentrations are more sensitive to changes, but they represent temporary adjustments rather than provide information as to the fetal tolerance.

Second, even obtaining information about such fundamental variables is not easy because the fetus is well protected from the human with relative ease. Most other functions, however, cannot be studied in humans because they require invasive techniques. In certain experimental animals chronic catheterization of the fetus can be used to study adaptive changes to a variety of stresses without the disadvantages of anesthesia or acute surgical stress.

Oxygen Consumption

Fetal oxygen consumption can be calculated from umbilical blood flow and umbilical arteriovenous O_2 content difference, and in the lamb during the third trimester it equals about 8.0 ml·min^{-1}·kg fetus^{-1} (14, 105). Moderate maternal hypoxia (Po$_2$=50 Torr) does not affect fetal O_2 consumption, but more severe maternal hypoxia reduces it markedly, resulting from a marked decrease in O_2 extraction without a change in umbilical blood flow (132). With short-term infusion of norepinephrine (106) or long-term infusion of triiodothyronine (107) into the fetus, O_2 consumpion increases about 25%. However, in contrast to hypoxia this is associated with an increase in umbilical blood flow but no change in O_2 extraction. To what extent catecholamine changes within the physiologic range affect fetal O_2 consumption has not been investigated. Nor have the effects of such large changes in O_2 consumption on fetal heat production, and

Table 3.1. Maximal Responses of Selected Maternal Physiologic Variables to Pregnancy, Exercise, and Training

	Near term Pregnancy[a]	Exercise[a]	Exercise during Pregnancy[b]	Training[b]	Training and Pregnancy[c]
O_2 consumption	↑ or ↑↑°	↑↑↑	↑	↑↑	↑ ?
Respiratory minute volume	↑ or ↑↑°	↑↑↑	↑ ?	↑	—
Tidal volume	↑	↑↑↑	↑ ?	— ?	— ?
Respiratory frequency	—	↑↑↑	— ?	↑	—
Cardiac output	↑ or ↑↑°	↑↑↑	↑ ?	↑ or ↑↑°	↑ ?
Stroke volume	↑	↑↑	↑ ?	↑ or ↑↑°	↑ ?
Heart rate	↑	↑↑↑	— ?	—	— ?
Mean arterial pressure	— or ↓°	↑	— ?	—	— ?
Plasma volume	↑ or ↑↑↑°	↓	— ?	—	— ?
Uterine blood flow	↑↑↑	↓↓↓ ?	↑ ?	— ?	— ?

[a] Change from nonpregnant, nontrained, resting values. ° = Marked species difference, ? = doubtful or unknown, — = change <5%, ↑ or ↓ increase or decrease of 6–20%, ↑↑ or ↓↓ 21–40%, ↑↑↑ or ↓↓↓ >40%.

[b] Change from nonpregnant, nontrained, exercise values.

[c] Change from pregnant, nontrained, exercise values.

consequently fetal temperature, been explored. This may be important for the interpretation of respiratory blood gas values, as will be discussed below. The observation that O_2 consumption by the uterus as a whole is constant during maternal exercise in sheep (17, 43, 45, 109) suggests the absence of major changes in fetal O_2 uptake. In addition, this has been demonstrated by observations of a constant umbilical uptake of oxygen during exercise (17, 43). Despite a 10% reduction in umbilical blood flow during exhaustive maternal exercise, O_2 extraction increased 13% (45).

According to the van't Hoff-Arrhenius law, the O_2 consumption of both total uterine contents and fetus should rise during exercise-induced hyperthermia. Assuming Q_{10} of 2–3, Lotgering and co-workers (109) calculated that with prolonged exercise O_2 consumption of the fetus should increase 9–16% and that of the placenta and uterine wall, 11–18%. However, they observed only a 6% increase in O_2 consumption of the total uterine contents. Although this result may not be significantly different from the value expected from the calculated Q_{10} effect, other changes in the fetus may also affect O_2 consumption. For instance, substrate limitation or pH changes may prevent increased enzymatic reaction rates as expected from the Q_{10} effect. In addition, the temperature effects on metabolism may be masked by central nervous system regulation, as occurs in poikilothermic species (35). Therefore it is impossible to assess accurately whether the fetal and placental O_2 requirements increased or not during maternal exercise.

Fetal Metabolism and Endocrinology

In the fetus, substrates are used not only for "basal" metabolism and heat production, but also for growth and muscular activities. Furthermore, it is conceivable that under certain conditions the fetus relies on anaerobic metabolism for short time periods (132).

According to Battaglia and Meschia (14) about 65% of the caloric expenditure in the sheep fetus is used for oxidative metabolism and 35% for growth. If one assumes that the O_2 consumption per kg tissue is the same in other species with different growth rates, it follows that fetal oxidative metabolism may vary considerably. The fetal respiratory quotient is 0.94 (78), indicating the predominant metabolism of carbohydrates and amino acids, but may be falsely low because relatively large amounts of carbon and nitrogen are incorporated in the growing organism.

Glucose crosses the placenta by facilitated diffusion; thus, the rate is dependent upon the concentration in maternal blood. The fetal blood glucose concentration, the umbilical glucose uptake, and the glucose-to-O_2 quotient decrease during maternal fasting, changes probably mediated by a lower fetal insulin concentration (154). Physical or verbal stress of the ewe does not affect the plasma glucose and insulin concentrations in mother or fetus (155). However, during prolonged moderate treadmill exercise in sheep, fetal blood glucose concentrations increase up to 75%, with less pronounced changes occurring during short-term or mild exercise (Fig. 3.2) (17, 43, 109). Uterine glucose extraction increases during prolonged exercise (43), probably because of the increased maternal-to-fetal glucose gradient (from about 2.0 to 3.1 mmol·l^{-1}) (16, 17, 43). Despite the hyperglycemia during exercise, fetal plasma insulin does not change significantly until after exercise (16), and thus may increase fetal glucose utilization during recovery. The fetal plasma concentrations of pancreatic glucagon, enteroglucagon and growth hormone were not affected significantly by maternal exercise (16). A gradual increase in fetal corticosteroid concentrations was observed during and following exercise in this study (16), an increase which in part may have resulted from the increased maternal concentrations, as cortisol crosses the sheep placenta at a slow rate (15).

Although fetal lactate concentration is about twice that of the maternal, under normal conditions this does not result from anaerobic metabolism (37). The placenta produces large quantities of lactate, and lactate metabolism may constitute 25% of fetal O_2 consumption (14). To what extent fetal anaerobic metabolism may produce lactate under stressed conditions is unknown. Although fetal lactate concentrations increase up to 50–70% during prolonged moderate exercise (16, 43, 45, 109), they do not change significantly during short-term or mild exercise (45, 109). Chandler and Bell (43) observed that during prolonged moderate exercise in sheep the normal placental release of lactate into the maternal circulation was reversed, with lactate being taken up by the pregnant uterus. Clapp (45) reported continued lactate uptake by the umbilical circulation during prolonged exhaustive exercise, but the data are inadequate for calculating quantitative changes. In contrast, Bell et al. (unpublished) have noted a significant decrease in umbilical net uptake of lactate during exercise. It is unlikely that increased fetal levels are due to increased maternal levels because the ovine placenta is highly impermeable to lactate at the relatively low maternal-fetal gradients observed. Calculations suggest that the increased fetal concentration during exercise would require only a modest increase in fetal glycolysis (16).

Amino acids are actively transported across the placenta, about 60% being used as fuel and 40% for growth in fetal sheep (14). Free fatty acids represent a negligible fraction of the total caloric intake in the sheep fetus, in which fat accounts for 2% of the body weight at term, but may be more important in other species, such as man, in which it constitutes 16% of birth weight. Another substrate, acetate, has been studied during maternal exercise in sheep, and its uterine uptake does not change significantly (43). It is unknown to what extent maternal exercise affects the relative contribution of the different substrates to fetal metabolism. The suggestion that physical training reduces fetal growth will be discussed below.

Body Temperature

Under normal resting conditions the fetal temperature in the human (2), baboon (122), and sheep (1, 141) is about 0.5°C higher than the maternal. When the maternal temperature rises, the fetal increases more slowly and the normal fetal-maternal temperature gradient diminishes (42) or reverses (2). When maternal temperature plateaus after artificial heating (2) or pyrogen injection (1), the temperature gradient returns to near normal values; and when maternal temperature falls during the recovery phase, the fetal temperature decrease is delayed, resulting in an increased fetal-to-maternal difference (2, 42). Fetal and maternal placental blood flows also can affect fetal temperature. The fetal-maternal temperature gradient increases with partial occlusion of the umbilical cord, the maternal aorta or the inferior vena cava, as well as with uterine contractions (122) and maternal heating, partly because of decreased uterine blood flow (42).

Lotgering et al. (109) demonstrated that during maternal exercise the fetal temperature changes (Fig. 3.1) are comparable to those observed during maternal heating (2), lagging behind the relatively rapidly changing maternal temperature at the onset and cessation of exercise. This results in a smaller or reversed temperature gradient during the onset and a larger gradient immediately following exercise (Fig. 3.1). The reversal of the temperature gradient is most pronounced soon after the exercise onset, when the maternal temperature increases rapidly, but becomes progressively less as the maternal temperature plateaus. With heavier exercise (100 vs. 70% $\dot{V}_{O_2max}$) the maternal temperature increases more rapidly, resulting in a larger reversal of the temperature gradient (Fig. 3.1). Following prolonged (40 min) exhaustive exercise at 70% $\dot{V}_{O_2max}$, return of the fetal temperature to normal required over one hour.

Heat is stored in the body core during exercise at rates proportional to exercise intensity. Because dissipation of fetal heat is by convection in blood and flow-limited diffusion, the fetal temperature will increase with that of the mother. A mathematical model of placental heat transfer developed by Schröder et al. (156) has predicted fetal temperature changes from changes in maternal temperature and uterine blood flow, when variables such as fetal metabolism are assumed constant (109). Further calculations (Schroder and Gilbert, unpublished data) suggest that maternal temperature is the major determinant, while changes in fetal metabolism or uterine blood flow of up to 50% will change fetal temperature by less than 0.3°C. Although the changes in fetal temperature suggest a passive dependence on the factors cited above, the constancy of the temperature gradient under steady state conditions suggests the presence of homeostatic mechanisms.

Temperature changes will affect placental and fetal respiratory gas transport, as a temperature increase shifts the oxyhemoglobin saturation curve to the right. This will tend to increase oxygen unloading in the fetal tissues. A mathematical model of placental O_2 transport (102) suggests that during maternal heating as in exercise, the larger shift in maternal than in fetal P_{50} will result in only a small increase in placental O_2 exchange and fetal O_2 tension. During exercise this effect is opposed by other factors, as fetal O_2 tension decreases. One such factor is uterine blood flow which is reduced not only by the sympathetic stimulation of exercise, but also by the temperature increase (42). The possible teratogenic effects of exercise hyperthermia are discussed below.

Respiration and Blood Gases

The fetus exchanges oxygen and carbon dioxide with the mother by passive diffusion across the placenta, a process affected by several factors, including maternal and fetal placental blood flows, arterial O_2 and CO_2 tensions, and hemoglobin concentrations (102).

Several studies in exercising sheep (43, 45, 54, 101), have reported significant decreases in fetal arterial O_2 tension and content of as much as 25%. However, in none of these reports were the respiratory blood gas values corrected for the fetal temperature changes in vivo, resulting in underestimates of fetal O_2 and CO_2 tensions and overestimates of pH values. As noted above, blood obtained anaerobically and analyzed at a temperature below that of the body shows a rise in pH and a fall in O_2 and CO_2 tensions (158). The failure to correct for a 1°C increase results in about a 1.9 and 2.7 Torr underestimate for fetal O_2 and CO_2 tensions respectively, while pH will be 0.015 unit too high (109). Failure to make temperature corrections largely explains the difference in blood gas values between the above studies and those of Lotgering et al. (109). In this latter study (109) fetal arterial O_2 and CO_2 tensions and O_2 content decreased with the level and the duration of exercise, but the values differed significantly from control only when the ewes were run to exhaustion. Near the end of prolonged (40 min) exercise at 70% $\dot{V}_{O_2 max}$, ascending aortic O_2 tension decreased 3.0 Torr, to 23.2 from 26.2 Torr at rest. CO_2 tension decreased 4.5 Torr from 54.1 Torr at rest, and O_2 content decreased 1.5 ml·dl^{-1} from 5.8 ml·dl^{-1} at rest, while pH increased 0.02 unit. Figure 3.5 shows the percent changes in fetal blood gases under these circumstances. With the exception of O_2 content, all blood gases returned to control values within 20 min of termination of exercise. The cause of the decrease in fetal O_2 tension and content during prolonged maternal exercise is not entirely clear. Theoretical calculations suggest that 30% of the decrease in O_2 saturation can be accounted for by the temperature and Bohr shifts of the oxyhemoglobin saturation curve (109). The remaining 70% of the decrease in O_2 saturation and the 3 Torr decrease in O_2 tension probably result largely from the decrease in placental blood flow.

The fetus makes respiratory-like movements (27, 28) in which episodes of breathing and apnea follow each other frequently but variably. They can be regarded as isometric muscular activity with a frequency of 30–70 bpm in humans and 60–120 bpm in sheep, occurring 75% of the time in humans and 40% of the time in sheep. They show a pronounced diurnal rhythm, with a rise during the day to a peak shortly after dusk, and in the fetal lamb they coincide

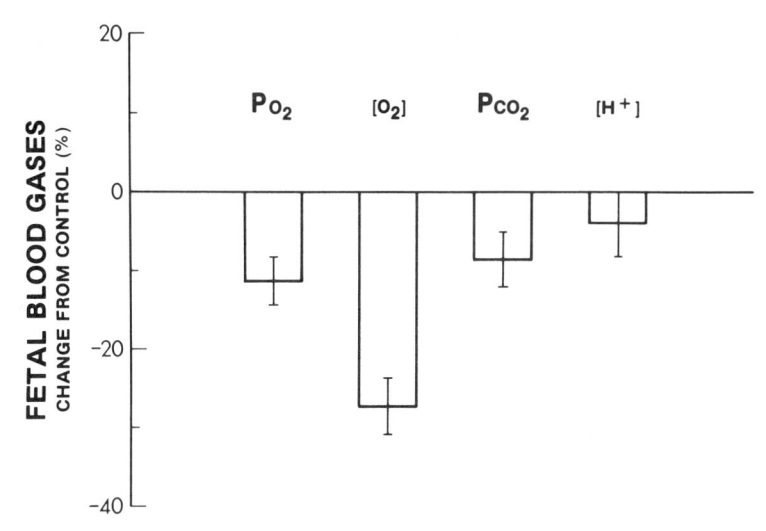

Figure 3.5. Percent changes in fetal sheep respiratory blood gases and hydrogen ion concentrations during prolonged (40 min) exercise at 70% $\dot{V}_{O_2 max}$. (From Lotgering et al. (110).)

with rapid eye movement EEG activity. Fetal breathing movements are less frequent with decreased O_2 tensions or glucose concentrations, and more frequent with increased CO_2 tensions or catecholamine concentrations.

Circulation

Fetal heart rate monitoring is widely used in clinical obstetrics to detect "distress" and to predict fetal outcome. Empirically associated with "fetal distress" are severe brady- and tachycardia (<100 or >180 bpm), loss of variability (bandwidth <5 bpm, zero crossings <2 per min), the absence of accelerations, and the presence of "late" or "variable" decelerations (59). Fetal heart rate usually decreases in response to catecholamines (47, 82, 106) and hypoxia (121) and increases in response to the pyrogen-induced rise in body temperature, but it is variable when the temperature plateaus (70).

Normally the fetal heart operates near the plateau of its Starling function curve with cardiac output near its maximum (61). Consequently, decreases in fetal heart rate directly affect cardiac output, whereas large increases do not increase it further (152). Fetal cardiac output is a function of body weight, being about 500 ml·min^{-1}·kg^{-1} in sheep (60, 151). Neither catecholamines (106) nor moderate degrees of hypoxia (104) appear to affect it, and it is not affected during short-term maternal exercise in sheep (109).

The increase in cardiac output with advancing gestation is associated with increases in whole blood (41) and plasma volumes, which in sheep are about 110 and 77 ml·(kg fetus)$^{-1}$ (32), respectively. Lotgering et al. (109) observed that fetal blood and plasma volumes are unaffected by prolonged, exhaustive treadmill exercise in the ewe, which confirms the absence of a change in hematocrit (43) and is indirect evidence of the absence of hypoxia (159).

The proportion of cardiac output distributed to the fetal organs is virtually constant until late gestation, when blood flows to the lung, brain, and intestines increase more markedly at the cost of flow to the placenta (151). About 40% of cardiac output (or about 200 ml·min^{-1}·kg^{-1}), the largest proportion to a single organ, is directed to the placenta in sheep (104, 115, 151). Measurements in human fetuses with the use of ultrasound have suggested a much lower flow (120 ml·min^{-1}·kg^{-1}) (62); however, this value depends critically upon an accurate measurement of the blood flow velocity and the vessel diameter, and further studies are needed to verify the technique. Catecholamines have been shown to increase umbilical flow in sheep (106), whereas hypoxia does not affect it (101, 136). However, changes in blood flow distribution to other organs (brain, heart, lungs, and adrenals) have been reported in response to hypoxia and norepinephrine infusion (104, 106, 136). Umbilical blood flow in sheep is unaffected by short-term exercise at 70 and 100% $\dot{V}_{O_2max}$ (109) and by prolonged but mild maternal exercise (45). In response to prolonged exhaustive exercise it has been reported to fall 10% (45), but this needs to be confirmed because the resting umbilical flow in these studies was 354 ml·min^{-1}·kg^{-1}, about 50% greater than accepted normal values. Lotgering et al. (109) found no change in cardiac output distribution to other organs during short-term maternal exercise, but this was not studied during prolonged exercise.

Fetal blood pressure gradually increases with advancing gestational age, reaching a value of about 40 mm Hg in near-term sheep when corrected for amniotic fluid pressure (57). Mean arterial pressure increases in response to norepinephrine infusion (106), whereas hypoxia may increase (104) or not affect it (121). Fetal arterial blood pressure was unaffected by short-term (109) as well as prolonged exercise in sheep (45, 54, 109, 131), suggesting no great release of catecholamines.

Table 3.2 summarized some of the fetal variables in relation to prolonged and strenuous exercise. Most of the results as shown in the table are derived from studies in sheep.

Although the studies of fetal cardiovascular responses during maternal exercise are limited, the available evidence suggests the absence of major changes. In turn, this suggests the absence of hypoxia or other "stress." In addition, only insignificant increases in fetal catecholamine concentrations have been noted in fetal sheep in response to both short-term (109) and prolonged exercise (71, 109, 131).

PLACENTAL RESPONSES

The placenta has a multitude of functions which are only partially understood. Barron (13) has recently reviewed the discovery of its respiratory function. As early as 1796 Erasmus Darwin inferred from the color difference of the umbilical vessels that the placenta is a respiratory organ for the fetus, and Zweifel established definitive proof in 1876 (for references, see Barron (13)). Placental physiology is difficult to study independently of the mother and fetus, because their functions are so interwoven.

One can measure the uptake of oxygen and nutrients simultaneously by the uterus as a whole as well as by the fetus. By subtraction one can calculate the O_2 and nutrient consumption of the uteroplacental mass. Meschia et al. (114) estimated that the myoendometrium and placenta consume 45% of the O_2 and 72% of the glucose metabolized by the uterus as a whole, indicating that the O_2 and glucose consumptions are respectively about 3 and 10 times as high as in the fetus on a per kg basis. With the available techniques one cannot separate placental metabolism from that of the myoendometrium under in vivo conditions. The myoendometrium has a mass about equal to the placenta, but is probably metabolically less active. Thus, the weight specific values for placental metabolism are probably even higher than the values presented above. The effect of exercise on pla-

Table 3.2. Maximal Response of Selected Fetal Physiologic Variables to Maternal Exercise

Variable	Response[a]
O_2 consumption	—
Cardiac output	—
Heart rate	— or ↑
Mean arterial pressure	—
Plasma volume	—
Umbilical blood flow	↓
Arterial O_2 tension	↓
Arterial O_2 content	↓↓
Arterial CO_2 tension	↓
Arterial H^+ concentration	—
Arterial catecholamine concentration	— ?

[a] ? = doubtful, — = change >5%, ↑ or ↓ = increase or decrease of 6–20%, ↓↓ = 21–40%.

cental metabolism is unknown. Because both total uterine (17, 43, 45, 109) and umbilical O_2 consumption (17, 45) do not change significantly during exercise, placental metabolism is probably not markedly affected.

The placenta uses several mechanisms to transport various substances: diffusion, facilitated diffusion, and active transport (97). Oxygen exchanges across the placenta by passive diffusion and may be considered flow limited. Theoretical analysis (102) suggests that both the magnitude and distribution of maternal and fetal placental blood flows, as well as maternal and fetal hemoglobin concentrations, will markedly affect placental O_2 transport, whereas only very large differences in the physical chemical characteristics of the membranes will affect oxygen diffusion. The placental diffusing capacity for O_2 cannot be quantified practically, but the diffusing capacity for carbon monoxide ($D_{P_{co}}$), a diffusion-limited gas, provides a method to measure steady-state gas exchange. The $D_{P_{co}}$ is sensitive to anatomical changes (exchange area and membrane thickness), but relatively insensitive to changes in blood flow per se and nonuniformity of distribution of maternal and fetal placental flows (103). Near term $D_{P_{co}}$ expressed in terms of fetal weight is relatively high in small species (24), but placental diffusing capacity per kg of fetal weight does not markedly decrease during the last two months of pregnancy in sheep (100).

In sheep acute exercise does not affect $D_{P_{co}}$ (109). However, this does not exclude the possibility that the amount of O_2 crossing the placenta per min is reduced during exercise, as this is affected by the increased maternal hemoglobin concentration, P_{50}, and temperature, as well as by reductions in uterine and umbilical blood flows. Thus, although it is not possible to assess experimentally the extent to which placental O_2 transfer will be affected, theoretical calculations can make predictions in this regard (see Chapter 12). The observation that total uterine and umbilical O_2 consumption do not decrease, even during prolonged exhaustive exercise (109) suggests the absence of major alterations in placental O_2 exchange.

In guinea pigs which were exercised throughout gestation, Gilbert and co-workers (61) and Nelson et al. (125) observed as much as 34% lower $D_{P_{co}}$ values than in controls, the decrease being a function of the amount of daily exercise. In other chronically exercised guinea pigs Smith and colleagues (163) demonstrated a linear relation between placental diffusing capacity and maternal and fetal surface area per unit volume of placenta. The reason for the smaller placental exchange areas in chronically exercised guinea pigs is unknown. Although theoretically O_2 transfer is affected by the decrease in surface area, it remains unclear whether O_2 transfer limitation caused the reduced birth weight observed in these fetuses.

Glucose diffuses across the placenta by facilitated diffusion, and the carrier system has been studied in detail (22, 23, 81, 182). Glucose uptake increases rapidly with increasing maternal blood concentrations until the concentration is reached where the "carriers" are saturated and above which the rate of transport is slower. Other D-monosaccharides compete for the same stereospecific carrier, and estrogens and progesterones inhibit the transport, but the system is sodium independent. In chronically catheterized sheep at rest, glucose uptake by the fetus and the uteroplacental mass equals 28% and 72%, respectively, of the total uterine glucose uptake (113, 162). Theoretical analysis (162) suggests that the net glucose transfer to the fetus is relatively insensitive to changes in uterine or umbilical blood flows. Despite a significant reduction in uterine flow, glucose uptake actually increased during prolonged exercise in sheep as the result of increased glucose extraction (43). This probably resulted largely from the increased transplacental glucose gradient during exercise (16, 43) (Fig. 3.2). In a preliminary report Bell et al. (16) showed that the increased uterine uptake of glucose during moderate exercise in sheep resulted largely (80%) from increased glucose uptake by the placenta plus myoendometrium.

Lactate is the second most important substrate for fetal metabolism (14). It also diffuses across the placenta by a facilitated process (119), but its carrier system has not been studied in the same detail as that of glucose, nor is it known whether or not glucose and lactate compete for the same carrier. In addition, rather than being transferred from maternal blood, most of the lactate metabolized by the fetus is produced by the placenta. In chronically catheterized near-term sheep uteroplacental lactate production was 11.8 mg·min^{-1}, 5.0 mg·min^{-1} of which was taken up by the placenta plus myoendometrium and 6.5 mg·min^{-1} (or 1.7 mg·min^{-1}·kg^{-1}) by the fetus (166). During prolonged exercise in sheep Chandler and Bell (43) observed only an insignificant reduction in maternal lactate uptake. It seems likely that this resulted from the increased maternal blood concentration and the resulting decreased placental-maternal lactate gradient. It is unknown to what extent placental lactate production is affected by exercise or what its physiological consequences might be.

Of the other substrates, acetate is an important fuel for the resting ewe. Its role in fetal-placental metabolism is largely unknown, but uterine acetate uptake is unaffected by exercise in sheep (43). Amino acids are also important for combustion by both the placenta and the fetus. They are actively transported by the placenta (14), but it is unknown whether this energy-requiring transport mechanism is affected by exercise.

Fetal body temperature is higher than that of the mother. Although little is known about the placenta as a heat exchanger, several groups (1, 2, 141) have concluded that the largest proportion of the heat produced by the fetus diffuses to the mother across the placenta, and a smaller proportion across the fetal skin, amniotic fluid, and uterine wall. In these calculations heat transfer is considered limited by blood flow, and there is some experimental evidence to support this concept (2, 122, 141). Therefore, during maternal exercise, fetal-to-maternal heat transfer will probably be affected by the decrease in uteroplacental flow.

In conclusion, the effects of acute and chronic exercise on metabolic and transport functions of the placenta have been investigated only to a limited extent; and exercise effects on placental endocrine functions are unknown.

FETAL OUTCOME

Adverse effects on fetal outcome have been reported in pregnant animals forced to exercise strenuously during pregnancy in a laboratory. Intrauterine growth retardation with 8% weight reduction was reported in mice (170) and guinea pigs (125). In the same mice Terada (170) noted an increased incidence of resorbed and macerated fetuses, but this observation has not been confirmed. In rats forced to swim (94) fetal weights were decreased 6%, but in rats that were forced to run (25) growth was not retarded. Dhindsa et al. (51) reported fetal growth retardation with 20% weight reduction in exercising pygmy goats with multiple pregnancies, but a 12% increase in goats with singleton pregnancy, however it is not clear whether the study included proper controls. In swine moderate daily exercise did not reduce fetal weight (66). In some of these studies the "stress" of fear and handling in a laboratory rather than the exercise per se may have contributed to the growth retardation.

Several studies have reported the organ weights and functional development in neonates born from exercised mothers. Nelson et al. (125) observed brain "sparing" in the growth retarded newborns of strenuously exercised guinea pigs. However, body and organ weights were not different from controls in neonatal rats born from exercised mothers (25, 80, 134, 135, 180). Wilson and Gisolfi (180) reported that $\dot{V}_{O_2 max}$, heart rate, blood pressure, myocardial blood flow, myocardial capillary density, and fiber-to-capillary ratio were not different from controls in male offspring of exercised rat mothers, although they did observe a lower fiber density in the right ventricle. These observations are in contrast with those of Parizková (133, 134), who reported increased capillary density and fiber-to-capillary ratio, and a decreased diffusion distance in hearts from neonatal rats born from exercised mothers. Bonner et al. (30) observed that cultured myocardial cells from offspring of exercised rat mothers were larger in size, showed an increased percentage of contracting cells, and beat at a slower rate than cells from controls. Other studies have reported altered lipid metabolism (135), decreased glucose and higher insulin concentrations (94), delayed ossification (170), poorer motor performance (80), and unchanged skeletal muscle myosin ATPase, succinate dehydrogenase and phosphofructokinase in offspring of mothers exercised repeatedly (48). However, the available evidence is insufficient to conclude that exercise of the mother affects the functional development of the neonate.

In conclusion, there is some evidence that strenuous, repetitive maternal physical activity is associated with a small reduction in birth weight in some species. However, further well controlled prospective studies are needed to confirm this. The mechanisms which might account for these effects are presently unresolved, but possibilities include decreases in uterine blood flow, substrate availability, or placental exchange area. Presently there is neither sufficient evidence nor a physiologic basis to suggest other adverse effects of maternal exercise on fetal and neonatal outcome.

SUMMARY

Exercise has numerous effects upon the pregnant mother, the developing fetus, and the placenta. In turn, pregnancy affects the ability to perform physical activity. Pregnancy affects maternal metabolism and the cardiovascular and respiratory systems. The increase in O_2 consumption of about 30% at rest results almost exclusively from the increased tissue mass. During pregnancy a higher cardiorespiratory effort is required to perform a given amount of external work. One would expect that the increase in energy requirements of a given task as induced by the weight gain would result in some training effect, unless a more sedentary life-style is adopted. However, the sedentary life-style commonly adopted in late pregnancy in most western societies may reflect a cultural rather than a physiological phenomenon. The possibility that maximal O_2 consumption may increase during pregnancy has not been studied extensively, yet it is a most important variable which puts other changes in perspective.

In contrast to the physiologic alterations in the mother, and despite reductions in uterine blood flow during maternal exercise, such changes in the fetus are small. During prolonged exhaustive exercise relatively minor changes occur in the blood concentrations of oxygen and substrates. In addition, despite a temperature increase of 1–2°C there is little evidence for significant alteration in fetal metabolism, cardiovascular hemodynamics, or blood catecholamine concentrations. This suggests that acute exercise normally does not represent a major stress for the fetus. Of course, most of the information concerning the fetus is derived from studies in experimental animals, particularly sheep. Conceivably, in humans the upright position, increased uterine contractility, and increased susceptibility to venous pooling may affect the fetal responses differently.

Virtually nothing is known about the physiologic effects of exercise training on the fetus. The most likely effect may be a relatively small reduction in birth weight, at least in some species; however, this needs to be further investigated. The data presently available do not allow any conclusions as to other possible fetal effects of physical training. Further studies are needed for a more complete understanding of the mechanisms involved in the remarkably effective mechanisms which account for the relative homeostasis of the fetus during maternal exercise.

APPENDIX: EXPERIMENTAL METHODS

The following description presents some of the experimental methods employed in the studies of maternal and fetal exercise effects in ewes. Although the details are those used by our group (108, 109), the basic techniques are similar to those used by others.

Principle of Method

Preliminary experiments determined $\dot{V}_{O_2max}$ in each ewe by measuring cardiac output and arteriovenous O_2 content difference during intermittent 10-min exercise periods at increasing levels. Subsequently, we measured uterine blood flow during three different exercise regimens: short-lasting exercise (10 min) at 70 and 100% $\dot{V}_{O_2max}$ and prolonged exercise (40 min) at 70% $\dot{V}_{O_2max}$. Blood and plasma volumes were measured during a single 40 min exercise period at 70% $\dot{V}_{O_2max}$.

The ewes were conditioned to walk on the treadmill at various speeds for short brief periods, totaling 10 min each per day for 1 week before surgery.

Surgery

Surgery was performed in two steps, using spinal anesthesia supplemented with pentobarbital sodium. First, through a midline abdominal and hysterotomy incisions, we inserted catheters into the fetal pedal artery and vein to study placental respiratory gas exchange and fetal oxygenation.

Immediately after the first phase of surgery, the ewe was placed in the right lateral position for a retroperitoneal approach to the distal branches of the aorta. Through a 15-cm hockeystick-shaped incision in the skin of the iliac crest, oblique and transverse abdominal muscles were incised parallel to the muscle fibers, and the distal branches of the aorta were exposed by blunt dissection. The right lateral and dorsal sacral arteries and the left lateral sacral artery were dissected free for about 2 cm and a Tygon catheter (1.5 mm OD) introduced, advancing the tip into the common internal iliac artery. An electromagnetic flow probe (Micron Instruments, Los Angeles) of appropriate size (8 mm ID) was then placed around the common internal iliac artery. Figure 3.6 illustrates the anatomy and nomenclature of the branches with the position of the flow probe, catheter and ligatures. The probe leads, catheter, and drain, as well as the catheters from the first phase of surgery were passed subcutaneously through a stab wound in the maternal flank into a nylon pouch attached to the skin for protection.

Measurement of Cardiac Output and $\dot{V}_{O_2}$

The experiments were begun 5–6 days postoperatively. A Swan-Ganz flow-directed thermodilution catheter (Edwards Laboratories, 93A-301-7F, Santa Ana, Calif.) was introduced into the right jugular vein, and the tip advanced into the pulmonary artery as shown by the pressure recording during inflation of the balloon (wedging). Cardiac output was measured by thermodilution using a cardiac output computer and recorder (Instrumentation Laboratory, model 601 and 601, Lexington, Mass.) in triplicate, employing the median value for calculations. In addition, 1-ml blood samples were taken simultaneously from the common internal iliac artery and right atrium, analyzed in duplicate for O_2 content (Lexington Instruments, Lex O_2 Con-K, Waltham, Mass.) and the mean value used for calculations.

The ewe was exercised at a room temperature of 22°C for 10-min periods, followed by 20 min of rest. Speed and inclination of the treadmill were gradually increased from initial values of 34 m·min^{-1} at 0° inclination to 99 m·min^{-1} at 10° until the ewe reached exhaustion within a 10-min exercise period. At this exhaustive level the animal operated at $\dot{V}_{O_2max}$, defined as that value when the $\dot{V}_{O_2max}$ had plateaued and did not rise further. Exercise was discontinued if it seemed no longer possible to prevent the animal from collapsing. Measurements were made during the 8th to 10th min of each exercise period and $\dot{V}_{O_2max}$ calculated according to the Fick principle, from cardiac output and arteriovenous O_2 difference. Heart rate was measured from the blood pressure pulse.

Uterine Blood Flow and Vascular Resistance

Uterine blood flow and vascular pressures were measured 1–4 days after the prelimi-

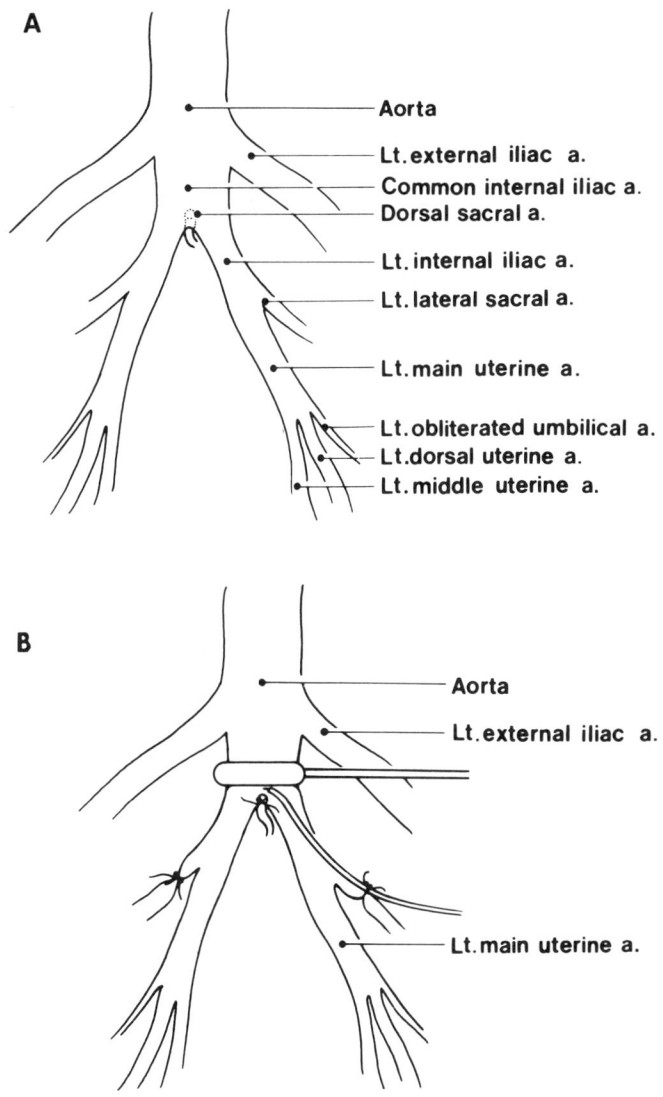

Figure 3.6. Schematic representation of distal branches of aorta in sheep, with position of electromagnetic flow probe, catheter, and ligatures. (From Lotgering (109).)

nary experiment, recording total uterine blood flow continuously from the flow probe around the common internal iliac artery. Flow was measured with an automatic-zeroing electromagnetic flowmeter (Dienco, model RF-2100, Los Angeles) and a DC amplifier and recorder (Gould models 13-4615-10 and 2800, Cleveland). Uterine arterial and venous pressures were recorded using pressure transducers and amplifiers (Gould, models P23 and 13-4615-50, Cleveland). One minute averages of all variables were calculated by computer (Texas Instruments, model 990/4, Houston) and stored on disk (Memorex, Markette, Santa Clara, Calif.)

Uterine blood flow was studied during three different exercise regimens (a) during 10 min of exercise with the treadmill at a speed and inclination similar to that which produced 70% $\dot{V}_{O_2 max}$ in the preliminary experiment, followed by 20 min of recovery; (b) during 10 min of exercise at 100% $\dot{V}_{O_2 max}$ which exhausted the ewe, followed by 2 hours of recovery; and (c) during prolonged (40 min) exercise at 70% $\dot{V}_{O_2max}$, which also exhausted the ewe and was followed by 2 hours of recovery. Three-minute mean values of uterine flow and blood pressure were calculated from 2 to 10 min of exercise and 4-min mean values from 2 to 5 min after exercise, as well as 5-min means for the control period before exercise, from 11 to 40 min of exercise, and from 6 to 60 min after exercise. One or more of the runs were repeated on separate days, up to 3 times (mean 1.5 times) in each ewe. The mean response to each exercise regimen was calculated for each individual animal and the values used for comparison between animals and for statistical analysis.

Blood and Plasma Volume

One to four days after determining the ewe's $\dot{V}_{O_2max}$, and in conjunction with the uterine blood flow studies, we measured blood volumes using ^{51}Cr-labeled erythrocytes in eight ewes. Eight milliliters of ^{51}Cr-labeled erythrocytes were injected into the maternal circulation 50 min before the beginning of exercise. Arterial samples were obtained (2 ml) 30, 20, 10, and 0 min before exercise, 3, 10, 20, 30, and 40 min after the beginning of a single 40-min exercise period at 70% $\dot{V}_{O_2max}$, and 3, 10, 30, and 60 min after stopping exercise. The samples and injection syringes (before and after injection) were counted for radioactivity in an Auto-Gamma scintillation spectrometer (Packard Instruments, model 5912, Downers Grove, Ill.) at a 285-357 keV window (peak 323 keV). Counts from samples taken 30, 20, 10, and 0 min before, and 30 and 60 min after exercise were used for linear regression analysis in each animal, extrapolating the counts to the time of injection by using the same regression for all samples of each individual animal. The microhematocrit of each sample was measured in triplicate and the median value used to calculate plasma and red cell volumes. Plasma protein was measured in triplicate using a refractometer (American Optical, Keene, N.H.) and median values used for comparison.

Temperatures

Maternal and fetal temperatures were measured continuously, using thermistors (Instrumentation Laboratory, model 601, Lexington, Mass.) and DC amplifier and recorder. The thermistors were calibrated before implantation and after removal and were found to vary by less than 0.02°C.

Respiratory Gases

Maternal and fetal respiratory blood gases were measured at rest, during the three exercise regimens (10 min at 70% $\dot{V}_{O_2max}$, 10 min at 100% $\dot{V}_{O_2max}$, and 40 min at 70% $\dot{V}_{O_2max}$, and during recovery. One-milliliter samples from the uterine artery and vein and the fetal ascending aorta were obtained 1–3 min before the beginning and end of each exercise period, and 18–20 min and 116–120 min after the cessation of exercise, for determination of P_{O_2}, P_{CO_2}, and pH (Radiometer, model BL2, Copenhagen) at 37°C. Corrections were made for body temperatures as measured by thermistors in the uterine artery and fetal inferior vena cava. O_2 content was measured in duplicate (Lexington Instruments, Lex O_2 CON-K, Waltham, Mass.) and mean values calculated. Differences between duplicate measurements were within 0.2 ml·dl^{-1}. Uterine $\dot{V}_{O_2max}$ was calculated from the uterine arteriovenous O_2 content difference and the simultaneously measured total uterine blood flow.

Placental Diffusing Capacity for Carbon Monoxide

We measured placental CO diffusing capacity was measured by having the ewe breath a loading dose of 125 ml CO in 10 liters room air for 1.5 min. Thereafter she breathed a mixture of 100 ppm CO in air for 70 min, supplied at a flow of 30 l·min^{-1} into a movable plastic bag fitted around the head and neck. The inspired CO concentration was monitored with a CO analyzer (Energetic Science, Ecolyzer, Elmsford, N.Y.). With the ewe standing quietly on the treadmill, we collected samples (1.5 ml) simultaneously from the uterine vein and fetal aorta 10, 25, and 40 min after the start of CO administration. Thereafter the ewe was exercised for 30 min at 70% $\dot{V}_{O_2max}$ and samples collected 15 and 30 min after the start of exercise. Mean placental diffusing capacity was calculated for the 30-min periods before and during exercise.

Fetal Heart Rate and Arterial Pressure

Fetal aortic pressure and amniotic fluid pressure were recorded using pressure transducers and amplifiers (Gould model P23 and 13-4615-50, Cleveland), and corrected the fetal arterial pressure for amniotic fluid pressure.

Fetal Cardiac Output and Blood Flow Distribution

Cardiac output and blood flow distributions were measured using microspheres 15 ± 1 μm in diameter labeled with ^{46}Sc, ^{51}Cr, ^{103}Ru, or ^{153}Gd (New England Nuclear, Boston). Injections were made at rest, during the last 3 min of exercise at 70% $\dot{V}_{O_2max}$. After sacrificing the ewe and fetus following the experiment, fetal organs as well as placental cotyledons and membranes were weighed, ashed, and counted for radioactivity. We calculated absolute organ blood flow per kg fetus and the percentage of cardiac output distributed to the different organs.

Acknowledgments—The authors wish to thank Mrs. S. Whitson, B. Kreutzer, and S. Taylor for preparing the manuscript.
This study was supported by USPHS Grants HD 03807 and HD 13949, and NATO grant N95-119 awarded by The Netherlands Organization for the Advancement of Pure Research (ZWO) to Fred K. Lotgering. Dr. Lotgering's present address is Erasmus University Rotterdam, Postbus 1738, 3000 DR Rotterdam, The Netherlands.

REFERENCES

1. Abrams R, Caton D, Clapp J, Barron DH: Thermal and metabolic features of life in utero. *Clin Obstet Gynecol* 13:549–564, 1970.
2. Adamsons K Jr: The role of thermal factors in fetal and neonatal life. *Pediatr Clin North Am* 13:599–619, 1966.
3. Annison EF, Brown RE, Leng RA, Lindsay DB, West CE: Rates of entry and oxidation of acetate, glucose, D(−)-α-hydroxybutyrate, palmitate, oleate and stearate, and rates of production and oxidation of propionate and butyrate in fed and starved sheep. *Biochem J* 104:135–147, 1967.
4. Artal R, Platt LD, Sperling M, Kammula RK, Jilek J, Nakamura R: Exercise in pregnancy; I. Maternal cardiovascular and metabolic responses in normal pregnancy. *Am J Obstet Gynecol* 140:123–127, 1981.
5. Asmussen E: Muscular exercise. In Fenn WO, Rahn H (eds): *Handbook of Physiology*, Sect 3: Respiration. Washington, D.C., American Physiological Society, 1965, vol II, pp 939–978.
6. Assali NS, Douglass RA Jr, Baird WW, Nicholson DB, Suyemoto R: Measurement of uterine blood flow and uterine metabolism; IV. Results in normal pregnancy. *Am J Obstet Gynecol* 66:248–253, 1953.
7. Assali NS, Rauramo L, Peltonen T: Measurement of uterine blood flow and uterine metabolism; VIII. Uterine and fetal blood flow and oxygen consumption in early human pregnancy. *Am J Obstet Gynecol* 79:86–98, 1960.
8. Åstrand PO, Rodahl K: *Textbook of Work Physiology*. New York, McGraw-Hill, 1977.
9. Atkins AFJ, Watt JM, Milan P, Davies P, Selwyn Crawford J: A longitudinal study of cardiovascular dynamic changes throughout pregnancy. *Eur J Obstet Gynecol Reprod Biol* 12:215–224, 1981.
10. Atkins AJF, Watt JM, Milan P, Davies P, Selwyn Crawford J: The influence of posture upon cardiovascular dynamics throughout pregnancy. *Eur J Obstet Gynecol Reprod Biol* 12:357–372, 1981.
11. Bader RA, Bader ME, Rose DJ, Braunwald E: Hemodynamics at rest and during exercise in normal pregnancy as studied by cardiac catheterization. *J Clin Invest* 34:1524–1536, 1955.
12. Baker CH: Blood reservoirs in the splenectomized dog. *Am J Physiol* 208:485–491, 1965.
13. Barron DH: A history of fetal respiration: from Harvey's question (1651) to Zweifels answer (1876). In Longo LD, Reneau DD (eds): *Fetal and Newborn Physiology*. New York, Garland, 1978, vol I, Developmental Aspects, pp 1–32.
14. Battaglia FC, Meschia G: Principal substrates of fetal metabolism. *Physiol Rev* 58:499–527, 1978.
15. Beitins IZ, Kowarski A, Shermeta DW, De Lemos RA, Migeon CJ: Fetal and maternal secretion rate of cortisol in sheep: diffusion resistance of the placenta. *Pediatr Res* 4:129–134, 1970.
16. Bell AW, Bassett JM, Chandler KD, Boston RC: Fetal and maternal endocrine responses to exercise in the pregnant ewe. *J Dev Physiol* 5:129–141, 1983.
17. Bell AW, Chandler KD, Leury BJ: Fetal and uteroplacental energy metabolism in the sheep: effects of maternal undernutrition and exercise. In *Proceedings of the 9th Symposium on Energy Metabolism*, Lillehammer, Norway, 1982 (in press).
18. Bell C: Autonomic nervous control of reproduction: circulatory and other factors. *Pharmacol Rev* 24:657–736, 1972.
19. Bell C: Control of uterine blood flow in pregnancy. *Med Biol* 52:119–228, 1974.

20. Berg A, Mross F, Hillemans HG, Keul J: Die Belastbarkeit der Frau in der Schwangerschaft. Med Welt 28:1267–1269, 1977.
21. Bird AR, Chandler KD, Bell AW: Effects of exercise and plane of nutrition on nutrient utilization by the hind limb of the sheep. Aust J Biol Sci 34:541–550, 1981.
22. Bissonnette JM, Black JA, Wickham WK, Acott KM: Glucose uptake into plasma membrane vesicles from the maternal surface of human placenta. J Membr Biol 58:75–80, 1981.
23. Bissonnette JM, Hohimer AR, Cronan JZ, Black JA: Glucose transfer across the intact guinea-pig placenta. J Dev Physiol 1:415–426, 1979.
24. Bissonnette JM, Longo LD, Novy MJ, Murata Y, Martin Jr CB: Placental diffusing capacity and its relation to fetal growth. J Dev Physiol 1:351–359, 1979.
25. Blake CA, Hazelwood RL: Effect of pregnancy and exercise on actomyosin, nucleic acid, and glycogen content of the rat heart. Proc Soc Exp Biol Med 136:632–636, 1971.
26. Blechner JN, Stenger VG, Prystowsky H: Uterine blood flow in women at term. Am J Obstet Gynecol 120:633–640, 1974.
27. Boddy K, Dawes GS: Fetal breathing. Br Med Bull 31:3–7, 1975.
28. Boddy K, Dawes GS, Robinson J: Intrauterine fetal breathing movements. In Gluck L (ed): *Modern Perinatal Medicine*. Chicago, Year Book, 1974, pp 381–389.
29. Bonica JJ: Maternal respiratory changes during pregnancy and parturition. In Marx GF (ed): *Clinical Anesthesia, Parturition & Perinatology*, Philadelphia, F. A. Davis, 1973, vol 10/2.
30. Bonner HW, Buffington CK, Newman JJ, Farrar RP, Acosta D: Contractile activity of neonatal heart cells in culture derived from offspring of exercised pregnant rats. Eur J Appl Physiol 39:1–6, 1978.
31. Bottger I, Schlein EM, Faloona GR, Knochel JP, Unger RH: The effect of exercise on glucagon secretion. J Clin Endocrinol Metab 35:117–125, 1972.
32. Brace RA: Blood volume and its measurement in the chronically catheterized sheep fetus. Am J Physiol 244:H487–H494, 1983.
33. Brengelman GL: Circulatory adjustments to exercise and heat stress. Ann Rev Physiol 45:191–212, 1983.
34. Bruce NW, Abdul-Karim RW: Mechanisms controlling maternal placental circulation. Clin Obstet Gynecol 17:135–151, 1974.
35. Brück K: Heat production and temperature regulation. In Stave U (ed): *Perinatal Physiology*. New York, Plenum, 1978, pp 455–498.
36. Brühl, Handovsky, and Möhle: Ermüdüngserscheinungen an Muskeln trächtiger Tiere. Klin Wochenschr 12:886, 1933.
37. Burd LI, Jones MD, Jr., Simmons MA, Makowski EL, Meschia G., Battaglia FC: Placental production and foetal utilisation of lactate and pyruvate. Nature 254:710–711, 1975.
38. Burwell CS: The placenta as a modified arteriovenous fistula, considered in relation to the circulatory adjustments to pregnancy. Am J Med Sci 195:1–7, 1938.
39. Burwell CS, Strayhorn WD, Flickinger D, Corlette MD, Bowerman EP, Kennedy JA: Circulation during pregnancy. Arch Intern Med 62:979–1003, 1938.
40. Buss DD, Bisgard GE, Rawlings CA, Rankin JHG: Uteroplacental blood flow during alkalosis in the sheep. Am J Physiol 228:1497–1500, 1975.
41. Caton D, Wilcox CJ, Abrams R, Barron DH: The circulating plasma volume of the foetal lamb as an index of its weight and rate of weight gain (g/day) in the last third of gestation. Q J Exp Physiol 50:45–54, 1975.
42. Cefalo RC, Hellegers AE: The effects of maternal hyperthermia on maternal and fetal cardiovascular and respiratory function. Am J Obstet Gynecol 131:687–694, 1978.
43. Chandler KD, Bell AW: Effects of maternal exercise on fetal and maternal respiration and nutrient metabolism in the pregnant ewe. J Dev Physiol 3:161–176, 1981.
44. Clapp III JF: Effect of epinephrine infusion on maternal and uterine oxygen uptake in the pregnant ewe. Am J Obstet Gynecol 133:208–212, 1979.
45. Clapp III JF: Acute exercise stress in the pregnant ewe. Am J Obstet Gynecol 136:489–494, 1980.
46. Clausen JP: Effect of physical training on cardiovascular adjustments to exercise in man. Physiol Rev 57:779–815, 1977.
47. Comline RS, Silver M: The release of adrenaline and noradrenaline from the adrenal glands of the foetal sheep. J Physiol 156:424–444, 1961.
48. Corbett K, Brassard L, Taylor AW: Skeletal muscle metabolism in the offspring of trained rats. Med Sci Sports Exerc 11:107, 1979.
49. Cugell DW, Frank NR, Gaensler EA, Badger TL: Pulmonary function in pregnancy. I. Serial observations in normal women. Am Rev Tuberc 67:568–597, 1953.
50. Curet LB, Orr JA, Rankin JHG, Ungerer T: Effect of exercise on cardiac output and distribution of uterine blood flow in pregnant ewes. J Appl Physiol 40:725–728, 1976.
51. Dhindsa DS, Metcalfe J, Hummels DH: Responses to exercises in the pregnant pygmy goat. Respir Physiol 32:299–311, 1978.
52. Dominguez De Costa C, Lerdo De Tejada A, Eisenberg De Smoler P, Carreno E, Briones E, Wionczek C, Karchmer S: Descenso en la excrecion de Ac. 5-HIA producido por el ejercicio en la embarazada. Ginecol Obstet Mex 44:347–353, 1978.
53. Eismayer G, Pohl A: Untersuchungen uber den

Kreislauf und den Gasstoffwechsel in der Schwangerschaft bei Arbeitsversuchen. *Arch Gynaekol* 156:428–453, 1934.
54. Emmanouilides GC, Hobel CJ, Yashiro K, Klyman G: Fetal responses to maternal exercise in the sheep. *Am J Obstet Gynecol* 112:130–137, 1972.
55. Erkkola R: The influence of physical training during pregnancy on physical work capacity and circulatory parameters. *Scand J Clin Lab Invest* 36:747–754, 1976.
56. Evans JW: Effect of fasting, gestation, lactation and exercise on glucose turnover in horses. *J Anim Sci* 33:1001–1004, 1971.
57. Faber JJ, Green TJ: Foetal placental blood flow in the lamb. *J Physiol (Lond)* 223:375–393, 1972.
58. Felig P, Wahren J, Hendler R, Ahlborg G: Plasma glucagon levels in exercising man. *N Engl J Med* 287:184–185, 1972.
59. Fischer WM, Stude I, Brandt H: Ein Vorschlag zur Beurteilung des antepartualen Kardiotokogramms. *Z Geburtshife Perinatol* 180:117–123, 1976.
60. Gilbert RD: Effects of afterload and baroreceptors on cardiac function in fetal sheep. *J Dev Physiol* 4:299–309, 1982.
61. Gilbert RD, Cummings LA, Juchau MR, Longo LD: Placental diffusing capacity and fetal development in exercising or hypoxic guinea pigs. *J Appl Physiol* 46:828–834, 1979.
62. Gill RW, Trudinger BJ, Garrett WJ, Kossof G, Warren PS: Fetal umbilical venous flow measured in utero by pulsed Doppler and B-mode ultrasound. I. Normal pregnancies. *Am J Obstet Gynecol* 139:720–725, 1981.
63. Greenleaf JE, Convertino VA, Stremel RW, Bernauer EM, Adams WC, Vignau SR, and Brock PJ: Plasma (Na^+), (Ca^{2+}), and volume shifts and thermoregulation during exercise in man. *J Appl Physiol* 43:1026–1032, 1977.
64. Greenleaf JE, Van Beaumont W, Brock PJ, Morse JT, Mangseth GR: Plasma volume and electrolyte shifts with heavy exercise in sitting and supine positions. *Am J Physiol* 236:R206–R214, 1979.
65. Greiss Jr FC: Differential reactivity of the myoendometrial and placental vasculatures: adrenergic responses. *Am J Obstet Gynecol* 112:20–30, 1972.
66. Hale OM, Booram CV, McCormick WC: Effects of forced exercise during gestation on farrowing and meaning performance of swine. *J Anim Sci* 52:1240–1243, 1981.
67. Hamilton HFH: The cardiac output in normal pregnancy as determined by the Cournand right heart catheterization technique. *J Obstet Gynaecol Br Emp* 56:548–552, 1949.
68. Hamilton HFH: Blood viscosity in pregnancy. *J Obstet Gynaecol Br Emp* 57:530–538, 1950.
69. Harbert GM: Biorhythms in the dynamics of a pregnant uterus (*Macaca mulatta*). *Am J Obstet Gynecol* 120:401–408, 1977.
70. Harris WH, Pittman QJ, Veale WL, Cooper KE, Van Petten GR: Cardiovascular effects of fever in the ewe and fetal lamb. *Am J Obstet Gynecol* 128:262–265, 1977.
71. Hobel CJ, Artal R, Emmanouilides G, Lam RW, Fisher DA: Maternal and fetal catecholamine responses to maternal exercise in the normal and compromised pregnant ewe. In Society for Gynecologic Investigation, Abstracts of 25th Annual Meeting, Atlanta, GA., March 15–18, 1978, p 5.
72. Hohimer AR, Bissonnette JM, Metcalfe J, Reppe M: The effect of mild maternal exercise on uterine blood flow in the pregnant pygmy goat. In Society for Gynecologic Investigation, Abstracts of 26th Annual Meeting, San Diego, Calif., March 21–24, 1979, p 26.
73. Hohimer AR, Bissonnette JM, Metcalfe J, McKean TA: Effect of exercise on uterine blood flow in the pregnant pygmy goat. *Am J Physiol* 246:H207–H212, 1984.
74. Huckabee WE, Crenshaw MC, Curet LB, Barron DH: Uterine blood flow and oxygen consumption in the unrestrained pregnant ewe. *Q J Exp Physiol* 57:12–23, 1972.
75. Hytten FE, Leitch I: *The Physiology of Human Pregnancy*. Oxford, Blackwell, 1964.
76. Issekutz Jr B, Miller HI, Paul P, Rodahl K: Aerobic work capacity and plasma FFA turnover. *J Appl Physiol* 20:293–296, 1965.
77. Issekutz Jr B, Miller HI, Rodahl K: Lipid and carbohydrate metabolism during exercise. *Fed Proc* 25:1415–1420, 1966.
78. James EJ, Raye JR, Gresham EL, Makowski EL, Meschia G, Battaglia FC: Fetal oxygen consumption, carbon dioxide production, and glucose uptake in a chronic preparation. *Pediatrics* 50:361–371, 1972.
79. Jarrett IG, Filsell OH, Ballard FJ: Utilization of oxidizable substrates by the sheep hind limb: effects of starvation and exercise. *Metabolism* 25:523–531, 1976.
80. Jenkins RR, Ciconne C: Exercise effect during pregnancy on brain nucleic acids of offspring in rats. *Arch Phys Med Rehabil* 61:124–127, 1980.
81. Johnson LW, Smith CH: Monosaccharide transport across microvillous membrane of human placenta. *Am J Physiol* 238:C160–C168, 1980.
82. Jones CT: Circulating catecholamines in the fetus, their origin, actions and significance. In Parvez H, Parvez S (eds): *Biogenic Amines in Development*. Amsterdam, Elsevier-North Holland, 1980, pp 63–86.
83. Judson GJ, Filsell OH, Jarrett IG: Glucose and acetate metabolism in sheep at rest and during exercise. *Aust J Biol Sci* 29:215–222, 1976.
84. Kalhan SC, D'Angelo LJ, Savin SM, Adam PAJ: Glucose production in pregnant women at term gestation. Sources of glucose for human fetus. *J Clin Invest* 63:388–394, 1979.
85. Kleiber M: Respiratory exchange and metabolic rate. In Fenn WO, Rahn H (eds): *Handbook of*

Physiology, Sect 3: Respiration. Washington, D.C., American Physiological Society, 1965, vol II, pp 927-938.
86. Knopp RH: Fuel metabolism in pregnancy. *Contemp Ob/Gyn* 12:83-90, 1978.
87. Knuttgen HG, Emerson Jr K: Physiological response to pregnancy at rest and during exercise. *J Appl Physiol* 36:549-553, 1974.
88. Krukenberg H: Arbeitsphysiologische Studien an graviden Frauen. 1. Mitteilung: Über den Einfluss der körperlichen Arbeit auf den Muskelstoffwechsel. *Arch Gynaekol* 149:250-277, 1932.
89. Krukenberg H: Arbeitsphysiologische Studien an Graviden. 2. Mitteilung: Der Einfluss der Korperarbeit auf Herz und Kreislauf. *Arch Gynaekol* 149:663-687, 1932.
90. Lanz E, Caton D, Schlereth H, Barron DH: Die Wirkung von Lokalanaesthetika auf Durchblutung und O_2-Verbrauch des Uterus von schwangeren Schafen. *Anaesthesist* 26:403-410, 1977.
91. Lees MM, Taylor SH, Scott DB, Kerr MG: A study of cardiac output at rest throughout pregnancy. *J Obstet Gynaecol Br Commw* 74:319-328, 1967.
92. Lehmann V, Regnat K: Untersuchung zur Körperlichen Belastungsfähigkeit schwangeren Frauen. Der Einfluss standardisierter Arbeit auf Herzkreislaufsystem, Ventilation, Gasaustausch, Kohlenhydratstoffwechsel und Säure-Basen-Haushalt. *Z Geburtshife Perinatol* 180:279-289, 1976.
93. Lehmann V: Die körperliche Leistungsfähigkeit während der Schwangerschaft. *Med Klin* 72:1313-1319, 1977.
94. Levitsky LL, Kimber A, Marchichow JA, Uehara J: Metabolic response to fasting in experimental intrauterine growth retardation induced by surgical and nonsurgical maternal stress. *Biol Neonate* 31:311-315, 1977.
95. Lindhard J: Über das Minutenvolum des Herzens bei Ruhe und bei Muskelarbeit. *Pflugers Arch* 161:233-283, 1915.
96. Lindheimer MD, Katz AI: Renal function in pregnancy. *Obstet Gynecol Annu* 1:139-176, 1972.
97. Longo LD: Disorders of placental transfer. In Assali NS (ed): *Pathophysiology of Gestation, Fetal-Placental Disorders.* New York, Academic Press, 1972, vol II, pp 1-76.
98. Longo LD: Maternal blood volume and cardiac output during pregnancy: a hypothesis of endocrinologic control. *Am J Physiol* 245:R720-729, 1983.
99. Longo LD, Ching KS: Placental diffusing capacity for carbon monoxide and oxygen in unanesthetized sheep. *J Appl Physiol* 43:885-893, 1977.
100. Longo LD, Hardesty JS: Maternal blood volume: measurement, hypothesis of control, and clinical considerations. *Rev Perinat Med* 5:1-28, 1984.
101. Longo LD, Hewitt CW, Lorijn RHW, Gilbert RD: To what extent does maternal exercise affect fetal oxygenation and uterine blood flow? *Fed Proc* 37:905, 1978.
102. Longo LD, Hill EP, Power GG: Theoretical analysis of factors affecting placental O_2 transfer. *Am J Physiol* 222:730-739, 1972.
103. Longo LD, Power GG, Forster II RE: Respiratory function of the placenta as determined with carbon monoxide in sheep and dogs. *J Clin Invest* 46:812-828, 1967.
104. Longo LD, Wyatt JF, Hewitt CW, Gilbert RD: A comparison of circulatory responses to hypoxic hypoxia and carbon monoxide hypoxia in fetal blood flow and oxygenation. In Longo LD, Reneau DD (eds): *Fetal and Newborn Cardiovascular Physiology.* New York, Garland, 1978, vol 2, pp 259-287.
105. Lorijn RHW, Longo LD: Clinical and physiological implications of increased fetal oxygen consumption. *Am J Obstet Gynecol* 136:451-457, 1980.
106. Lorijn RHW, Longo LD: Norepinephrine elevation in the fetal lamb: oxygen consumption and cardiac output. *Am J Physiol* 239:R115-R122, 1980.
107. Lorijn RHW, Nelson JC, Longo LD: Induced fetal hyperthyroidism: cardiac output and oxygen consumption. *Am J Physiol* 239:H302-H307, 1980.
108. Lotgering FK, Gilbert RD, Longo LD: Exercise responses in pregnant sheep: oxygen consumption, uterine blood flow, and blood volume. *J Appl Physiol* 55:834-841, 1983.
109. Lotgering FK, Gilbert RD, Longo LD: Exercise responses in pregnant sheep: blood gases, temperatures and fetal cardiovascular system. *J Appl Physiol* 55:842-850, 1983.
110. Lundvall J, Mellander S, Westling H, White T: Fluid transfer between blood and tissues during exercise. *Acta Physiol Scand* 85:258-269, 1972.
111. Makowski EL, Meschia G, Droegemueller W, Battaglia FC: Distribution of uterine blood flow in the pregnant sheep. *Am J Obstet Gynecol* 101:409-412, 1968.
112. Maršál K, Gennser G, Löfgren O: Effects on fetal breathing movements of maternal challenges. Cross-over study on dynamic work, static work, passive movements, hyperventilation and hyperoxygenation. *Acta Obstet Gynecol Scand* 58:335-342, 1979.
113. McKeown T, Record RG: The influence of placental size on foetal growth in man, with special reference to multiple pregnancy. *J Endocrinol* 9:418-426, 1953.
114. Meschia G, Battaglia FC, Hay WW, Sparks JW: Utilization of substrates by the ovine placenta in vivo. *Fed Proc* 39:245-249, 1980.
115. Meschia G, Cotter JR, Makowski EL, Barron DH: Simultaneous measurement of uterine and umbilical blood flows and oxygen uptakes. *Q J Exp Physiol* 52:1-18, 1967.
116. Metcalfe J, McAnulty JH, Ueland K: Cardiovascular physiology. *Clin Obstet Gynecol* 24:693-710, 1981.
117. Metcalfe J, Parer JT: Cardiovascular changes dur-

ing pregnancy in ewes. *Am J Physiol* 210:821–825, 1966.
118. Metcalfe J, Romney SL, Ramsey LH, Reid DE, Burwell CS: Estimation of uterine blood flow in normal human pregnancy at term. *J Clin Invest* 34:1632–1638, 1955.
119. Moll W, Girard H, Gros G: Facilitated diffusion of lactic acid in the guinea-pig placenta. *Pflugers Arch* 385:229–238, 1980.
120. Morishima HO, Bruce SL, Dyrenfurth I, Sakuma K, Stark RI, James LS: The effect of stress on uterine blood flow and plasma cortisol level in the pregnant sheep. In Society for Gynecologic Investigation, Abstracts of 26th Annual Meeting, San Diego, Calif., March 21–24, 1979, p 170.
121. Morishima HO, Yeh M, James LS: Reduced uterine blood flow and fetal hypoxemia with acute maternal stress: experimental observation in the pregnant baboon. *Am J Obstet Gynecol* 134:270–275, 1979.
122. Morishima HO, Yeh M, Niemann WH, James LS: Temperature gradient between fetus and mother as an index for assessing intrauterine fetal condition. *Am J Obstet Gynecol* 129:443–448, 1977.
123. Morris N, Osborn SB, Wright HP, Hart A: Effective uterine blood-flow during exercise in normal and pre-eclamptic pregnancies. *Lancet* 2:481–484, 1956.
124. Morriss Jr FH, Rosenfeld CR, Resnik R, Meschia G, Makowski EL, Battaglia FC: Growth of uterine oxygen and glucose uptakes during pregnancy in sheep. *Gynecol Invest* 5:230–241, 1974.
125. Nelson PS, Gilbert RD, Longo LD: Fetal growth and placental diffusing capacity in guinea pigs following long-term maternal exercise. *J Dev Physiol* 5:1–10, 1983.
126. Nielsen M: Die Regulation der Körpertemperatur bei Muskelarbeit. *Scand Arch Physiol* 79:193–230, 1938.
127. Novotna J, Pros JR, Tučková H: Průběh těhotenství výkonnostních sportovkyň se zřetelem k disciplínám a některým psychologickým faktorům. *Cesk Gynekol* 42:730–733, 1977.
128. Oakes GK, Walker AM, Ehrenkranz RA, Cefalo RC, Chez RA: Uteroplacental blood flow during hyperthermia with and without respiratory alkalosis. *J Appl Physiol* 41:197–201, 1976.
129. Orr J, Ungerer T, Will J, Wernicke K, Curet LB: Effect of exercise stress on carotid, uterine, and iliac blood flow in pregnant and nonpregnant ewes. *Am J Obstet Gynecol* 114:213–217, 1972.
130. Palmer AJ, Walker AHC: The maternal circulation in normal pregnancy. *J Obstet Gynaecol Br Emp* 56:537–547, 1949.
131. Palmer SM, Oakes GK, Hobel CJ, Hawkins PM, Fisher DA: The role of hypocapnea on acute exercise (EX) induced catecholamine (CAT) release in chronically catheterized ovine pregnancy. In Society for Gynecologic Investigation, Abstracts of 27th Annual Meeting, Denver, Col., March 19–22, 1980, p 62.
132. Parer JT: Fetal oxygen uptake and umbilical circulation during maternal hypoxia in the chronically catheterized sheep. In Longo LD, Reneau RR (eds): *Fetal and Newborn Cardiovascular Physiology*, New York, Garland, 1978, vol 2, pp 231–247.
133. Pařízková J: Impact of daily work-load during pregnancy on the microstructure of the rat heart in male offspring. *Eur J Appl Physiol* 34:323–326, 1975.
134. Pařízková J: Cardiac microstructure in female and male offspring of exercised rat mothers. *Acta Anat* 104:382–387, 1979.
135. Pařízková J, Petrásek R: The impact of daily work load during pregnancy on lipid metabolism in the liver of the offspring. *Bibl Nutr Dieta* 27:57–64, 1979.
136. Peeters LLH, Sheldon RE, Jones Jr. MD, Makowski EL, Meschia G: Blood flow to fetal organs as a function of arterial oxygen content. *Am J Obstet Gynecol* 135:637–646, 1979.
137. Pethick DW, Lindsay DB, Barker PJ, Northrop AJ: Acetate supply and utilization by the tissues of sheep in vivo. *Br J Nutr* 46:97–110, 1981.
138. Pernoll ML, Metcalfe J, Paul M: Fetal cardiac response to maternal exercise. In Longo LD, Reneau DD (eds): *Fetal and Newborn Cardiovascular Physiology*. New York, Garland, 1978, vol 2, pp 389–398.
139. Pernoll ML, Metcalfe J, Schlenker TL, Welch JE, Matsumoto JA: Oxygen consumption at rest and during exercise in pregnancy. *Respir Physiol* 25:285–293, 1975.
140. Power GG, Longo LD, Wagner Jr HN, Kuhl DE, Forster RE: Uneven distribution of maternal and fetal placental blood flow, as demonstrated using macroaggregates, and its response to hypoxia. *J Clin Invest* 46:2053–2063, 1967.
141. Power GG, Schröder H, Gilbert RD: Measurement of fetal heat production using differential calorimetry. *J Appl Physiol* 57:917–922, 1984.
142. Probst: Funktionsprüfung des Kreislaufes gesunder Schwangerer. *Arch Gynaekol* 166:59–62, 1938.
143. Pruett EDR: Plasma insulin concentrations during prolonged work at near maximal oxygen uptake. *J Appl Physiol* 29:155–158, 1970.
144. Rankin JHG, McLaughlin MK: The regulation of the placental blood flows. *J Dev Physiol* 1:3–30, 1979.
145. Rose DJ, Bader ME, Bader RA, Braunwald E: Catheterization studies of cardiac hemodynamics in normal pregnant women with reference to left ventricular work. *Am J Obstet Gynecol* 72:233–246, 1956.
146. Rosenfeld CR: Distribution of cardiac output in ovine pregnancy. *Am J Physiol* 232:H231–H235, 1977.
147. Rosenfeld CR, Morriss FH Jr, Makowski EL, Meschia G, Battaglia FC: Circulatory changes in the reproductive tissues of ewes during pregnancy.

Gynecol Invest 5:252–268, 1974.
148. Rosenfeld CR, West J: Circulatory response to systemic infusion of norepinephrine in the pregnant ewe. *Am J Obstet Gynecol* 127:376–383, 1977.
149. Rowell LB: Human cardiovascular adjustments to exercise and thermal stress. *Physiol Rev* 54:75–159, 1974.
150. Rubler S, Damani PM, Pinto ER: Cardiac size and performance during pregnancy estimated with echocardiography. *Am J Cardiol* 40:534–540, 1977.
151. Rudolph AM, Heymann MA: Circulatory changes during growth in the fetal lamb. *Circ Res* 26:289–299, 1970.
152. Rudolph AM, Heymann MA: Cardiac output in the fetal lamb: the effects of spontaneous and induced changes of heart rate on right and left ventricular output. *Am J Obstet Gynecol* 124:183–192, 1976.
153. Saltin B, Blomquist G, Mitchell JH, Johnson Jr RL, Wildenthal K, Chapman CB: Response to exercise after bed rest and after training. *Circulation* 38 (suppl 7):1–78, 1968.
154. Schreiner RL, Burd LI, Douglas Jones Jr M, Lemons JA, Sheldon RE, Simmons MA, Battaglia FC, Meschia G: Fetal metabolism in fasting sheep. In Longo LD, Reneau DD (eds): *Fetal and Newborn Cardiovascular Physiology*. New York, Garland, 1978, vol 2, pp 197–222.
155. Schreiner RL, Lemons JA, Gresham EL, Nolen PA, Bohnke RA, Reyman DS: Effect of acute nonsurgical stress on fetal and maternal plasma glucose, glucagon and insulin concentration in sheep. *Biol Neonate* 39:86–90, 1981.
156. Schröder H, Gilbert RD, Power GG: Fetal heat dissipation: A computer model and some preliminary experimental results from fetal sheep. In Society for Gynecologic Investigation, Abstracts of 29th Annual Meeting, Dallas, Tex., March 24–27, 1982, p 113.
157. Secher NJ, Arnsbo P, Heslet Andersen L, Thomsen A: Measurements of cardiac stroke volume in various body positions in pregnancy and during Caesarean section: a comparison between thermodilution and impedance cardiography. *Scand J Clin Lab Invest* 39:569–576, 1979.
158. Severinghaus JW: Blood gas calculator. *J Appl Physiol* 21:1108–1116, 1966.
159. Shelley HJ: The use of chronically catheterized foetal lambs for the study of foetal metabolism. In Comline RS, Cross KW, Dawes GS, Nathanielsz PW (eds): *Foetal and Neonatal Physiology*. Cambridge, Cambridge University Press, 1973, pp 360–381.
160. Shnider SM, Wright RG, Levinson G, Roizen MF, Wallis KL, Roblin SH, Craft JB: Uterine blood flow and plasma norepinephrine changes during maternal stress in the pregnant ewe. *Anesthesiology* 50:524–527, 1979.

161. Sibley L, Ruhling RO, Cameron-Foster J, Christensen C, Bolen T: Swimming and physical fitness during pregnancy. *J Nurse Midwif* 26:3–12, 1981.
162. Simmons MA, Battaglia FC, Meschia G: Placental transfer of glucose. *J Dev Physiol* 1:227–243, 1979.
163. Smith AD, Gilbert RD, Lammers RJ, Longo LD: Placental exchange area in guinea pigs following long-term maternal exercise: a stereological analysis. *J Dev Physiol* 5:11–21, 1983.
164. Smith EE, Guyton AC, Manning RD, White RJ: Integrated mechanisms of cardiovascular response and control during exercise in the normal human. In Sonnenblick EH, Lesch M (eds): *Exercise and Heart Disease*. New York, Grune & Stratton, 1977, pp 1–23.
165. Soiva K, Salmi A, Grönroos M, Peltonen T: Physical working capacity during pregnancy and effect of physical work tests on foetal heart rate. *Ann Chir Gynaecol* 53:187–196, 1963.
166. Sparks JW, Hay Jr WW, Bonds D, Meschia D, Battaglia FC: Simultaneous measurements of lactate turnover rate and umbilical lactate uptake in the fetal lamb. *J Clin Invest* (submitted).
167. Sparks JW, Pegorier J-P, Girard J, Battaglia FC: Substrate concentration changes during pregnancy in the guinea pig studied under unstressed steady state conditions. *Pediatr Res* 15:1340–1344, 1981.
168. Spetz S: Peripheral circulation during normal pregnancy. *Acta Obstet Gynecol Scand* 43:309–329, 1964.
169. Steel JW, Leng RA: Effect of plane of nutrition and pregnancy on glucose entry rates in sheep. *Proc Aust Soc Anim Prod* 7:242, 1968.
170. Terada M: Effect of physical activity before pregnancy on fetuses of mice exercised forcibly during pregnancy. *Teratology* 10:141–144, 1974.
171. Tulchinski D, Hobel CJ, Yaeger E, Marshall JR: Plasma estrone, estradiol, estriol, progesterone, and 17-hydroxyprogesterone in human pregnancy. *Am J Obstet Gynecol* 112:1095–1100, 1972.
172. Turner AW, Hodgetts VE: The dynamic red cell storage function of the spleen in sheep. I. Relationship to fluctuations of jugular hematocrit. *Aust J Exp Biol* 37:399–420, 1959.
173. Ueland K, Novy MJ, Metcalfe J: Cardiorespiratory responses to pregnancy and exercise in normal women and patients with heart disease. *Am J Obstet Gynecol* 115:4–10, 1973.
174. Ueland K, Novy MJ, Peterson EN, Metcalfe J: Maternal cardiovascular dynamics; IV. The influence of gestational age on the maternal cardiovascular response to posture and exercise. *Am J Obstet Gynecol* 104:856–864, 1969.
175. Wade L: Splenic sequestration of young erythrocytes in sheep. *Am J Physiol* 224:265–267, 1973.
176. Walker AM, Oakes GK, McLaughlin MK, Ehrenranz RA, Alling DW, Chez RA: 24-Hour rhythms in uterine and umbilical blood flows of conscious pregnant sheep. *Gynecol Invest* 8:288–298, 1977.

177. Wallenburg HCS: Modulation and regulation of uteroplacental blood flow. *Placenta* 2 (suppl 1):45–64, 1981.
178. Weinberger SE, Weiss ST, Cohen WR, Weiss JW, Johnson TS: Pregnancy and the lung. *Am Rev Respir Dis* 121:559–581, 1980.
179. Widlund G: The cardio-pulmonal function during pregnancy. A clinical-experimental study with particular respect to ventilation and oxygen consumption among normal cases in rest and after work tests. *Acta Obstet Gynecol Scand* 25 (suppl 1):1–125, 1945.
180. Wilson NC, Gisolfi CV. Effects of exercising rats during pregnancy. *J Appl Physiol* 48:34–40, 1980.
181. Young DR, Pelligra R, Shapira J, Adachi RR, Skrettingland K: Glucose oxidation and replacement during prolonged exercise in man. *J Appl Physiol* 23:734–741, 1967.
182. Yudilevich DL, Eaton BM, Short AH, Leichtweiss H-P: Glucose carriers at maternal and fetal sides of the trophoblast in guinea pig placenta. *Am J Physiol* 237:C205–C212, 1979.

4
The Effect of Exercise on the Menstrual Cycle

The central nervous system (CNS)-hypothalamic-pituitary regulatory center appears to be very sensitive to changes in its environment. In animals reduced reproductive capacity secondary to poor nutrition (weight loss) is well documented (1, 2). There is also evidence suggesting that the attainment and maintenance of normal menstrual cycle and reproductive function may be dependent upon a certain weight to height ratio (3, 4). Furthermore, it is well established that girls engaged in vigorous physical training such as in ballet dancing have a dichotomy in development in that they have a normal onset of pubarche but a marked delay in thelache and menarche (3). This observation supports the theoretical model that an increase in adrenal androgen production which occurs at the beginning of puberty is unaffected by strenous exercise and weight loss, while breast development and menarche, both being estrogen-dependent events, are suppressed.

There is documented evidence that frequency of amenorrhea increases in women athletes who undergo strenuous training (5). It was reported that the incidence of amenorrhea was approximately 20% in a group of women running 20 miles/week as compared to an incidence of 43% in a group of women running 70–80 miles/week ($P < 0.01$).

Since starvation is a known cause of reproductive failure (anorexia nervosa) the question comes up as to whether the amenorrhea seen in athletes is related to low body weight or due to CNS-hypothalamic dysfunction as a result of stress (6). Feicht et al. (5) found that the amenorrheic and regularly menstruating runners were of equal weight and height. Abraham et al. (7) reported that, in 79% of young women training at a professional ballet school, the menstrual cycles either completely stopped or became irregular. None of these menstrual cycle disturbances were related to significant change in body weight. The menstrual irregularly improved during periods of long rest (due to injury) or long vacations. It therefore appears that exercise does cause disturbances in the normal menstrual cycles and that this alteration is not only due to body weight loss but in many instances due to alterations in the regulatory mechanism of the reproductive centers in the brain. It must be noted that this CNS dysfunction is not an universal accepted finding. Cumming and Rebar (18) have published data supporting their postulate that exercise-induced amenorrhea results from some alterations "originating in the periphery that only secondarily affects the CNS-hypothalamic-pituitary function (8).

EFFECT OF EXERCISE ON NEUROTRANSMITTER-HYPOTHALAMIC FUNCTION

The major effects of regular and strenous exercise may result in the following menstrual abnormalities: (*a*) delayed menarche, (*b*) oligomenorrhea, and (*c*) possible inadequate luteal phase inadequacy.

Since many of these patients have demonstrated an exaggerated response of gonadotropins following administration of gonadotropin-releasing hormone (GnRH) it has been suggested that the menstrual dysfunction is mediated at the hypothalamic level (9). Endogenous opioid peptides are known to inhibit pulsatile gonadotropin release (10) and have been implicated by Howlett et al. (11) as the major contributing factor in exercise-induced menstrual irregularities. Fraoli et al. (12) and Farrell et al. (13) have reported that the opioid peptide, β-endorphin, and its precursor lipotropin (both derived from pro-opiomelanocortin) are released from the anterior pituitary in response to stress. In addition, Carr et al. (14) reported the same changes seen as result of exercise. Recently Howlett et al. (11) reported plasma β-endorphin and met-enkephalin concentration changes seen before and after treadmill exercise (Fig. 4.1). This report clearly demonstrated the release of both β-endorphin in response to acute physical exertion induced by treadmill exercise. The release of β-endorphin presumably is the result of its release from the anterior pituitary and occurs in conjunction with release of ACTH a known "stress" hormone. These authors also found a more variable but never-the-less demonstrable release of met-enkephalin in response to treadmill exercise. The source of met-enkephalin remains unknown although Howlett did postuate that it may be released from the adrenal medulla, sympathetic nerve endings or gut. The source may be also in part due to decreased rate of degradation or release of a immunoreactive met-enkephalin from its precursor in plasma (15). Since opioid receptors in the median eminence of the hypothalamus are known to exist and have been reported to inhibit pulsatile release of GnRh (16) it becomes very tempting to develop a pathophysiological model supporting the hypothesis that release of exercise induced opioids into plasma contributes to the menstrual disturbances seen in athletes. However, the role of other substances such

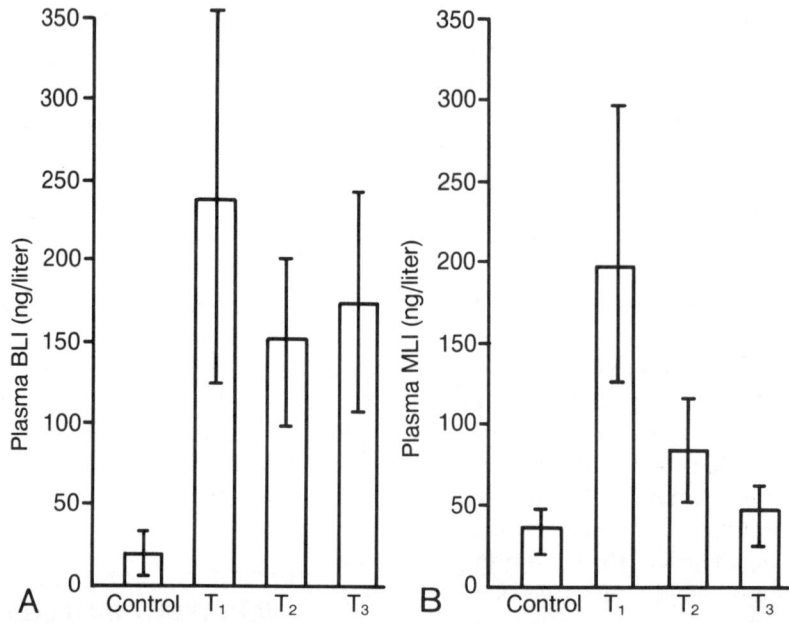

Figure 4.1. (*A*) Peak plasma β-endorphin-like immunoreactivity (*BLI*) during three treadmill runs compared with control day. Values are means. Bars are SEM. (*B*) Peak plasma met-enkephalin-like immunoreactivity (*MLI*) during three treadmill runs compared with control day. Values are means. *Bars* are SEM. (From Howlett et al. (11).)

as melatonin secreted from the pineal gland and prolactin secreted from the pituitary must also be seriously considered (17).

EFFECT OF EXERCISE ON PITUITARY FUNCTION

From the above data the alterations seen in the menstrual cycle of normal exercising women is generally considered to be CNS-hypothalamic in origin. However, to get an overall view of the endocrinopathy produced by physical activity, changes in pituitary hormone secretion and resultant changes in gonadal and adrenal hormones must be considered. In reviewing the literature dealing with this subject it becomes obvious that contradictions exist and absolute or dogmatic statements cannot be made. However, trends are identifiable and should be reviewed.

Cumming and Rebar (18) have published extensive data dealing with effect of acute short-term exercise (cycling) on pituitary hormones, and ovarian and adrenal steroids. These authors compared the circulating levels of LH, FSH (also T, E_1, E_2, cortisol, A, DHEA, PRL, GH, TSH) in three groups of subjects. The control group consisted of untrained women. The second group was made up of women who were runners and were having normal menstrual cycles. The third group consisted of women who were engaged in running and were amenorrheic. The basal LH and FSH concentrations were similar in all three groups (Fig. 4.2A). All three groups showed an unexpected increase in LH just prior to exercise which is most likely a neuroendocrine event. The gonadotropin levels continued to rise and peaked 15–20 min after onset of cycling in the controls and menstruating runners but showed a drop in the amenorrheic runners. This is most likely secondary to alteration in the neurotransmitter-GnRH axis. Not all investigators have found that exercise has the same effect on LH as the above authors. Baker et al. (19) reported lower plasma levels of LH in amenorrheic runners compared with the levels in both running and nonrunning controls. Jurkowski et al. (20) reported that LH was unchanged with exercise in normal subjects. These reported disagreements may be suggesting that exercise-induced amenorrhea is a distinct entity with a heterogenous etiology.

Cumming and Rebar (18) found that prolactin levels increased during exercise in nonexercising and normal menstruating runners but do not increase in amenorrheic runners (Fig. 4.3A). There was a decrease in PRL levels in the amenorrheic group when compared to the PRL rise seen in controls and in the normal cycling runners. This difference may be due to difference in levels of dopamine secreted by the amenorrheic group. GH was noted to increase in controls, menstruating and amenorrheic runners but the increase was significantly less in the nonexercising women (Fig. 4.3B). TSH was noted to be significantly greater in its rise after completion of exercise in the menstruating runners but not so in the amenorrheic runners. In both the menstruating and amenorrheic women, the TSH increment was higher than the nonexercising controls (Fig. 4.3C).

EFFECT OF EXERCISE ON STEROID HORMONES

Basal levels of testosterone (T) appear to increase in anticipation of exercise in controls as well as menstruating and amenorrheic runners (Fig. 4.2B). This finding was explained by the authors as a possible secondary effect in response to elevated LH levels. The latter increment being a dopamine-norepineprine mediated neuroendocrine event. It is also postulated that changes in T and other steroids may be a result of hemoconcentration, altered binding, production or decreased in renal clearance during exercise. Jurkowski et al. (20) have reported that there is an increase in E_2 and progesterone (P) levels which occurs in all levels of exercise intensity when normal subjects were evaluated in the luteal phase and that only E_2 is increased when samples are obtained and measured during the follicular phase. Since these authors did not find any changes in the LH levels (FSH did

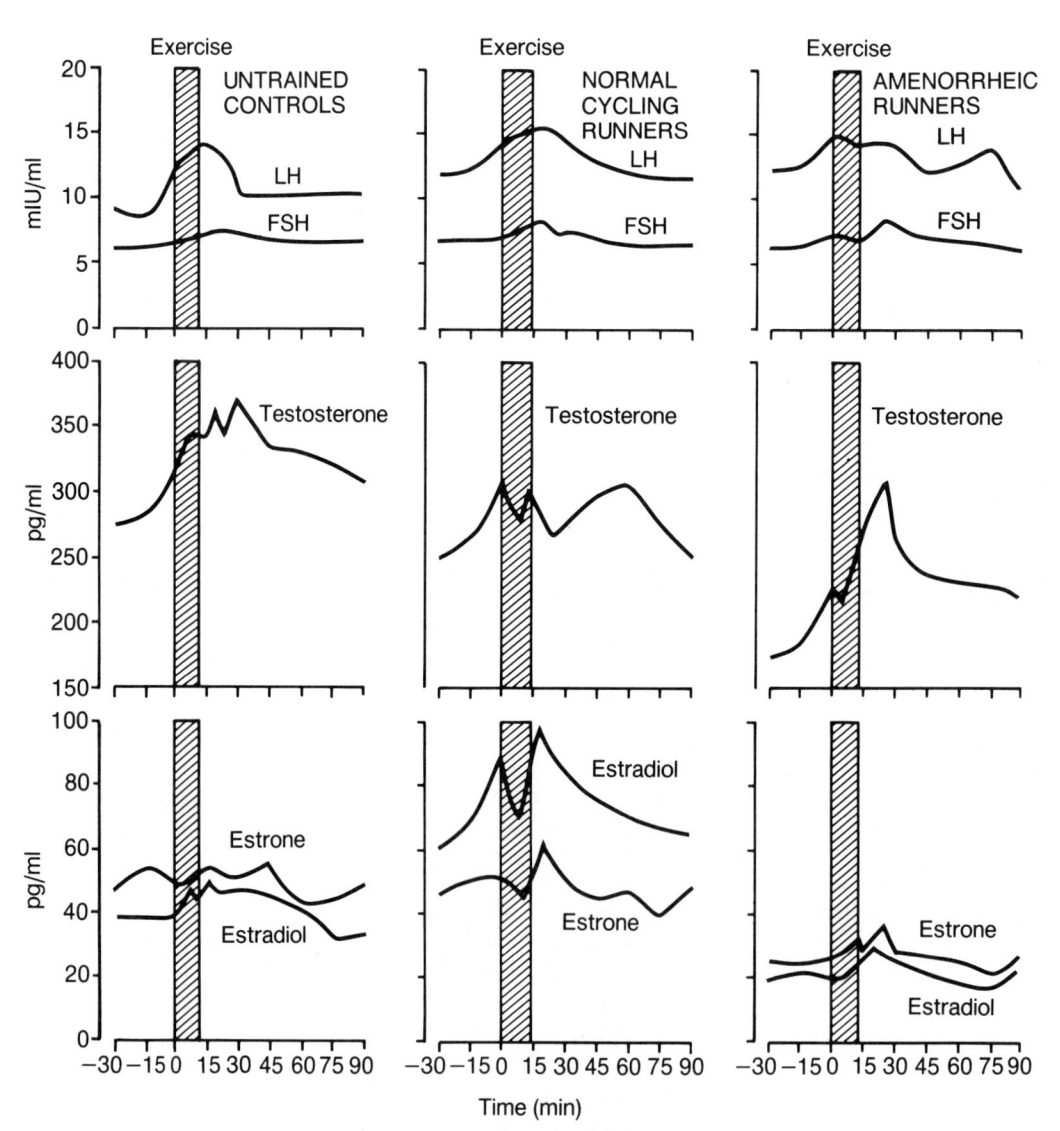

Figure 4.2. Levels of LH, FSH, T, E_1, E_2 before, during and after symptom-limited incremental exercise on a bicycle ergometer showing responses of normally cycling untrained women, normally cycling women runners and amenorrheic runners. (*Smoothed curves* from data accumulated by Cumming et al. (8).) (From Cumming and Rebar (18).)

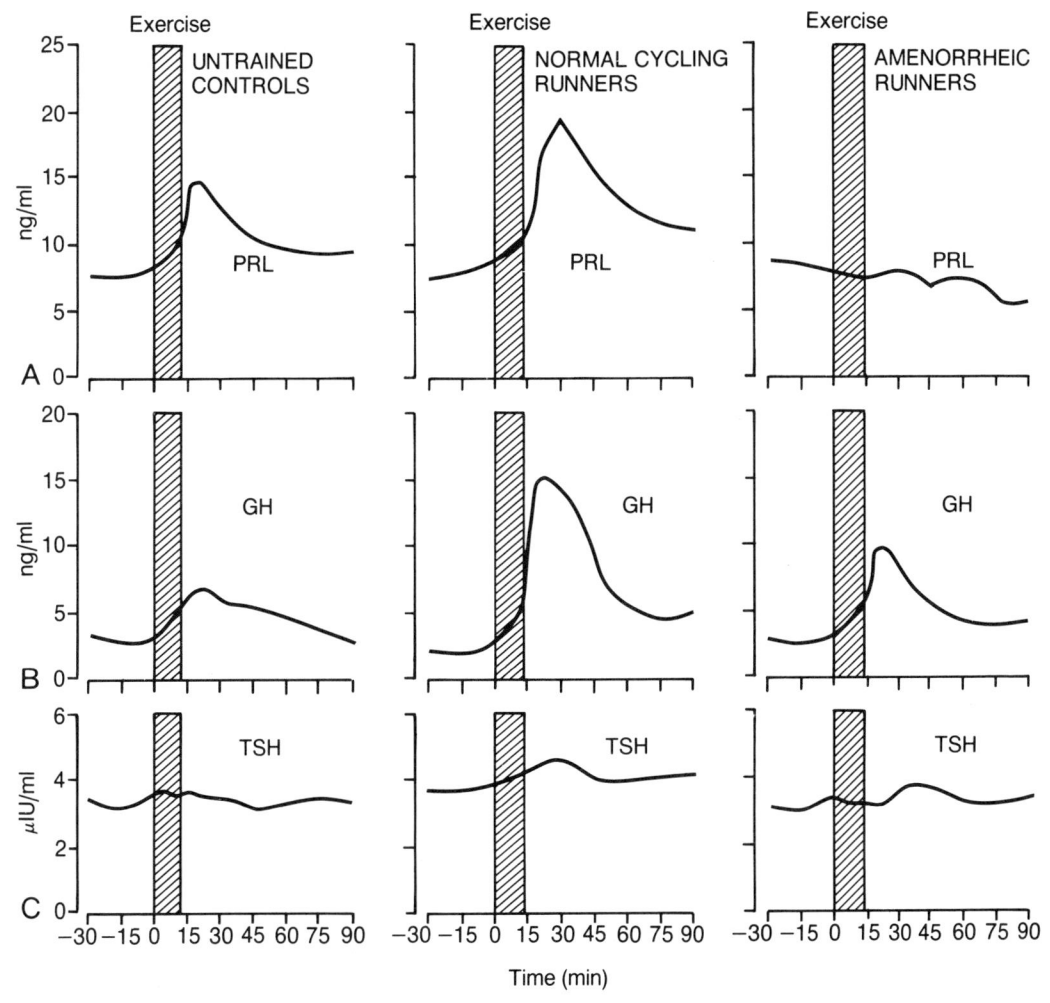

Figure 4.3. Levels of prolactin (*PRL*), growth hormone (*GH*), and thyroid-stimulating hormone (*TSH*) before, during, and after symptom-incremental exercise on a bicycle ergometer showing responses of normally cycling women runners, and amenorrheic runners. (Smoothed curves from data accumulated by Cumming et al. (8).) (From Cumming and Rebar (18).)

increase in the follicular phase), they concluded that exercise is a physiological stimulus to E_2 and that the P increases were related to intensity of exercise and probably independent of pituitary control (20). No significant increase in E_1 or E_2 was noted in immediate postexercise period in response to exercise in amenorrheic runners as compared to menstruating runners. The latter group were found to have an increment significantly higher than the controls. The authors could not explain this difference by the findings of LH or FSH secretions in these two groups of subjects.

Basal levels of cortisol were reported by Cumming and Rebar (18) to elevated in both the menstruating runners and amenorrheic runners. The cortisol was noted to decline initially in nonrunner controls. In all subjects the cortisol significantly increased after the exercise was discontinued. The cortisol levels in amenorrheic runners declined during exercise which also was noted in the nonrunners but remained flat in the menstruating runners. These differences were not explained by the authors.

These findings all point to the fact that exercise does alter the pituitary-adreno-gonadal system and that these changes in turn in some women lead to the amenorrheic states. It is unclear why under the same exercise condition some have normal levels of E_2 and some have low E_2. Most authors do seem to agree that the amenorrhea seen among women who are exercising is most likely a neurotransmitter-hypothalamic induced phenomena with evidence that some of the alteration in ovarian and adrenal steroids are peripheral which in turn have central effect. The alteration of the hypothalamic-pituitary-adrenal-ovarian axis is almost always reversible and does not appear to have permanent consequence.

MANAGEMENT

From the above data presented, it appears that exercise-induced amenorrhea has a multifactorial etiology. It is also apparent that in most instances this specific endocrinopathy is reversible when the exercise program is discontinued. Certain findings appear to be identifiable and associated factors which lead to menstrual irregularities in women who get involved in rigorous physical activity. These factors include previous menstrual abnormalities (before starting the exercise routine), endurance type exercise rather than acute exercise, amount of weight loss and stress encountered by the women athletes. There is no specific amount of training, body fat loss, or critical weight loss that appears to cause menstrual abnormalities in all women. Women react differently to exercise and appear to have individualized thresholds, which when crossed, lead to oligomenorrhea.

In establishing a protocol for the workup of women who develop menstrual abnormalities related to exercise, the major factors to be dealt with include establishing the degree to hypoestrogenicity that may exist and whether there is an undetected pathological state independent of exercise which may be the major etiological factor. With these two points in mind we have been utilizing the following protocol in working up women with oligomenorrhea associated with exercise. The initial step after a complete history and physical is to obtain a serum prolactin (PRL). If the PRL level is less than 20 ng/ml, the status of the sella turcica is not evaluated. However, if the woman has hyperprolactinemia she deserves a complete endocrinological evaluation in order to determine whether she has or does not have a prolactin secreting adenoma. If the amenorrheic woman is found to have a normal serum PRL level, then her estrogen status should be determined, since it has been reported that hypoestrogen status can be associated with decreased regional bone mass and early onset of osteoporosis (21). We have utilized IM progesterone-in-oil (100–200 mg/ml) challenge test as the first test to determine the estrogen status. If the patient has any amount of uterine bleeding, it can be assumed that her serum estradiol (E_2) level is above 40 pg/ml and no estrogen replacement is therefore required. However, if the patient does not have withdrawal uterine bleeding following 200 mg of progesterone IM, then a serum E_2 level should be obtained and if the level is noted to be below 40 pg/ml then estrogen/progestin replacement therapy should be instituted. We recommend conjugated estrogen replacement of 0.625 mg/day given from day 1 to 25 of the month. On the day 14–25 of the month, medroxyprogesterone acetate (Provera) 10 ng/ml should be given in order to avoid an unopposed estrogen effect on the endometrium and breast tissue. It is not clear when replacement therapy should be started. Arbitrarily, we have decided to start all young hypoestrogenic women on E/P therapy at age 17, an age when most normal young women have gone through menarche. At this institution, the rather vigorous and early start of E/P replacement therapy is a new approach based on the most recent published but rather limited information.

REFERENCES

1. Fries H, Nillus SJ, Pettersson F: Epidemiology of secondary amenorrhea: a retrospective evaluation of etiology with special regard to psychogenic factors and weight loss. *Am J Obstet Gynecol* 118:473, 1974.

2. Frisch RE: Nutrition, fatness and fertility: the effect of food intake on reproductive ability. In Mosley WH (ed): *Nutrition and Human Reproduction*. New York, Plenum, 1978, p 106.
3. Warren MP: The effects of exercise on pubertal proression and reproductive function in girls. *J Clin Endocrinol Metab* 51:1156, 1980.
4. Frisch RE, McArthur JW: Menstrual cycles: fatness as a determinant of minimum weight for height necessary for their maintenance or onset. *Science* 185:949, 1974.
5. Feicht CB, Johnson TS, Martin BJ, Sparkes KE, Wagner Jr WW: Secondary amenorrhea in athletes. *Lancet* 2:1145–1146, 1978.
6. Thorn GW et al (eds): *Harrison's Principles of Internal Medicine*. New York, McGraw-Hill, 1977.
7. Abraham SF, Beaumont PJV, Fraser IS, Llewellyn-Jones D: Body weight, exercise and menstrual status among ballet dancers in training. *Br J Obstet Gynaecol* 89:507, 1982.
8. Cumming DC, Strich G, Brunsting L, Greenberg L, Ries AL, Yen SC, Rebar RW: Acute exercise related endocrine changes in women runners and nonrunners. *Fertil Steril* 36:421, 1981.
9. McArthur JW, Bullen BA, Bettins IZ, Pagane M, Bader TM, Klianski A: Hypothalamic amenorrhea in runners of normal body distribution. *Endocr Res Commun* 7:13, 1980.
10. Moult PA, Grossman A, Evans JM, Reese LH, Beser GM: The effect of naloxone on pulsatile gonadotropin release in normal subjects. *Clin Endocrinol (Oxf)* 14:321, 1981.
11. Howlett TA, Tomlin S, Ngahfoony L, Rees LH, Bullen BA, Skrinar GS, McArthur JW: Release of β-endorphin and met-enkephalin during exercise in normal women: response to training. *Br Med J* 288:1950, 1984.
12. Fraioli F, Morett C, Paolucci D, Alicicco E, Crescenzi F, Fortunio G: Physical exercise stimulates marked concomitant increase of β-endorphin and adrenocorticotrophin (ACTH) in peripheral blood in man. *Experientia* 36:987, 1980.
13. Farrell PA, Gates WK, Maksud MG, Morgan WP: Increase in plasma β-endorphin/β-lipotropin immunoreactivity after treadmill running in humans. *J Appl Physiol* 52:1245, 1982.
14. Carr DB, Bullen BA, Skrinar GS: Physical conditioning facilitates the exercise-induced secretion of β-endorphin and β-lipothrophin in women. *N Engl J Med* 305:560, 1981.
15. Smith R, Grossman A, Gaillard R: Studies on circulating met-enkephalin and β-endorphin. Normal subjects and patients with renal and adrenal disease. *Clin Endocrinol (Oxf)* 15:291, 1981.
16. Grossman A, Moult PJA, Gailard RC: The opioid control of LH and FSH release. effects of met-enkephalin analogue and naloxone. *Clin Endocrinol (Oxf)* 14:41, 1981.
17. Carr DM, Reppert SM, Bullen BA: Plasma melatonin increases during exercise in women. *J Clin Endocrinol Metab* 53:224, 1981.
18. Cumming DC, Rebar RW: Exercise and reproductive function in women. *Am J Indust Med* 4:113, 1983.
19. Baker EM, Mather RS, Kirk RF, Williamson HO: Female runners and secondary amenorrhea: correlation with age, parity, mileage and plasma hormonal and sex hormone binding globulin concentrations. *Fertil Steril* 36:183, 1981.
20. Jurkowski JE, Jones JL, Walker WC, Younglai EV, Sutton JR: Ovarian hormonal response to exercise. *J Appl Physiol* 44:109, 1978.
21. Drinkwater BL, Nilson K, Chesnut CH, Bremner WJ, Shainholtz S, Southworth MB: Bone mineral content of amenorrheic and eumenorrheic athletes. *N Engl J Med* 311:277, 1984.

5
Physiological and Endocrine Adjustments to Pregnancy

Pregnancy is distinguished by a multitude of physiological and endocrine adjustments directed toward the creation of an optimal environment for the fetus. Every organ system in the expectant mother as well as her personality are intimately involved in this complex process.

The sequence of events is not yet completely elucidated, and many times limited to descriptive terms. The changes in the reproductive system must be supported by secondary adjustments of other systems. Because of the complexity of the mechanisms involved, no seemingly ideal adjustment can be achieved. But, by and large, the side effects of the pregnant state do require adjustments and do not constitute a threat to maternal health if properly achieved. Conversely, inadequate adjustment or an imbalance among various body systems results in pathology.

In summarizing the above adjustments, our intention is to focus on those systems that can be affected by exercise.

Exercise is a process in which chemical energy is transformed into a movement (or muscular tension in isometric exercise), and inevitably into heat. The human body can be compared to a sophisticated engine, equipped with very sensitive sensors and an immense macroprocessor, that is in continuous need of a mechanism to process fuel (food), dispose of waste products, and dissipate heat. With this somewhat mechanistic view in mind, we divided our description into four sections:

1. Locomotive system (neuromusculoskeletal)
2. Energy generating system (gastrointestinal, respiratory, cardiovascular)
3. Disposal system (urinary tract, skin)
4. The endocrine system.

LOCOMOTIVE SYSTEM (NEUROMUSCULOSKELETAL)

The physical fitness of any individual is the result of his motor fitness and his physical working capacity defined as the maximum level of metabolism (power) of which an individual is capable (1). Listing the elements of motor fitness: strength, speed, agility, endurance, power, coordination, balance, flexibility, and body control, it is clear that these are the results of the performance and integration of the musculoskeletal and neurologic systems.

Musculoskeletal System

The protruding abdomen, waddling gait and exaggerated lordosis are familiar features of normal pregnancy.

The constantly growing uterus, although a muscular organ not belonging to the musculoskeletal system per se, is the main cause for the changes occurring in the statics and dynamics of the skeleton in the gravida.

From a strictly pelvic organ at 12 weeks, the uterus becomes an abdominal organ displacing the intestines and coming into direct contact with the abdominal wall. Its dimensions increase 150-fold throughout pregnancy and the capacity more than 1000-fold (2). Its weight increases up to 20 times at term, not taking into account the weight of the fetus. Altogether, at term, the pregnant uterus with its content contributes an average of 6 kg to the maternal weight gain (3, 4).

The anterior orientation of the uterus expanding into the abdominal cavity displaces the woman's center of gravity, resulting in progressive lumbar lordosis and rotation of the pelvis on the femur. This shifts the center of the gravity back over her pelvis preventing a forward fall (Fig. 5.1).

In order to maintain the line of vision and also compensate for the lumbar lordosis, the gravida increases the anterior flexion of the cervical spine in addition to slumping abduction of the shoulders. Exaggeration of this position can lead to increased paresthesias over the distribution of the ulnar and/or median nerve with increasing motor weakness (the hand syndrome of pregnancy) (5) (see Chapter 16).

In addition, the growing uterus rotates on its long axis, usually to the right. The movement of the uterus is restricted anteriorly by the abdominal wall and posteriorly by the vertebral column. Even in the absence of laxity in an abdominal wall, as in most primigravidas, there is still enough room for displacement. Because the displacement is always in the direction of the inclination, the result is increased instability. The enlarging breasts (500 g at term), as well, contribute to the change in the center of gravity. As a result of the above changes, the center of gravity in pregnant women is high, rising and unstable. If those were the characteristics of a ship, there could be a constant threat of capsizing.

A pregnant woman's stability is obtained at the expense of an increased burden upon the muscles and ligaments of the vertebral column. No wonder low back pain is so common in pregnancy.

In addition to its content, the pelvic girdle itself changes profoundly during pregnancy. The bones which comprise the pelvis are held together by fibrocartilage with small synovial articular cavities and reinforced with pelvic ligaments: the pubic and sacrosciatic.

Early in pregnancy, secondary to the release of estrogens and/or relaxin, there is increasing relaxation of ligaments. Softening of the cartilage and increase in the synovia and synovial fluid widens the pelvic joints. The result is increased joint mobility and an unstable pelvis reflected in a waddling gait. Changes similar to the one in the pelvis occur in the other joints and muscles.

In the third trimester of pregnancy, the gravida experiences reduced mobility of ankle joints and wrists in spite of increased relaxation of the ligaments. These changes

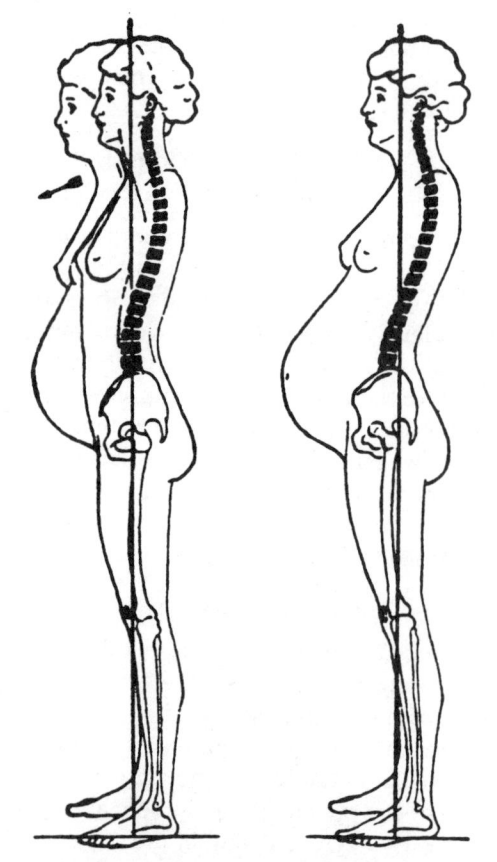

Figure 5.1. Statics of the nonpregnant woman (*left*) and pregnant woman (*right*). (From J. P. Greenhill: *Obstetrics*, ed. 13, Philadelphia, W. B. Saunders, 1965, p. 183.)

are caused by water retention mainly in the ground substance of connective tissue resulting in visible ankle edema in the majority of pregnant women and paraesthesias in the hands, and even muscular weakness, the carpal tunnel syndrome (6, 7).

It is clear from this description that sports requiring agility, balance and strength, especially of hands, like skiing, horse riding, gymnastics, and tennis can be more injury producing to the pregnant woman, particularly after the first trimester of pregnancy, whereas swimming is not affected in a similar way.

Neurologic System

From the very scanty literature, it appears that the pregnant woman has significant changes in perception senses. In a rather old report (1930), but still the most comprehensive, J. P. Johns (8) describes the definite concentric contraction of form and color fields and also enlargement of the blind spot during pregnancy with a return to normal about 10 days postpartum.

The corneal sensitivity as well as the corneal topography changes, most probably secondary to edema. That is the rationale for not prescribing new optical corrections until some weeks after delivery (9).

It is common knowledge, although not validated in strictly scientific terms, that heightening or dulling of the senses of taste and smell may account for the cravings and aversions toward certain food during pregnancy (10,11).

There is a paucity of data about other senses and their adaptations during pregnancy.

There is evidence that even the most sophisticated activities controlled by the central nervous system, namely the emotional and cognitive processes, may be altered in pregnancy with a tendency toward insomnia, lability of mood, anxiety, as well as slightly impaired cognitive functions (12).

ENERGY GENERATING SYSTEMS

The energy utilized by the body is chemical and released in the process of oxygenation. The oxygen serves as an oxidant, via the pulmonary tract, and the distribution system for both is the cardiovascular system.

The energetic cost of pregnancy is estimated at about 80,000 kcal or 300 kcal/day (13). This is required to cover the growth and development of the fetus, buildup of maternal tissue such as the uterus, breasts, fat, and to compensate for the increased metabolism due to increased activity of the cardiovascular, respiratory and urinary systems, and the addition of the fetal metabolism (Table 5.1). The demand is unevenly distributed, being at maximum during the two middle quarters of pregnancy, an extra need of about 390 kcal/day. It is mainly caused by fat storage during that period. The last quarter of pregnancy is less demanding, only an additional 250 kcal/day is needed for the growing fetus, while the fat storage ceases (Table 5.2; Fig. 5.2).

There are two ways to meet this energetic cost of pregnancy, either by increased intake or reduced expenditure of energy.

It seems that both ways are utilized during pregnancy. The average pregnant woman eating an unrestricted diet probably increases her total daily energy consumption by approximately 150–300 kcal due to increased appetite (14).

Conversely, it is common to pregnant women to reduce their physical activity, not only because of the demands imposed by the growing fetus, and the mechanical instability and laxity of joints, but also because of the feeling of lassitude and somnolence caused by the surge in hormones, mainly progesterone (15, 16).

If dietary intake is inadequate to meet the caloric and nutrient needs of the expectant mother, protein will be catabolized. Since pregnancy is, in essence, an anabolic state with positive nitrogen balance throughout, increased breakdown of proteins to combat the inadequate energy supply will reduce the availability of amino acids for maternal buildup and fetal growth, with adverse results (17). Similar adverse effects on the fetus will most probably occur with a diet

Table 5.1. The Extra Components of Estrogen Consumption in Pregnancy[a]

Source of Extra Energy Output	Increment at Weeks of Pregnancy 10	20	30	40	Estimated Cost (ml O_2/min)	Increment of O_2 Consumption (ml/min) Weeks of Gestation 10	20	30	40
Cardiac output (l/min)	1.0	1.5	1.5	1.5	About 20 at 4.5 l/min. Increase pro rata	4.5	6.8	6.8	6.8
Respiration (l/min)	0.75	1.50	2.25	3.00	1.0 per l ventilation	0.8	1.5	2.3	3.0
Uterine muscle (g)	140	320	600	970	3.7 per kg	0.5	1.2	2.2	3.6
Placenta (g)									
Wet	20	170	430	650	3.3 per 100 g dry weight	0	0.5	2.2	3.7
Dry	2	17	65	110					
Fetus (g)	5	300	1500	3400	3.65 per kg	0	1.1	5.5	12.4
Breasts (g)	45	180	360	410	3.3 per kg	0.1	0.6	1.2	1.4
Kidneys (mEq Na reabsorbed)	7	7	7	7	1.0 per meq	7	7	7	7
					Total ml per min	12.9	18.7	27.2	37.9

[a] From F. E. Hytten: Nutrition. In F. E. Hytten and G. Chamberlain (eds): *Clinical Physiology in Obstetrics*, Oxford, Blackwell, 1980, p. 167.

Table 5.2. Cumulative Energy Cost of Pregnancy Computed for the Energy Equivalents of Protein and Fat Increments and the Energy Cost of Maintaining the Fetus and Added Maternal Tissues[a,b]

	Equivalent (kcal/day) per Weeks of Pregnancy: 0–10	10–20	20–30	30–40	Cumulative Total (kcal)[c]
Protein	3.6	10.3	26.7	34.2	5,186
Fat	55.6	235.6	207.6	31.3	36,329
Oxygen consumption	44.8	99.0	148.2	227.2	35,717
Total net energy	104.0	344.9	382.5	292.7	77,234
Metabolizable energy (total net energy + 10%)	114	379	421	322	84,957

[a] The total is derived from oxygen consumption figures (Table 5.1) and assumes an RQ of 0.90. Note: For the first 10-week period total increment is divided by 56 since pregnancy is dated from the last menstrual period.

[b] From F. E. Hytten: Nutrition. In F. E. Hytten and G. Chamberlain (eds.): *Clinical Physiology in Obstetrics*, Oxford, Blackwell, 1980, p. 165.

[c] Taken as 5.6 kcal/g for protein and 9.5 kcal/g for fat.

restricted in proteins in spite of adequate caloric intake. This issue is compounded because of the close relationship between optimal protein use and the adequacy of the energy sources (18).

Adequate weight gain is the most practical indicator of caloric intake. It is estimated that a healthy primigravida, eating without restriction, will gain an average of 27.5 lb (12.5 kg) (19). This estimation served as a baseline for the compilation of the Recommended Daily Dietary Allowance (RDAs) for Pregnancy. Yet, it is important to keep in mind that the RDAs published by the Committee on Maternal Nutrition, Food and Nutrition Board, National Research Council (Table 5.3) are intended as guidelines for average population, not individuals. Additional information on these topics can be found in Chapters 6 and 7.

Gastrointestinal System

It is rather controversial whether the anatomic and physiologic changes in the gastrointestinal tract encourage the efficiency of the food intake or the increased caloric intake occurs in spite of it.

The main change in the function of the

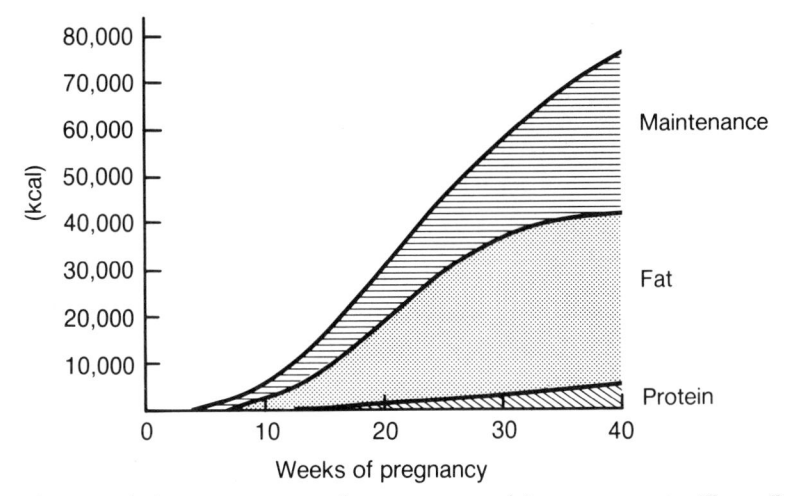

Figure 5.2. The cumulative energy cost of pregnancy and its components. (From F. E. Hytten: Nutrition. In F. E. Hytten and G. Chamberlain (eds.): *Clinical Physiology in Obstetrics*, Oxford, Blackford, 1980, p. 166.)

Table 5.3. Recommended Daily Dietary Allowance (RDAs) for Pregnancy[a]

Energy (kcal)	2,400 (2,300)[b]
Protein (gm)	78 (76)[b]
Vitamin A (IU)	5,000
Vitamin D (IU)	400
Vitamin E activity (IU)	15
Ascorbic acid (mg)	60
Folic acid (mg)	800
Niacin (mg)	16
Riboflavin (mg)	1.7
Thiamine (mg)	1.4
Vitamin B_6 (mg)	2.5
Vitamin B_{12} (μg)	4.0
Calcium (mg)	1,200
Phosphorus (mg)	1,200
Iodine (μg)	125
Iron (mg)	18[c]
Magnesium (mg)	450
Zinc (mg)	20

[a] Source: Committee on Maternal Nutrition, Food and Nutrition Board, National Research Council: *Recommended Dietary Allowances*, ed 9, publication 2216. Washington, D.C., National Academy of Sciences, 1980.
[b] Recommended for gravidas more than 23 years old.
[c] Recommended for gravidas more than 19 years old. The increased requirement cannot be met by the diet; supplemental iron is recommended.

gastrointestinal tract in pregnancy is its decline in activity. The esophageal peristalsis has a slower wave speed and lower amplitude. The lower esophageal sphincter responses to hormonal pharmacological and physiological stimuli are reduced. In addition, the intraesophageal pressure is reduced while the intragastric pressure is slightly elevated compared to the nonpregnant state, lowering the barrier pressure (20, 21).

As pregnancy progresses, the growing uterus displaces the stomach and the intestines. The relatively common displacement of the lower esophageal sphincter upward into the negative pressure region of the thorax contributes to its reduced compliance (22). In all, these changes favor gastroesophageal reflux and result in frequent indigestion and regurgitation.

There is a decrease in the tone and motility of the gastrointestinal tract which results in prolongation of the gastric emptying time (23) and delayed intestinal passage (24). As a result of the reduced intestinal motility and the slow passage of the food through the large bowel, with increased absorbtion of water, the feces are dry, hard, and difficult to expel; constipation is a common complaint (25).

In pregnancy, the oropharynx is affected by excessive salivation and hyperemia with softening of the gums, which are easily traumatized and bleed. The gallbladder is usually hypotonic and distended with thick and tarry bile, emptying slower in pregnancy (26, 27).

Respiratory System

The changes in the respiratory system are extensive, including anatomic and functional alterations. These changes occur very early due to hormonal influence, mainly progesterone, even before the growing uterus mechanically impairs ventilation. Actually, in spite of the space occupied by the uterus, the total lung capacity (TLC) shows relatively little change (reduction of 300 ml) in pregnancy (28–30). The rise of the diaphragm by about 4 cm caused by flaring of the lower ribs, as is seen observing the progressively increasing subcostal angle from about 68° in early pregnancy to 103° in late pregnancy, is compensated by increasing the transverse diameter of the chest (Fig. 5.3) (31). The net result is that the thoracic cavity is not reduced. More than that, the diaphragmatic excursion is increased with breathing (32).

Significant respiratory functional changes are observed in pregnancy. The respiratory center has a reduced threshold for P_{CO_2} and increased sensitivity to any increase in P_{CO_2}.

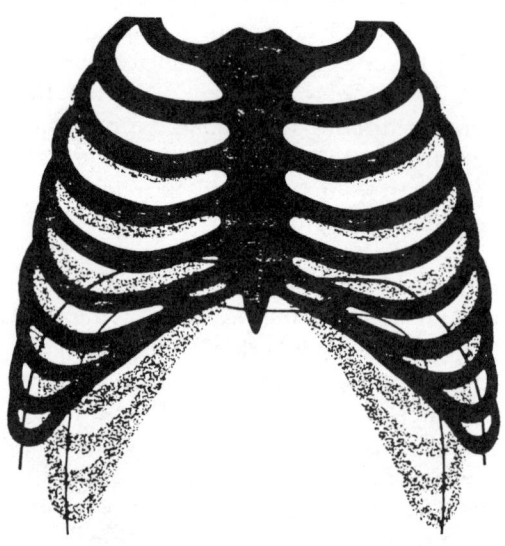

Figure 5.3. The ribcage in pregnancy (*black*), and the nonpregnant state (*strippled*) showing the increased subcostal angle, the increased transverse diameter, and the raised diaphragm in pregnancy. (From M. deSwiet: The respiratory system. In F. E. Hytten and G. Chamberlain (eds.): *Clinical Physiology in Obstetrics*, Oxford, Blackwell, 1980, p. 86.)

For a given increase in P_{CO_2}, the induced increase in pulmonary ventilation rate is about 4 times greater during pregnancy (33). The increased ventilation is achieved by breathing more deeply and not more frequently.

There is a gradual increase up to 40% in tidal volume (V_T), from 500 ml in the nonpregnant state to about 700 ml in late pregnancy (34). Because the vital capacity is changed very little during pregnancy (increase of about 100 ml), the change in V_T must come at the expense of other functional lung volume, namely the expiratory reserve volume, as illustrated in Figure 5.4. The expiratory reserve volume (ERV) decreases by about 200 ml while residual volume (RV) decreases by 300 ml, reducing the functional reserve capacity (RV + ERV) by 500 ml. It means that, at the end of quiet expiration, there is a smaller oxygen reserve in the lung (35) and, thus, a reduced ability to withstand periods of apnea, a factor that should be taken into account when considering participation in sports like diving or short sprints. The cause for the reduction in the residual volume is unclear and the answer may lie with the increased central blood volume (CBV) which includes the lung, heart, and great vessels. The CBV rises by 20% or 260 ml and is illustrated on chest radiographs by the increased prominence of the pulmonary vasculature (36, 37).

The increased minute ventilation which is directly related to the increased V_T and rises, as expected, by 40% from 7.5 liters/min to 10.5 liters/min, results in a significant decrease in P_{CO_2} from about 39 mm Hg in the nonpregnant state to 31 mm Hg during pregnancy (38, 39).

Obviously, it increases the oxygen supply by at least 40% and even more, up to 50% because the alveolar ventilation increases proportionally more than expected with increased pulmonary ventilation as expressed by the minute volume. One additional explanation is that the fixed respiratory dead space caused by the increased V_T, as the sole promoting factor for increased minute volume, involves a relatively smaller dilu-

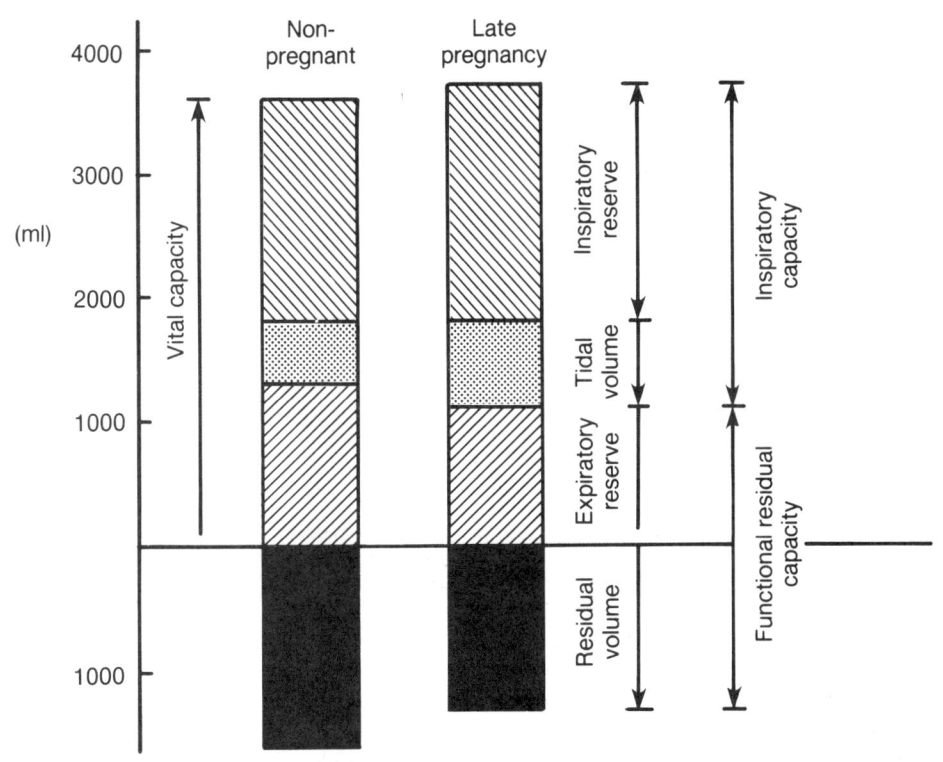

Figure 5.4. Subdivisions of lung volume and their alterations in pregnancy. (From M. deSwiet: The respiratory system. In F. E. Hytten and G. Chamberlain (eds.): *Clinical Physiology in Obstetrics*, Oxford, Blackwell, 1980, p. 81.)

tional effect of the unventilated air trapped in the dead space.

The adaptation of the respiratory system should be viewed from two different perspectives: Does it meet the increased oxygen demand of pregnancy? And what portion of the inborn functional reserve is utilized in the adaptation process?

The basal oxygen consumption increases through pregnancy by about 40 ml/min (39, 40). The main consumers being the heart and the kidney in addition to the fetus and the placenta (Fig. 5.5).

The approximately 20% increase in oxygen consumption is facilitated by the 40–50% increase in ventilation.

The increase in ventilation may be the cause of the common subjective feeling of dyspnea in pregnancy in spite of the increased oxygen supply. The usual explanations for dyspnea, i.e., mechanical restriction or airways resistance were not validated in pregnancy (41).

Additional stress like the one caused by exercise is easily compensated within the respiratory system with the capacity to increase tenfold (42). (See Chapter 11 for additional information.)

Cardiovascular System

The goal of the adaptation of the cardiovascular system, teleologically speaking, is to provide increased amounts of oxygen and fuel to all the organs with increased activity. The cardiovascular performance augments more than physiologically needed as reflected by the increased oxygen consumption. In addition, whereas the cardiac output increases about 40%, there is an increase of only 13% in body mass to be supplied by maternal blood. The major increase in cardiac output occurs early in pregnancy at the end of the first trimester (43) during which period the oxygen consumption only starts to rise (Fig. 5.5). Furthermore, the arterial-venous oxygen difference is reduced re-

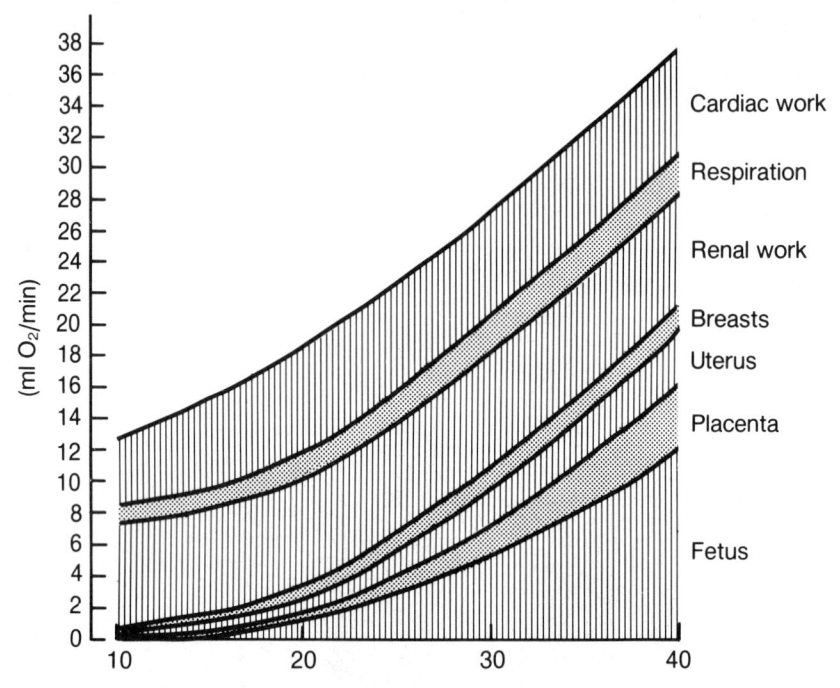

Figure 5.5. Partition of the increased oxygen consumption in pregnancy amongst the organs concerned. (From M. deSwiet: The respiratory system. In F. E. Hytten and G. Chamberlain (eds.): *Clinical Physiology in Obstetrics*, Oxford, Blackwell, 1980, p. 91.)

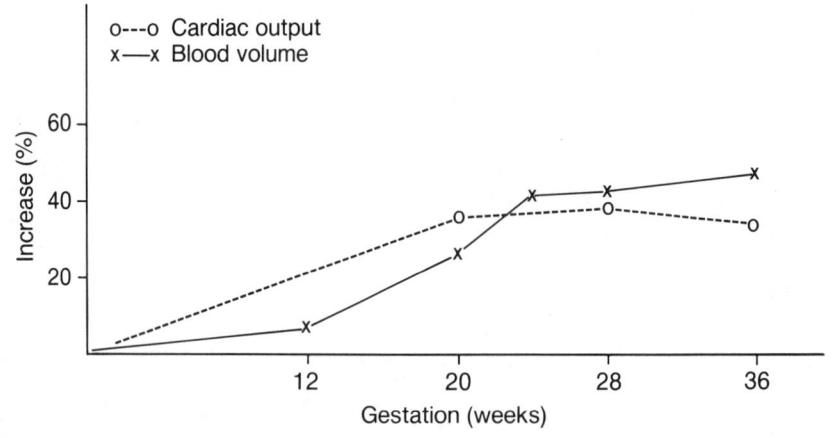

Figure 5.6. Changes in cardiac output and blood volume throughout pregnancy. Based on data from Pyorala (48) and Lund and Donovan (47).

markably at the beginning of pregnancy and reaches prepregnant levels only at term (43–45).

The aforementioned facts defy the teleologic explanations for the increased cardiovascular performance. A more plausible hypothesis is that the increase in cardiac output follows the increase in blood volume either in time or magnitude; both rise as early as 6–8 weeks of gestation, reaching the peak toward the end of the second trimester. Cardiac output and blood volume both increase in the range of 40–50% (Fig. 5.6).

The increase in the blood volume is a result of an increase in plasma volume up to 50% and red cell volume up to 20% (46, 47). This discrepancy between the increase in plasma volume and the red cell volume has a dilutional effect causing a drop in hematocrit from about 40% in the nonpregnant state to 35% at term, if not treated with iron. Therefore, the term "physiologic anemia" is a misnomer, implying only negative connotations. Actually, the relative reduction in red cell mass does not interfere with oxygen distribution to the various organs as evidenced by decreased A-V difference, which shows that more oxygen is carried to the tissues than is necessary.

Both components of cardiac output, the stroke volume and the heart rate, contribute to this increase. The former contributing more during early pregnancy. The stroke volume increases at mid-pregnancy, up to 30% declining toward term (43, 48, 49). The resting heart rate rises up through pregnancy reaching a plateau by 32 weeks, about 20 beats/min (bpm) higher than in the nonpregnant state (Fig. 5.7) (50).

The increased cardiac output is achieved at the expense of the enlargement of the heart. The mean end-diastolic volume of the heart increases between 70 and 80 ml during pregnancy due to increased diastolic filling and, most probably, also by muscle hypertrophy (51, 52). The contractility of the myocardium is changed in pregnancy, whether increased or decreased is still a matter of controversy (53–55). The increased excitability of the heart leads to more frequent atrial and ventricular extrasystoles (56). Such individuals must be closely supervised during exercise.

The 40% increase in cardiac output of about 1.5 liters/min is similar in percentage to the increase in pulmonary function, but it represents a much higher proportion in the cardiac function reserve. Taking into consideration that the maximum cardiac output can be increased no more than 3-fold (57) in comparison to 10-fold increase in pulmonary function, the cardiovascular performance is therefore lagging and constitutes a limiting factor in work capability.

There are some other very specific phenomena concerning the cardiovascular system in pregnant women:

As stated, the cardiac output rises significantly in pregnancy while, at the same time, the mean arterial pressure (MAP) drops. The decrease in MAP occurs as early as the first trimester, being lowest at mid-pregnancy and rising toward the nonpregnant state values at term (Fig. 5.8). The systolic blood pressure changes relatively insignificantly (58). As a result, pregnant women have an increased pulse pressure with a throbbing pulse. The inevitable conclusion from the rising cardiac output concomitantly with the drop in blood pressure is that the peripheral resistance of the circulation in pregnancy

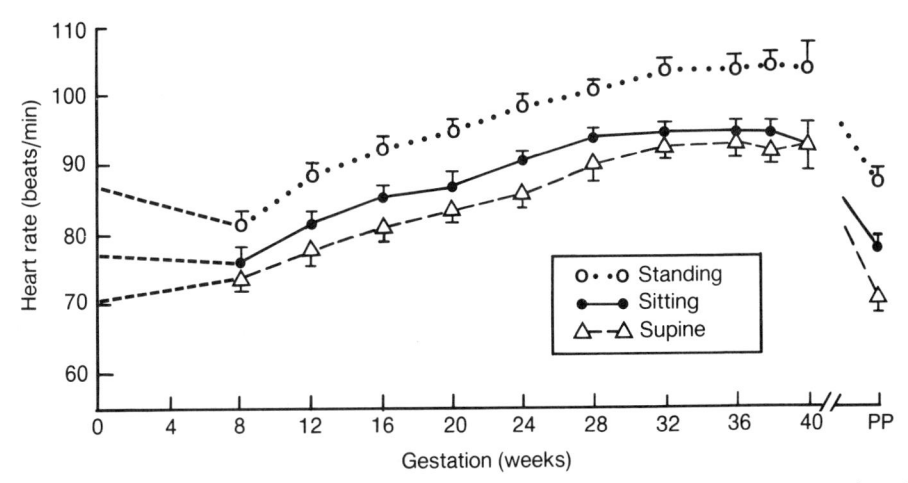

Figure 5.7. Serial changes in heart rate during pregnancy. (From M. Wilson et al.: *American Journal of Medicine*, 68:97, 1980 (50).)

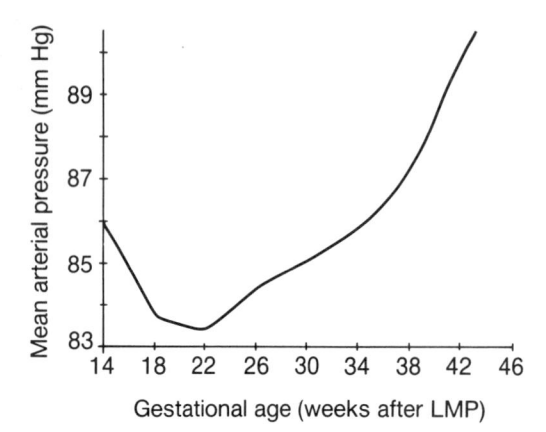

Figure 5.8. Mean arterial pressure by gestational age for single white term live births (nulliparas, 25–34 years of age). (From E. W. Page and R. Christianson: *American Journal of Obstetrics & Gynecology*, 125:740, 1976.)

must be significantly reduced. Indeed, it was found that peripheral resistance in mid-pregnancy of 979 dyne sec/cm^5 rose to 1200–1300 toward term gestation, compared to over 1200 for the nonpregnant state (45, 48).

The cardiovascular clinical state as we find it in pregnancy: throbbing, rapid pulse, increased cardiac output, increased oxygen consumption, and decreased peripheral resistance, is that of a hyperkinetic state similar to hyperthyroidism.

An important factor which should be taken into consideration when advising physical activity to pregnant women is the change in cardiac output and arterial blood pressure that may occur with changes in posture. Because of uterine mobility, change in posture changes its axis. In an upright position, the uterus falls forward, while supine, it falls backward and rests upon the vertebral column, often compressing the inferior vena cava and the abdominal aorta. The result is reduced cardiac output and supine hypotension (48, 59–61).

DISPOSAL SYSTEMS

By-products of increased metabolism in pregnancy result in increased heat and waste production, which need to be disposed. Changes occurring in pregnancy in skin and kidneys facilitate these functions.

The mechanism for heat dissipation has particular relevance in the gravida who engages in physical activities. There are three ways to dissipate heat: radiation, conduction, and evaporation. Heat is produced mainly in the core of the body and must be conducted to the outer layer, the skin, in order to be effectively dissipated. We have to keep in mind that the subcutaneous tissue abundant in fat is a very efficient insulator, therefore, direct conduction is impaired (62).

It is the capillary network of the skin which serves as a radiator for the body, with the blood serving as a coolant. The abundant sweat glands are instrumental in exploiting the mechanism of evaporation to loose heat.

The significant increase of blood flow to the skin starts at the beginning of the second trimester, reaching the highest level at about 30 weeks of gestation when it levels off until delivery (63, 64). It is accomplished via peripheral vasodilatation (65), which is also evident in congestion of the nasal mucous membranes (66, 67), leading to occasional nose bleeding or snoring.

Along with increased hyperemia of the skin, there is an increase in the activity of the sebaceous and sweat glands which causes increased evaporation.

The mechanism of radiation and conduction are effective only under conditions where the temperature of the surroundings is less than that of the skin. Otherwise, the only means by which the body can rid itself of the heat is by evaporation. Any disruption in proper functioning of the protective mechanisms described above as in the case of dehydration with arrest of perspiration, or mainstay in high humidity areas, has immediate repercussions on the fetus. The fetus depends totally on the mother for his heat dissipation. Any increase in maternal core temperature is immediately reflected in elevated fetal body temperature. It has been suggested by experimental teratology and retrospective studies that hyperthermia is teratogenic and may lead to neural tube defects in the offspring. These reports have to be viewed very cautiously since they linked such effects to maternal temperatures in excess of 38.9°C. These temperatures are reached fairly easily during exercise activities (68, 69).

The kidneys have an intrinsic large functional capacity as exemplified by the fact that an individual may lose 50% function (unilateral nephrectomy) and yet maintain normal creatinine values. Furthermore, within 1–2 weeks of the nephrectomy, the remaining kidney attains a compensatory increase in function only slightly below the preoperative value for both kidneys (70).

It seems, therefore, that the expectant mother is well equipped to deal with the burden of having to clear additional waste products of metabolism of the fetus added to her own. Changes imposed by pregnancy are in direct proportion to the increase in the kidney's functional capability. Anatomically, the urinary system enlarges during pregnancy. The kidneys increase in weight and size, but the main change is seen in the collecting system, with dilatation of calyces, renal pelvis, and ureters (71).

The functional equivalent of the anatomical changes is the 30–50% increase in glomerular filtration rate (GFR) as expressed by creatinine clearance (72). The increase in GFR facilitates not only the filtration of waste products, but, in the process, other vital elements are lost. The most significant of those is the sodium. It is the increased tubular reabsorbtion of sodium, which is responsible for a considerable proportion of the specific metabolic cost of pregnancy, that prevents the critical process of sodium depletion (73).

Still, there are other important constituents of plasma which are filtered and lost because of the increased GFR: the glucose, amino acids, and water-soluble vitamins.

In pregnancy the tubular reabsorbtion of glucose, amino acids, and water-soluble vitamins (nicotinic acid, ascorbic acid, and folate) is less than optimal, with greater excretion in the urine as compared to the nonpregnant state. The loss of amino acids may reach 2 g per day (74, 75). Although a regular, well-balanced diet provides an ample substitute for the urinary loss, in cases of increased demand, as in exercise, this particular point should be taken into account. (For additional information, see Chapters 8 and 9.)

ENDOCRINE SYSTEM

The endocrine system is involved in significant changes in pregnancy. These changes are modulated, in part, by the ovaries and the fetoplacental unit and by the maternal endocrine glands.

The main source for pregnancy sustaining hormones during the first 6–8 weeks of gestation is the ovarian corpus luteum.

From the very beginning, and most probably the day of conception, the trophoblast produces the human chorionic gonadotropin (hCG) which prevents the corpus luteum from involution (76).

At a gestational age of 6–8 weeks, the placenta becomes the main source for hormone production (77).

Contrary to the common belief, the corpus luteum activity persists until term (78). Two kinds of hormones are produced by the corpus luteum: the steroids, and a unique polypeptide, relaxin. The ovaries appear to be the only source for production of relaxin during pregnancy. Relaxin is a 6500 low molecular weight peptide, structurally similar, in part, to the insulin molecule. By present assay techniques, it is detectable only in pregnancy. Plasma levels are highest at the end of the first trimester and maintained somewhat lower throughout pregnancy (79). The function of relaxin is still unclear, but as the name suggests, its main functions are thought to be relaxation of ligaments, softening and stretching of fibrocartilage by collagenolytic activity in preparation for delivery. Such functions have been demonstrated in animals (80).

Among the steroids secreted by the corpus luteum, progesterone is the most essential and vital for the maintenance of pregnancy. Throughout pregnancy, the bulk, about 90%, originates from the placenta. But during the first 6–8 weeks of gestation, the corpus luteum is the principal source for progesterone (77).

The production of steroids by the corpus luteum reaches its peak 3–4 weeks after

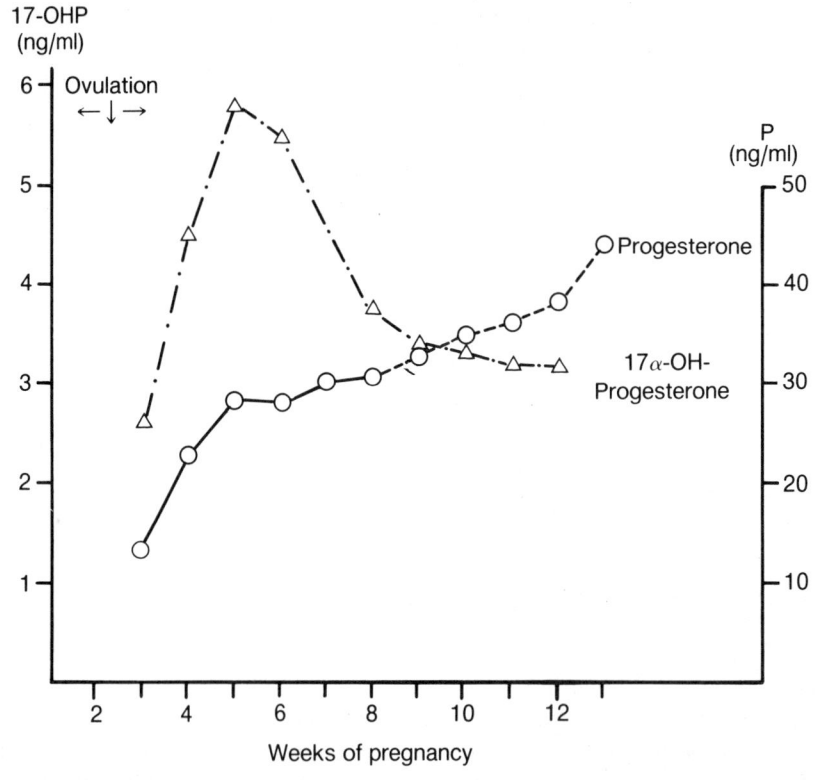

Figure 5.9. Mean plasma values of progesterone (*P*), and 17α-hydroxyprogesterone (*17-OHP*) of 10 normal patients followed weekly from the 3rd to 13th week of pregnancy. ↓ indicates the presumed time of ovulation. (From D. Tulchinsky and C. J. Hobel: *American Journal of Obstetrics & Gynecology*, 117:884, 1973.)

ovulation and then decreases, but does not entirely stop until the end of pregnancy. This pattern of production can be detected by monitoring the production of 17-hydroxyprogesterone, a metabolite of progesterone secreted almost exclusively by the ovarian tissue until late mid-pregnancy (Fig. 5.9) (81).

Two other groups of steroids secreted by the corpus luteum are the estrogens and androgens. Of the estrogens, only estradiol and estrone are secreted by the corpus luteum in significant amounts. Estriol, the estrogen most commonly associated with pregnancy, is produced almost exclusively by the fetoplacental unit (82).

The androgen production by the corpus luteum is noticeable only when in excess, as in the case of pregnancy luteoma, causing virilization of the expectant mother (83). It is conceivable that androstenedione, dehydroepiandrosterone, and testosterone significantly add to the anabolic changes of pregnancy, yet the pregnant woman is relatively protected from excessive influence of androgens, whatever their source, by an increased level of sex binding globulins generated by high levels of estrogens. The high efficiency of the placenta to convert androgens into estrogens acts as a protective barrier for the fetus against virilization by androgens originating from the mother (84).

Placenta

The placenta can be seen as the major endocrine organ of pregnancy. Either alone or in conjunction with the fetus, it modulates the physiological homeostasis of the mother and fetus.

The protein hormones of the placenta are closely related in their structure and function to the pituitary hormones. The human placental lactogen (hPL) and human chorionic gonadotropin (hCG) share a common unit with the luteinizing hormone (LH), human growth hormone (hGH) and thyrotropic stimulating hormone (TSH), thus, the similarities in biological function of LH and hCG. The same can be stated for the hPL, prolactin and hGH.

hCG functions and regulation is enigmatic, it rises rapidly in the early stages of pregnancy, reaching a peak between 8 and 10 weeks of gestational age. Following, there is a relatively rapid decline up to 18 weeks, and, thereafter, the levels remain constant with a slight increase toward term. This type of pattern is in total contrast to those of other protein hormones of the placenta and does not simulate placental growth (Fig. 5.10).

Undoubtedly, hCG has a key role in the maintenance of the corpus luteum of pregnancy, but its mainstay after 8 weeks of gestation is poorly understood. It is speculated that hCG has a role in fetal development like induction of fetal testosterone secretion from the Leydig cells of the testis, or some regulatory function for the adrenal fetal zone (85, 86).

In pathological conditions, (trophoblastic diseases, hyperemesis gravidarium), the high levels of hCG highlight thyrotropic properties and increase the body metabolic rates (87). One common complication of early pregnancy, "morning sickness," is attributed to the high hCG levels (88).

hPL follows a more predictable pattern, with concentrations in direct proportion to the growth of the placenta (Fig. 5.10). Being closely related to hGH, the hPL activities involve lypolysis, nitrogen retention, hyperinsulinism, and peripheral resistance to insulin in pregnancy, all known to have diabetogenic effects (89). The pregnant woman, even when not affected by diabetes mellitus, is more prone to develop metabolic acidosis and hypoglycemia in the event of relative starvation or increased energy consumption not supported by appropriate caloric intake (90) as is likely to occur in diet-minded pregnant compulsive joggers.

Recently, a new group of proteins produced by the placenta has been discovered. These are the schwangerschaftsprotein I (SP1), the pregnancy associated plasma protein A (PAPP-A), the pregnancy associated plasma protein B (PAPP-B), and the placental protein 5 (PP5). The distribution of these proteins throughout pregnancy resembles that of the hPLs, however, their function is as yet unknown (91) (Fig 5.10).

Placental Steroids

ESTROGENS

Three estrogens, among a large amount of hormones, are known to be produced by the placenta and have been the target of attention for both researchers and clinicians: the estradiol, estriol, and estetrol. Estriol, produced in large quantities by the fetoplacental unit and secreted via maternal circulation, therefore, has been used as a predictor of fetal well-being (92).

The concentration of estrogens in plasma rises constantly, reaching levels up to and in excess of 15 ng/ml, increasing 2–5-fold throughout pregnancy (Fig. 5.11).

PROGESTAGENS

There are three biologically active progestagens produced in the placenta, the major one, progesterone, is the most abundant and biologically active, the other two being the 20-alpha (α)- and 20-beta (β)-hydroxylated derivatives of progesterone much less active and produced in small amounts. Unlike estrogens, their production is independent of the fetus. Progesterone levels increase from 40 ng/ml during the first trimester of pregnancy to 160 ng/ml during the third trimester (Fig. 5.12).

The effects of the steroidal hormones can be divided into two groups: those promoting growth and those having mixed effects, mainly metabolic.

The primary target cells for the steroids that promote growth are the reproductive organs: the uterus and the breasts.

Under estrogenic and progestative influence, the uterus alters in size from 7.5 × 5 × 2.5 cm with a capacity of 4 ml to 28 × 24

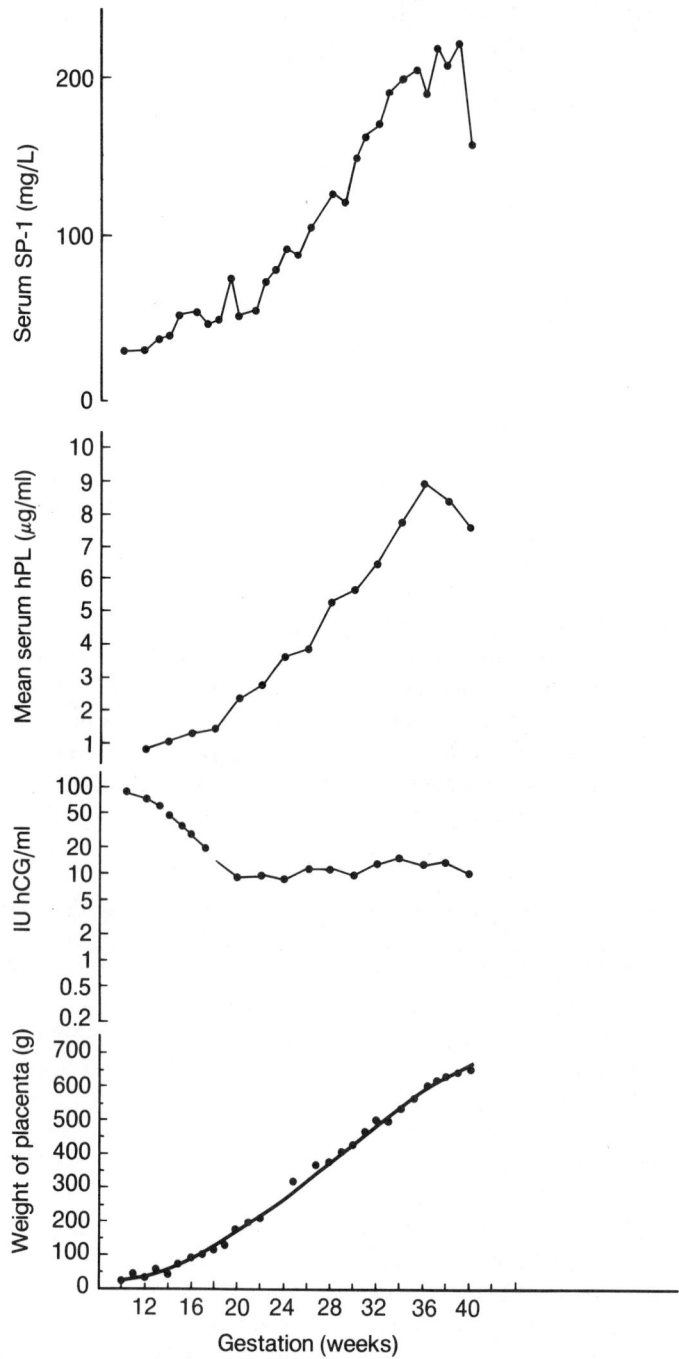

Figure 5.10. Relationship of placental weight to plasma concentration of hormones through pregnancy.

× 21 cm and capacity of about 4000 ml at term. The weight increases from 30–60 g before pregnancy to 750–1000 g at term (2).

The increase of the uterine mass is accompanied by significant vascular changes. The arteries and the veins increase both in diameter and length. The net result is that, at term, the uterus and the associated blood vessels contain one-sixth or more of the total maternal blood volume. The uterine blood flow increases from about 50 ml/min at 10 weeks of gestation to a maximum of 500–700 ml/min at term (93, 94). This change could be seen as equivalent to implanting an additional kidney (renal plasma flow equals 700–800 ml/min).

The estrogens also change the functional properties of the uterine muscle, increasing the elastic properties and the contractility, while the progesterone has a quiescent effect keeping the uterus in a nonactive state (95).

The breasts, another specific target organ for estrogens and progesterone, enlarge through the process of hypertrophy and hyperplasia of the gland and, at the same time, increasing the fat content and vascularity. The estrogens influence the ductal growth, whereas the progesterone the alveolar (96). The nipples which progressively enlarge become more pigmented and erectile, while the breast seems to be less sensitive to tactile stimulation (97).

Progesterone generates an overall systemic smooth muscle relaxation effect in pregnancy and is the principal cause for venous dilatation, and atony of the bowel (98).

Progesterone also has a profound effect on the hypothalamic control centers. Progesterone resets the respiratory center, lowering the threshold for P_{CO_2} as a consequence causing hyperventilation and decrease in P_{CO_2}. The insignificant increase in

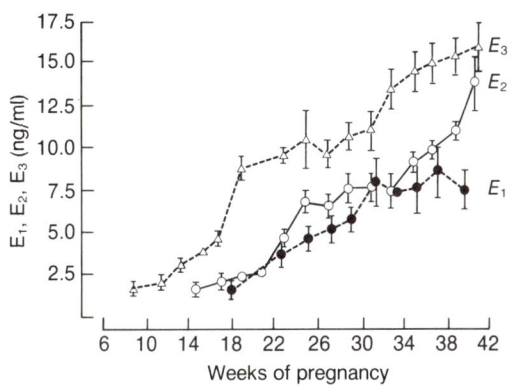

Figure 5.11. Mean plasma concentrations of estrogens during pregnancy. E_1 = estrone; E_2 = estradiol; E_3 = estradiol. The *bars* represent the standard error of the means. (From D. Tulchinsky et al.: *American Journal of Obstetrics & Gynecology*, 112:1095, 1972.)

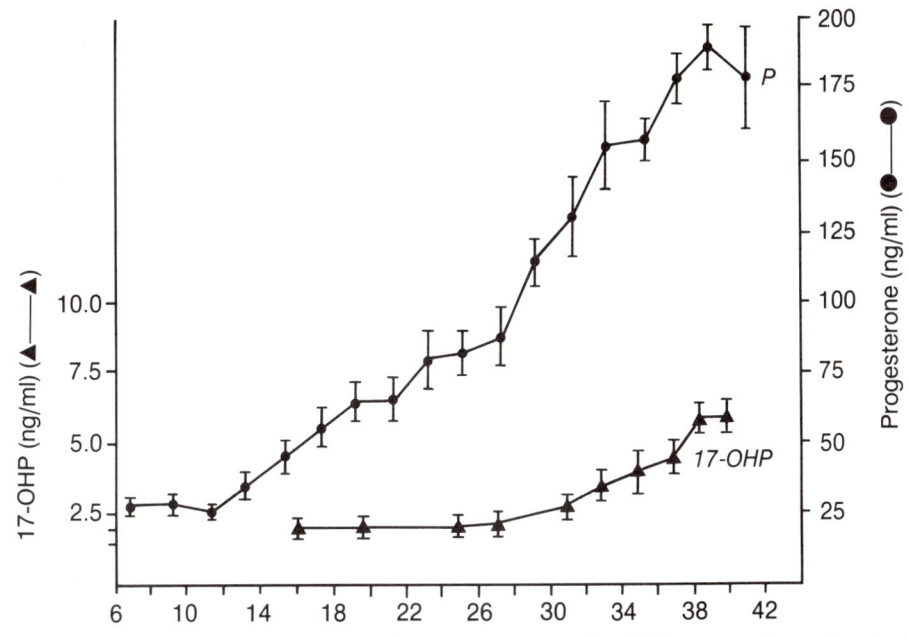

Figure 5.12. Progesterone (*P*) and 17-hydroxyprogesterone (*17-OHP*) mean plasma levels during human pregnancy. (From D. Tulchinsky et al.: *American Journal of Obstetrics & Gynecology*, 112:1095, 1972; and M. C. MacNaughton, in A. Klopper: *Plasma Hormone Assays in Evaluation of Fetal Well-being*, Edinburgh, Churchill Livingstone, 1976 (81).)

pH is due to compensatory and concomitant decrease in bicarbonate (33, 99). Resetting of the "lipolytic center" involves fat deposition, mainly during the first and second trimesters of pregnancy.

There is change in the appetite-satiety center toward increased ingestion of food, a contributing factor to the weight gain, while there is some evidence that progesterone engenders a feeling of lassitude, acting as an additional factor for energy saving (15, 16, 100).

An additional important effect of progesterone is resetting of the thermoregulatory control center with an elevation of at least 0.5°F (101) in addition to the increase in body temperature because of a higher metabolic rate.

Changes in ground substance of the connective tissue which may underlie the increased laxity of the joints, or water retention in the interstitial space, are felt to be caused by direct estrogenic activity (102).

The indirect influences of steroidal hormones are transmitted by changes exerted on the maternal endocrine system as described below.

Pituitary

High levels of estrogens have various effects on the anterior pituitary. The production of follicular stimulating hormone (FSH) and luteinizing hormone (LH) declines in pregnancy to luteal phase levels of menstrual cycle causing an anovulatory state (103, 104). The suppression of FSH and LH production is potentiated by the inhibitory influence of high levels of the placental analog for those hormones, the hCG (105).

In spite of the stimulatory effect of estrogens on hGH levels in the nonpregnant state, in pregnancy hGH levels are lower than in the nonpregnant state, because of the prevailing inhibitory effect of placental lactogen (106).

Conversely, prolactin levels, in spite of the inhibitory effect of high levels of its placental analog, the hPL, rise in pregnancy and are 10–20 times higher at term than in the nonpregnant state (107). There is a well-recognized function for prolactin to prepare the breast for lactation. The remainder of functions remain to be elucidated. There are animal studies to support that osmoregulation in the fetus is modulated by prolactin (108). In addition, it also appears that prolactin has a role in the maternal metabolism of calcium by enhancing the transformation of 25-hydroxycholecalciferol to its most active form the 1,25-dihydroxycholecalciferol (109).

The actions of corticotrophin (ACTH) and thyrotropin (TSH), two other hormones originating in the anterior pituitary, do not appear to change during pregnancy.

Thyroid

Tachycardia, up to 100 beats per minute, elevated basal metabolic rate, intolerance to heat and, very often, emotional lability are common features of the pregnant state. Falsely, it can be deduced that these are results of a hyperactive thyroid, but measurements of free T_3 and T_4 levels that modulate the metabolic state, reveal no change from the nonpregnant state (110). The elevation of total T_3 and T_4 are caused by increases in thyroxin-binding globulin (TBG), a known effect of estrogenic hormones (111). The elevated BMR is actually normal if we take into account in the equation the increased metabolic activity of the mother secondary to the enlarged uterus, increased work of lung and heart, and the metabolism of the products of conception (112).

Parathyroid and Calcium Metabolism

The parathyroid gland is the source of two hormones involved in the regulation of calcium metabolism: the parathyroid hormone (PTH) and the calcitonin (CT). In addition, the regulatory mechanism involves vitamin D and its metabolites, phosphorous and magnesium. From a teleological point of view, there is a sound rationale for a complex regulatory system, because of the multiple inflow and outflow sources for calcium in plasma. Absorption of calcium is accomplished through the gastrointestinal tract and bone reabsorption, and is lost in urine, feces, and bone deposition.

Certain changes occurring in pregnancy, such as an increase in maternal extracellular fluid volume, maternal glomerular filtration and calcium transfer across the placenta in the amount of about 30 g throughout pregnancy (113), result in a progressive reduction in serum calcium as pregnancy advances. The total serum Ca concentration in pregnant women reflects the significant decline in Ca which is bound to plasma protein, primarily albumin (Fig. 5.13). The ionic Ca, the functional fraction, does not change, except for a slight decline in the third trimester. Concurrently, in the third trimester, the fetus incorporates calcium at the maximal rate of 200–300 mg/day (114).

The increase in demand is met by: increased digestive tract absorption, reduction in urinary loss, increased bone mobilization, or any combination of the above.

The homeostasis of Ca in pregnancy is maintained mainly by increased levels of the parathyroid hormone (PTH) (Fig. 5.14). The PTH affects the increased production in the kidneys of the most active vitamin D derivative, the 1,25-hydroxycholecalciferol whose role is to enhance intestinal absorption and reduce renal excretion.

Contrary to the common belief, the positive Ca balance in pregnancy is not at the expense of maternal bone tissue loss. Selective blocking of PTH activity on bone tissue prevents the resorption activated by the hormone.

Protection of the maternal skeleton is achieved, most probably, through the effects of high levels of estrogen and progesterone which inhibit PTH activity and promote bone deposition. CT levels in pregnancy tend to decline (115).

Although the recommended daily allowance (RDA) for Ca is 1200 mg, the ideal minimal dose is 400–600 mg (116). That amount is easily acquired by regular diet. In cases of starvation, when maternal diet is

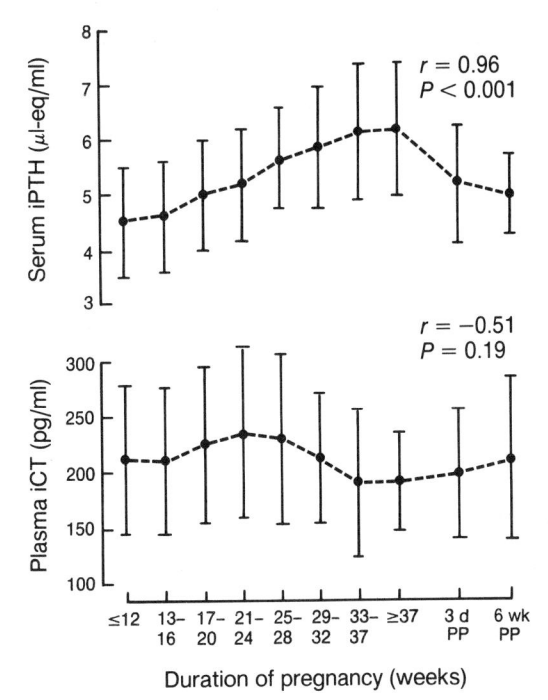

Figure 5.14. Mean (±SD) levels of inhibitory parathyroid hormone (*iPTH*) and calcitonin (*iCT*) during pregnancy and the puerperium. (From R. M. Pitkin et al.: *American Journal of Obstetrics & Gynecology*, 133:181, 1979 (115).)

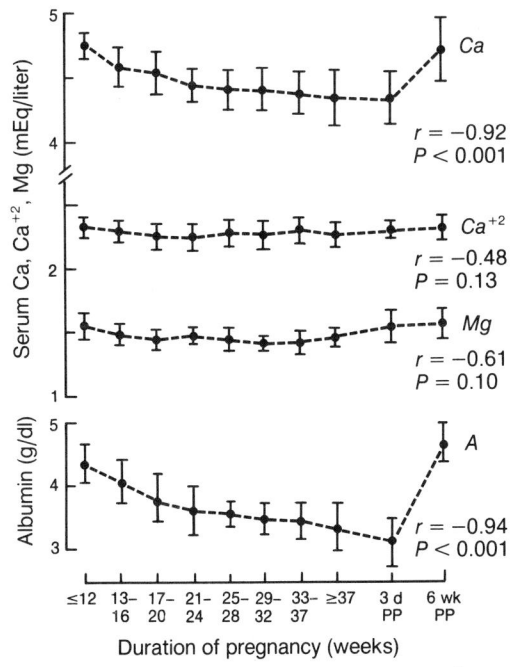

Figure 5.13. Mean (±SD) levels of Ca, Ca^{+2}, Mg, and A during pregnancy and the puerperium. (From R. M. Pitkin et al.: *American Journal of Obstetrics & Gynecology*, 133:781, 1979 (115).)

lacking calcium or vitamin D and there is lack of exposure to sun and/or renal disease, the fetal calcium demands will be met by demineralization of the maternal skeleton. Phosphorus (P) and magnesium (Mg) metabolism are intimately related to the metabolism of Ca.

P and Ca are both regulated by the same intestinal, renal, and skeletal factors and PTH modulates their activity in a similar fashion mobilizing effects on bone tissue for both. The mechanism of intestinal absorption is similar with the exception that vitamin D is not essential for P absorbtion.

The kidney is the regulatory organ for P plasma levels. The kidney has a P transport maximum (T_m) which means that, under certain levels in plasma, all filtrated P will be reabsorbed. This particular mechanism is influenced by PTH, CT, estrogens, and adrenal steroids resulting in an increased urinary loss of P.

The GH and, most probably, hPL due to its GH-like effect, increase the T_m, reducing the P urinary loss. The net result of these various factors activities in pregnancy is a tendency toward decline in P levels during the first two-thirds of pregnancy with a nadir at about 30 weeks of gestational age, and therafter a slight rise (115).

An important aspect is that an increase in P blood levels promotes the Ca incorporation into the bone tissue (117), lowering the plasma Ca level.

Because of a very efficient intestinal absorbtion and renal recovery, and abundant amounts of P found in any food there is no P deficiency recognized in pregnancy, and it is believed that high levels of P are the cause for leg cramps (115).

Little is known about magnesium (Mg) homeostasis. By and large, it is influenced by the same factors as Ca and P, including PTH.

Adrenal Gland and Water Metabolism

Despite increased concentrations of hormones originating in the adrenal, no anatomic enlargement is found in pregnancy (118). Specific binding proteins, like sex hormones, globulins, or transcortin increase in pregnancy secondary to high levels of estrogens.

It is believed that steroids play a crucial role in the homeostasis of pregnancy by modulating the activity of other hormones and by their own direct action. The adrenal estrogen production is negligible compared to the large amount produced in the fetoplacental unit or the ovary. Testosterone is found in higher concentration during pregnancy, but is less active because of the diminished free fraction and reduced peripheral conversion to dihydrotestosterone, the more potent derivative (119).

Dehydroepiandrosterone (DHEA) and its sulfate derivative, the most abundant of androgens, are produced almost exclusively by the adrenals, are very efficiently metabolized by the placenta and aromatized to estradiol and estrone (84).

Circulating catecholamines: epinephrine and norepinephrine are not changed in pregnancy compared to the nonpregnant state, but they increase significantly during labor and delivery (120).

The plasma levels of cortisol are elevated in the first trimester and rise thereafter until delivery. This elevation is caused largely by the estrogen-mediated increase in transcortin. More significantly, there is also an increase in the free fraction which is the active part of the hormone (Fig. 5.15). The free cortisol concentration in plasma, during pregnancy, reaches levels encountered in pathologic states such as Cushing syndrome (121, 122). The reason for this rise is only partially understood. The increase in free cortisol appears not to be related to pituitary ACTH, which levels, although rising, are within the normal range during pregnancy (123), but subject to other sources of stimulating hormones. There is some evidence that the placenta is capable of producing ACTH-like hormone (124). Indirect evidence for the extrapituitary source of the stimulating hormone is the inability to suppress cortisol production after stimulation with corticosteroids (125).

The additional mechanism responsible for

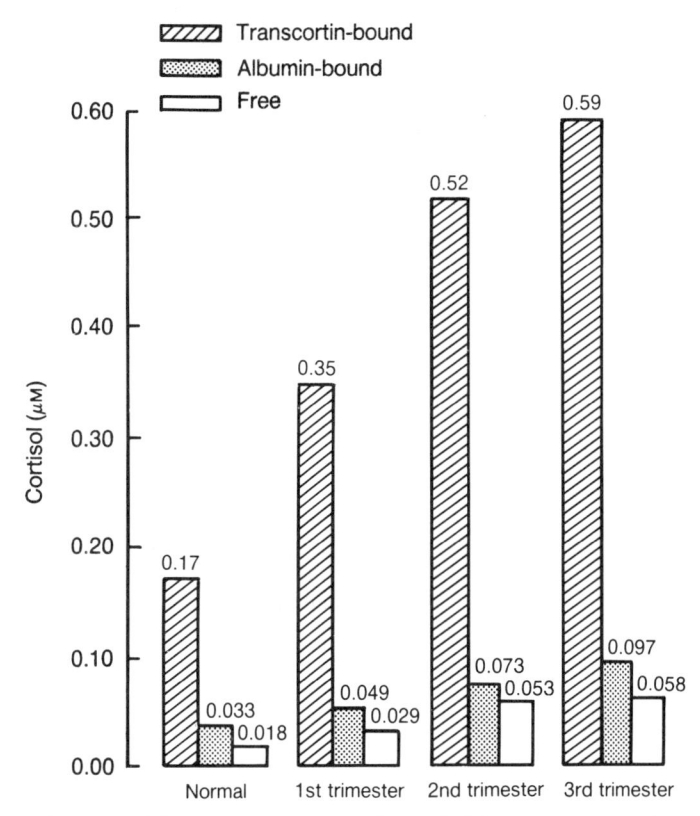

Figure 5.15. Distribution of bound and unbound cortisol in pregnancy plasma. (From H. E. Rosenthal et al.: *Journal of Clinical Endocrinology & Metabolism*, 29:352, 1969.)

elevated cortisol levels is reduced elimination with a half-life that is double compared to the nonpregnant state (126). It is not clear why, despite high levels of cortisol, there is no clinical, Cushing-like manifestation. The reason could be attributed to the competitive actions of other hormones, particularly progesterone, that has a high affinity to cytosol receptors for cortisol (127).

Mineralocorticoids and Water Metabolism

The two potent mineralocorticoids produced by the zona glomerulosa of the adrenal cortex, aldosterone and 11-deoxycorticosterone (DOC) are elevated during pregnancy, and a clear distinction can be made between the two. Plasma levels of aldosterone increase significantly at about 12 weeks of gestation, and reach a plateau at 30 weeks of gestation, 3–5-fold higher than in the nonpregnant state (Fig. 5.16). Increased levels of sodium suppress aldosterone production while ACTH increases it (128). Conversely, plasma levels of DOC rise progressively, mainly during the third trimester of pregnancy, increasing at term 10–15-fold from the nonpregnant state (Fig. 5.16). DOC levels are unresponsive to changes in salt intake or ACTH (129, 130). A significant portion of DOC originates during the third trimester from peripheral extra-adrenal 21-hydroxylation of maternal progesterone and the fetus (131, 132).

Aldosterone production is modulated by various systems: The renin angiotensin, which responds to changes in mean arterial pressure, sodium and potassium levels, and by direct stimulation of ACTH. As previously maintained, ACTH levels do not change significantly during pregnancy. The sodium and potassium levels are the result rather than the cause to aldosterone changes.

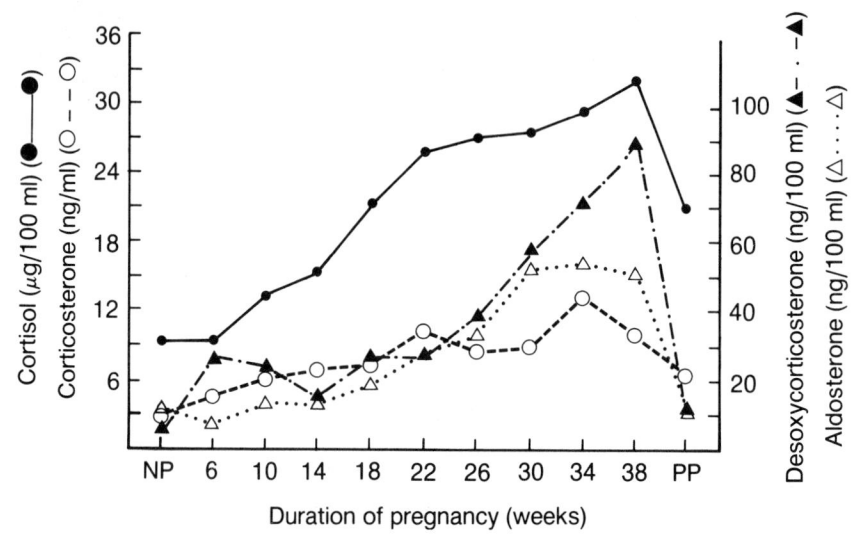

Figure 5.16. Mean steroid levels in 11 women throughout pregnancy and postpartum (*PP*) compared to levels in nonpregnant (*NP*) women. (Data from E. M. Wintour et al.: *Clinical and Experimental Pharmacology and Physiology*, 5:399, 1978.)

High estrogen levels stimulate liver production of angiotensinogen, the substrate for renin to produce angiotensin II. Angiotensin II, in turn, stimulates aldosterone production.

Reduced mean arterial pressure in pregnancy is a trigger for the increased release of renin. The cumulative effect of this phenomenon is sodium retention expressed as fluid retention and intravascular fluid expansion. It happens in spite of increased glomerular filtration rate and reduction in colloid osmotic pressure (133, 134).

Theoretically, the changes described of elevated aldosterone and angiotensin II levels should have harmful effects: i.e., depletion of potassium, excessive retention of sodium, and hypertension. The fact is that usually neither depletion of potassium with excessive sodium retention, nor hypertension occur in pregnancy. The counteractive action is believed to be secondary to progesterone, which guards for stable potassium concentration and prevents excess of sodium retention (135). The hypertensive effects of angiotensin II are counteracted by reduced responsiveness of the renal and systems vasculature under the influence of high levels of prostaglandins, and high estrogen activity (136).

Toward the end of pregnancy, the expectant mother accumulates an excess of 8.5 liters of water. Up to 30 weeks of gestation, the measured gain is close to the expected one from added maternal blood, tissue, and products of conception. However, at term, only part of the total extracellular fluid gain (6.5 liters) can be recovered by computation of the volume added in the known sites (4.0 liters) (137). The excess 2.5 liters are most probably distributed in the ground substance of the connective tissue visible as pitting ankle edema in about 40–50% of otherwise normal pregnant women.

As a whole, the adaptive anatomical and physiological changes in pregnancy are having a significant impact on the ability of the pregnant woman to maintain physical fitness or to participate in certain sports activities. It is important to recognize those limiting factors whenever attempting to prescribe exercise programs in pregnancy.

REFERENCES

1. DeVries HA: *Physiology of Exercise*, ed. 3. Dubuque, Iowa, William C. Brown, 1980, p 246.
2. Davey AD: Normal pregnancy: physiology and management. In Dewhurst J (ed): *Integrated Obstetrics and Gynecology for Postgraduates*, 3rd Ed. Oxford, Blackwell, 1981, p 105.
3. Hytten FE, Cheyne GA: The size and composition

of the human pregnant uterus. *J Obstet Gynaecol Br Commonw* 76:400, 1969.
4. Hytten FE: Weight gain in pregnancy. In Hytten FE, Chamberlain G (eds): *Clinical Physiology in Obstetrics.* Oxford, Blackwell, 1980, pp 208–209.
5. Crisp WE, DeFrancesco S: The hand syndrome of pregnancy. *Obstet Gynecol* 23:433, 1964.
6. Tobin SM: Carpal tunnel syndrome in pregnancy. *Am J Obstet Gynecol* 97:493, 1967.
7. Voitk AJ, Mueller JC, Farlinger DE, Johnson RU: Carpal tunnel syndrome in pregnancy. *Can Med Assoc J* 128:277, 1983.
8. Johns JP: The influence of pregnancy on the visual field. *Am J Ophthalmol* 13:956, 1930.
9. Millodot M: The influence of pregnancy on the sensitivity of the cornea. *Br J Ophthalmol* 61:646, 1977.
10. Jacobs WH, Janowitz HD: The digestive tract. In Rovinsky JJ, Guttmacher AF (eds): *Medical, Surgical and Gynecologic Complications of Pregnancy,* Baltimore, Williams & Wilkins, 1965, p 177.
11. Hansen R, Langer W: Über geschmacks Veränderung in der Schwangershaft. *Klin Wochenschr* 14:1173, 1935.
12. Jarrahi-Zadeh A, Kane Jr FJ, Van de Castlf RL, Lachenbruch PA, Ewing JA: Emotional and cognitive changes in pregnancy and early puerperium. *Br J Psychiatry* 115:797, 1969.
13. Hytten FE: Nutrition. In Hytten FE, Chamberlain G (eds): *Clinical Physiology in Obstetrics.* Oxford, Blackwell, 1980, p 165.
14. Bruce NH: Gestational adaption: major systems. In Iffy L, Kaminetzky HA (eds): *Principles and Practice of Obstetrics and Perinatology.* New York, John Wiley & Sons, 1981, p 688.
15. Merryman M, Borman R, Barnes L, Rothchild I: Progesterone "anasthesia" in human subjects. *J Clin Endocrinol Metab* 14:1567, 1954.
16. Selye HJ: Studies concerning anesthetic action of steroid hormones. *J Pharmacol Exp Ther* 73:127, 1941.
17. Kaminetzky HA, Baker H: Nutritional needs in pregnancy. In Iffy L, Kaminetzky HA (eds): *Principles and Practice of Obstetrics and Perinatology.* New York, John Wiley & Sons, 1981, p 665.
18. Pitkin RM: Nutritional support in obstetrics and gynecology. *Clin Obstet Gynecol* 19:489, 1976.
19. Thompson AM, Billewicz WZ: Clinical significance of weight trends during pregnancy. *Br Med J* 1:243, 1957.
20. Ulmsten U, Sundström G: Esophageal manometry in pregnant and non-pregnant women. *Am J Obstet Gynecol* 132:260, 1978.
21. Fisher RS, Roberts GS, Grabowski CJ, Cohen S: Altered lower esophageal sphincter function during early pregnancy. *Gastroenterology* 74:1233, 1978.
22. Bassey OO: Pregnancy heartburn in Nigerians and Caucasians with theories about aetiology based on manometric recordings from oesophagus and stomach. *Br J Obstet Gynaecol* 84:439, 1977.
23. Davison JS, Davison MC, Hay DM: Gastric emptying time in late pregnancy and labour. *J Obstet Gynaecol Br Commonw* 77:37, 1970.
24. Parry E, Shields R, Turnbull AC: Transit time in the small intestine in pregnancy. *J Obstet Gynaecol Br Commonw* 77:900, 1970.
25. Parry E, Shields R, Turnbull AC: The effect of pregnancy on the colonic absorption of sodium potassium and water. *J Obstet Gynaecol Br Commonw* 77:616, 1970.
26. Gerdes MM, Boyden EA: The rate of emptying of the human gallbladder in pregnancy. *Surg Gynecol Obstet* 66:145, 1938.
27. Potter MG: Observations of the gallbladder and bile during pregnancy at term. *JAMA* 106:1070, 1936.
28. Gazioglu K, Kaltreider NL, Rosen M, Yu PN: Pulmonary function during pregnancy in normal women and in patients with cardiopulmonary disease. *Thorax* 25:445, 1970.
29. Alaily AB, Carrol KB: Pulmonary ventilation in pregnancy. *Br J Obstet Gynaecol* 85:518, 1978.
30. Knuttgen HG, Emerson K: Physiological response to pregnancy at rest and during exercise. *J Appl Physiol* 36:549, 1974.
31. Thomson KJ, Cohen ME: Studies on the circulation in pregnancy; II. Vital capacity observations in normal pregnant women. *Surg Gynecol Obstet* 66:591, 1938.
32. McGinty AP: The comparative effects of pregnancy and phrenic nerve interruption on the diaphragm and their relation to pulmonary tuberculosis. *Am J Obstet Gynecol* 35:237, 1938.
33. Prowse CM, Gaensler EA: Respiratory and acid-base changes during pregnancy. *Anaesthesiology* 26:381, 1965.
34. Lehmann V, Fabel H: Lungen funktionsuntersuchungen an schwangeren feil; II. Ventilation, Atemmechanik und Diffisionkapazitat. *Z Geburtshilfe Perinatol* 177:397, 1973.
35. Archer GW, Marx GF: Arterial oxygen tension during apnoea in parturient women. *Br J Anaesth* 46:358, 1974.
36. Adams JQ: Cardiovascular physiology in normal pregnancy: Studies with the dye-dilution technique. *Am J Obstet Gynecol* 67:741, 1954.
37. Rovinsky JJ, Jaffin H: Cardiovascular hemodynamics in pregnancy; III. Cardiac rate, stroke volume, total peripheral resistance, and antral blood volume in multiple pregnancy. Synthesis of results. *Am J Obstet Gynecol* 95:787, 1966.
38. Bouterline-Young H, Bouterline-Young E: Alveolar carbon dioxide levels in pregnant parturient and lactating subjects. *J Obstet Gynaecol Br Emp* 63:509, 1956.
39. Pernoll ML, Metcalfe J, Schlenker TT, Welch JE, Matsumoto JA: Oxygen consumption at rest and during exercise in pregnancy. *Respir Physiol* 25:285, 1975.
40. Knuttgen HG, Emerson K: Physiological response

to pregnancy at rest and during exercise. *J Appl Physiol* 36:549, 1974.
41. Campbell EJM, Howell JBL: The sensation of breathlessness. *Br Med Bull* 19:36, 1963.
42. Comroe J, Forster RE, Dubois AB, Briscoe WA, Carlsen E: *The Lung: Clinical Physiology and Pulmonary Function Tests*. Chicago, Year Book, 1962.
43. Walters WAW, MacGregor WG, Hills M: Cardiac output at rest during pregnancy and the puerperium. *Clin Sci* 30:1, 1966.
44. Lees MM, Taylor SH, Scott DB, Kerr MG: A study of cardiac output at rest throughout pregnancy. *J Obstet Gynaecol Br Commonw* 74:319, 1967.
45. Bader RA, Bader ME, Rose PJ, Braunwald E: Haemodynamics at rest and during exercise in normal pregnancy as studied by cardiac catheterization. *J Clin Invest* 34:1524, 1955.
46. Pirani BBK, Campbell DM: Plasma volume in normal first pregnancy. *J Obstet Gynaecol Br Commonw* 80:884, 1973.
47. Lund CJ, Donovan JC: Blood volume during pregnancy. *Am J Obstet Gynecol* 98:393, 1967.
48. Pyorala T: Cardiovascular response to the upright position during pregnancy. *Acta Obstet Gynecol Scand* 45(suppl):5, 1966.
49. Ueland K, Novy MJ, Peterson EN, Metcalfe J: Maternal cardiovascular dynamics; IV. The influence of gestational age on the maternal cardiovascular response to posture and exercise. *Am J Obstet Gynecol* 104:856, 1969.
50. Wilson M, Morganti AG, Zervoudakis I, Letcher RL, Romney BM, Von Oeyon P, Papera S, Sealey JE, Laragh JH: Blood pressure, the unine-aldosterone system and sex steroids throughout normal pregnancy. *Am J Med* 68:97, 1980.
51. Gemzell CA, Robbe H, Strom G: Total amount of haemoglobin and physical working capacity in normal pregnancy and the puerperium. *Acta Obstet Gynecol Scand* 36:93, 1957.
52. Ihrman K: A clinical and physiological study of pregnancy in material from northern Sweden; VII. The heart volume during and after pregnancy. *Acta Soc Med Upsala* 65:326, 1960.
53. Rubler S, Schneebaum R, Hammer N: Systolic time intervals in pregnancy and the post-partum period. *Am Heart J* 86:182, 1973.
54. Burg JR, Dodek A, Kloster FE, Metcalfe J: Alterations of systolic time intervals during pregnancy. *Circulation* 49:560, 1974.
55. Liebson PR, Mann LI, Evans MI, Duchin S, Arditi L: Cardiac performance during pregnancy: serial evaluation using external systolic time intervals. *Am J Obstet Gynecol* 122:1, 1975.
56. Szekely P, Snaith L: *Heart Disease and Pregnancy*. Edinburgh, Churchill Livingstone, 1974.
57. Ueland K, Novy MJ, Metcalfe S: Hemodynamic responses of patients with heart disease to pregnancy and exercise. *Am J Obstet Gynecol* 113:47, 1972.
58. MacGillivray I, Rose GA, Rowe B: Blood pressure survey in pregnancy. *Clin Sci* 37:395, 1969.
59. Vorys N, Ullery JC, Hanusek GE: The cardiac output changes in various positions in pregnancy. *Am J Obstet Gynecol* 82:1312, 1961.
60. Kerr MG, Scott DB, Samuel E: Studies of the inferior vena cava in late pregnancy. *Br Med J* 1:532, 1964.
61. Bieniarz J, Crottongini JJ, Curuchet E, Romero-Salinas G, Yoshida T, Poseiro JJ, Caldeyro-Barcia R: Aortocaval compression by the uterus in late human pregnancy. An angiographic study. *Am J Obstet Gynecol* 100:203, 1968.
62. Guyton AC: *Medical Physiology*, Ed. 6. Philadelphia, W. B. Saunders, 1981, p 887.
63. Spetz S, Jansson I: Forearm blood flow during normal pregnancy studied by venous occlusion plethysmography and 133-xenon muscle clearance. *Acta Obstet Gynaecol Scand* 48:285, 1966.
64. Katz M, Sokal MM: Skin perfusion in pregnancy. *Am J Obstet Gynecol* 137:30, 1980.
65. Melbard SM: Valeur diagnostique de la capillaroscopie dans la grossesse et dans la sepsie puerperale. *Gynecol Obstet* 37:100, 1938.
66. Scott JH: Heat-regulating function of the nasal mucose membrane. *J Laryngol Otol* 65:308, 1954.
67. Fabricant ND: Sexual functions and the nose. *Am J Med Sci* 239:498, 1960.
68. Miller P, Smith DW, Shepard TH: Maternal hyperthermia as a possible cause of anencephaly. *Lancet* 1:519, 1978.
69. Pleet HB, Graham JM, Harvey MA: Patterns of malformations resulting from the teratogenic effects of trimester hyperthermia. *Pediatr Res* 14:587, 1980.
70. Davison JM: The urinary system. In Hytten FE, Chamberlain G (eds): *Clinical Physiology in Obstetrics*. Oxford, Blackwell, 1980, p 302.
71. Marchant DJ: Alterations in anatomy and function of the urinary tract during pregnancy. *Clin Obstet Gynecol* 21:855, 1978.
72. Davison JM, Hytten FE: Glomerular filtration during and after pregnancy. *J Obstet Gynaecol Br Commonw* 8:583, 1975.
73. Lindheimer MD, Katz AI, Nolten WE, Oparil S, Ehrlich EN: Sodium and mineralocorticoids in normal and abnormal pregnancy. *Arch Nephrol* 7:33, 1977.
74. Davison JM: Renal nutrient excretion with emphasis on glucose. *Clin Obstet Gynecol* 2:365, 1975.
75. Hytten FE, Cheyne GA: The aminoaciduria of pregnancy. *J Obstet Gynaecol Br Commonw* 63:509, 1972.
76. Mishell Jr. DR, Nakamura RM, Barberia JM, Thorneycroft IH: Initial detection of human chorionic gonadotropin in serum in normal human gestation. *Am J Obstet Gynecol* 118:990, 1974.
77. Csapo AI, Pulkkinen M: Indispensability of the human corpus luteum in maintenance of early pregnancy. Lute-ectomy evidence. *Obstet Gynecol Surv* 33:69, 1978.
78. Mikhail G, Allen WM: Ovarian function in hu-

man pregnancy. *Am J Obstet Gynecol* 99:308, 1967.
79. Quagliarello J, Szlachter N, Steinetz BG, Goldsmith LT, Weiss MD: Serial relaxin concentrations in human pregnancy. *Am J Obstet Gynecol* 135:43, 1979.
80. Porter DG, Amoroso EC: The endocrine functions of the placenta. In Philipp E, Barnes J, Newton M (eds): *Scientific Foundation of Obstetrics and Gynaecology*. Chicago, Year Book, 1977, p 700.
81. MacNaughton MC: Hormone assays in early pregnancy. In Klopper A (ed): *Plasma Hormone Assays in Evaluation of Fetal Well-Being*. Edinburgh, Churchill Livingstone, 1976, p 42.
82. Lauritzen C, Klopper A: Estrogens and androgens. In Fuchs F, Klopper A (eds): *Endocrinology of Pregnancy*. Ed. 3. Philadelphia, Harper & Row, 1983, p 80.
83. Garcia-Bunuel R, Berek JS, Woodruff JD: Luteomas of pregnancy. *Obstet Gynecol* 45:407, 1975.
84. Bolte E, Mancuso S, Eriksson G, Wigust N, Diczfalusy E: Studies on the aromatization of neutral steroids in pregnant women; 3. Overall aromatization of dehydroepiandrosterone sulphate circulating in the fetal and maternal compartments. *Acta Endocrinol* 45:576, 1964.
85. Wilson JD, Griffith JE, George FW, Leshin M: The role of gonadal steroids in sexual differentiation. *Recent Prog Horm Res* 37:1, 1981.
86. Lauritzen C, Lehman WD: Levels of chorionic gonadotropin in the newborn infant and their relationship to adrenal dehydroepiandrosterone. *Acta Endocrinol (suppl) Kbh* 100:112, 1965.
87. Nisula BC, Morgan FJ, Caufield RE: Evidence that chorionic gonadotropin has intrinsic thyrotropic activity. *Biochem Biophys Res Commun* 59:86, 1974.
88. Fairweather DVI: Nausea and vomiting in pregnancy. *Am J Obstet Gynecol* 102:135, 1968.
89. Osathanondh R, Tulchinsky D: Placental polypeptide hormones. In Tulchinsky D, Ryan KJ (eds): *Maternal-Fetal Endocrinology*. Philadelphia, W. B. Saunders, 1980, p 29.
90. Felig P, Lynch V: Starvation in human pregnancy: hypoglycemia, hypoinsulinemia and hyperketonemia. *Science* 170:990, 1970.
91. Klopper A: The new placental proteins. *Biol Med* 1:89, 1979.
92. Curet LB, Olson RW: Oxytocin challenge tests and urinary estriols in the management of high risk pregnancies. *Obstet Gynecol* 55:196, 1980.
93. Assali NS, Rauramo L, Peltonen T: Uterine and fetal blood flow and oxygen consumption in early human pregnancy. *Am J Obstet Gynecol* 79:86, 1960.
94. Metcalfe J, Romney SL, Ramsey LH, Burwell CS: Estimation of uterine blood flow in normal human pregnancy at term. *J Clin Invest* 34:1632, 1955.
95. Klopper A: The ovary. In Hytten FE, Chamberlain G (eds): *Clinical Physiology in Obstetrics*. Oxford,

Blackwell, 1980, p 434.
96. Guyton AC: *Textbook of Medical Physiology*, Ed. 6. Philadelphia, W. B. Saunders, 1981, p 1033.
97. Robinson JE, Short RV: Changes in breast sensitivity at puberty, during the menstrual cycle and at parturition. *Br Med J* 1:1188, 1977.
98. Kumar D: In vitro inhibitory effect of progesterone on extrauterine human smooth muscle. *Am J Obstet Gynecol* 84:1300, 1962.
99. Lyons HA, Antonio R: The sensitivity of the respiratory center in pregnancy and after the administration of progesterone. *Trans Assoc Am Physicians* 72:173, 1959.
100. Harvey GR: Regulation of energy balance. *Nature* 222:629, 1969.
101. Moghissi KS, Syner FN, Evans TN: A composite picture of the menstrual cycle. *Am J Obstet Gynecol* 114:405, 1972.
102. Langgard H, Hvidberg E: The composition of oedema fluid provoked by estradiol and of acute inflammatory oedema. *J Reprod Fertil* 9(suppl):37, 1969.
103. Faiman C, Ryan RJ, Jarrck SJ, Rubin ME: Serum FSH and hCG during human pregnancy and puerperium. *J Clin Endocrinol Metab* 28:1323, 1968.
104. Jeppsson S, Rannevik G, Thorell JI: Pituitary gonadotropin secretion during first weeks of pregnancy. *Acta Endocrinol* 85:177, 1977.
105. Miyake A, Tanizawa O, Aono T, Yasuda M, Kurachi K: Suppression of luteinizing hormone in castrated women by the administration of human chorionic gonadotrophin. *J Clin Endocrinol Metab* 43:928, 1976.
106. Mochizuki M, Morikawa H, Kawaguchi K, Tojo S: Growth hormone, prolactin and chorionic somatomammotropin in normal and molar pregnancy. *J Clin Endocrinol Metab* 43:614, 1976.
107. Rigg LA, Lein A, Yen SSC: The pattern of decrease in circulating prolactin levels during human gestation. *Am J Obstet Gynecol* 129:454, 1977.
108. Tyson JE: The evolutionary role of prolactin in mammalian osmoregulation: effects on fetoplacental hydromineral transport. *Semin Perinatol* 6:216, 1982.
109. Spanos E, Pike JW, Haussler MR, Colston KW, Evans IMA, Goldner AM, McCain TA, MacIntyre I: Circulating 1-alpha-25-dihydroxy vitamin D in the chicken: enhancement by injection of prolactin and during egg laying. *Life Sci* 19:1751, 1976.
110. Souma JA, Niejadlik DC, Cottrell S, Rankel S: Comparison of thyroid function in each trimester of pregnancy with the use of triiodothyronine uptake, thyroxine iodine, free thyroxine, and free thyroxine index. *Am J Obstet Gynecol* 116:905, 1973.
111. Dowling JT, Freinkel N, Ingbar SH: The effect of oestrogens upon peripheral metabolism of thyroxine. *J Clin Invest* 39:1119, 1960.
112. Sandiford I, Wheeler T: Basal metabolism before,

during and after pregnancy. *J Biol Chem* 62:329, 1924.
113. Pitkin RM: Calcium metabolism in pregnancy: a review. *Am J Obstet Gynecol* 121:724, 1975.
114. Irwin MI, Kienholtz WW: A conspectus of research on calcium requirements of man. *J Nutr* 103:1019, 1973.
115. Pitkin RM, Reynolds WA, Williams GA, Hargis GG: Calcium metabolism in normal pregnancy: A longitudinal study. *Am J Obstet Gynecol* 133:781, 1979.
116. Reeve J: Calcium metabolism. In Hytten FE, Chamberlain G (eds): *Clinical Physiology in Obstetrics*. Oxford, Blackwell, 1980, p 263.
117. Slatopolsky E, Rutherford E, Hruska K, Martin K, Klahr S: How important is phosphate in the pathogenesis of renal osteodystrophy? *Arch Intern Med* 138:848, 1978.
118. Whiteley HJ, Stoner HB: The effect of pregnancy on the human adrenal cortex. *J Endocrinol* 14:325, 1957.
119. Saez JM, Forest MG, Morera AM, Bertrand J: Metabolic clearance rate and blood production rate of testosterone and dehydrotestosterone in normal subjects during pregnancy and in hyperthyroidism. *J Clin Invest* 51:1226, 1972.
120. Lederman RP, Lederman E, Work Jr, BA, McCann PS: The relationship of maternal anxiety, plasma catecholamines and plasma cortisol to progress in labor. *Am J Obstet Gynecol* 132:495, 1978.
121. Burke CW, Roulet F: Increased exposure of tissues to cortisol in late pregnancy. *Br Med J* 1:657, 1970.
122. Rosenthal HE, Slaunwhite WRJ, Sandberg AA: Transcortin: a corticosteroid-binding protein of plasma; X. Cortisol and progesterone interplay and unbound levels of these steroids in pregnancy. *J Clin Endocrinol Metab* 19:352, 1969.
123. Carr BR, Parker Jr, CR, Madden JD, MacDonald PC, Porter JC: Maternal plasma adrenocorticotroph and cortisol relationships throughout human pregnancy. *Am J Obstet Gynecol* 139:416, 1981.
124. Genazzani AR, Fraioli F, Hurlimann J, Fioretti P, Felber JP: Immunoreactive ACTH and cortisol plasma levels during pregnancy. Detection and partial purification of corticotropin-like placental hormone: The human chorionic corticotropin (hCC). *Clin Endocrinol* 4:1, 1975.
125. Nolten WE, Rueckert PA: Elevated free cortisol index in pregnancy: Possible regulatory mechanisms. *Am J Obstet Gynecol* 138:492, 1981.
126. Cohen M, Stiefel M, Reddy WJ, Saidlaw JC: The secretion and disposition of cortisol during pregnancy. *J Clin Endocrinol Metab* 18:1076, 1958.
127. Nolten WE, McKenna MV, Rueckert PA, Ehrlich EN: Inhibition of 3H-dexamethasone binding to lymphocytes in vitro; relevance to the apparent development of refractoriness to cortison in pregnancy. *Clin Res* 28:7624, 1980.
128. Erlichs EN, Lindheimer MD: Effect of administered mineralocorticoid or ACTH in pregnant women: Attenuation of kaliuretic influence of mineralcorticoids during pregnancy. *J Clin Invest* 51:1301, 1972.
129. Ehrlich EN, Nolten WE, Oparil S, Lindheimer MD: Mineralocorticoids in normal pregnancy. In Lindheimer MD, Katz AI and Zuspan FP (eds): *Hypertension in Normal Pregnancy*. New York, John Wiley & Sons, 1976, p 1989.
130. Nolten WE, Lindheimer MD, Opard S, Erlich EN: Desoxycortisterone in normal pregnancy; 1. Sequential studies of the secretory patterns of desoxycarbiosterone, aldosterone and cortisol. *Am J Obstet Gynecol* 132:414, 1978.
131. Winkel CA, Milewich L, Gant NF, Parker Jr, CK, Gant NF, Simpson ER, MacDonald PC: Conversion of plasma progesterone to deoxycorticosterone in men, nonpregnant and pregnant women and adrenalectomized subjects. Evidence for steroid II-hydroxylase activity in nonadrenal tissues. *J Clin Invest* 66:803, 1980.
132. Nolten WE, Holt LH, Rueckert PA: Desoxycorticosterone in normal pregnancy; III. Evidence of a fetal source of desoxycorticosterone. *Am J Obstet Gynecol* 139:477, 1981.
133. Davidson JM, Hytten FE: Glomerular filtration. during and after pregnancy. *J Obstet Gynaecol Br Commonw* 81:583, 2975.
134. Robertson EG: Increased erythrocyte fragility in association with osmotic changes in pregnancy serum. *J Reprod Fertil* 16:323, 1968.
135. Landau RL, Lugibihl K: Inhibition of the sodium retaining influence of aldosterone by progesterone. *J Clin Endocrinol Metab* 18:1237, 1958.
136. Everett RB, Worley RJ, MacDonald PC, Gant NF: Effect of prostaglandin synthetase inhibitors on pressor response to angiotensin II in human pregnancy. *J Clin Endocrinol Metab* 46:1007, 1978.
137. Hytten FE: Weight gain in pregnancy. In *Clinical Physiology in Obstetrics*. Oxford, Blackwell, 1980, p 216.

6
Fuel Metabolism in Pregnancy

There is no other period in adult life in which such major physiological changes occur as in pregnancy. All available resources are channeled to the fetus without harming the mother. These functions are regulated by a variety of hormones, including the specific gestational hormones secreted by the placenta.

Fats, proteins, and carbohydrates are recognized as fuels since they are capable of supplying energy requirements. They are also the major building blocks of the body. Their demand during pregnancy is increased to supply the above functions.

FUEL COMPONENTS AND STORAGE

All of the three major food components, proteins, carbohydrates, and fats, can be utilized as fuels since they can be oxidized for energy (ATP) production. The rate of utilization varies and depends on the metabolic state of an individual at a given moment and on the specific need of the organ. The most selective organ is the brain which under normal conditions utilizes glucose almost exclusively.

The supply of fuels is derived from either external sources, namely diet, or from internal stores. Of the three possible fuels, only fat is stored in significant amounts in the adipose tissues. A nonpregnant 60-kg woman stores about 18 kg of fat which can generate 160,000 kcal. Carbohydrates stored as glycogen are very limited and are estimated as 800–1000 kcal, about half stored in the liver, the other half is stored in the skeletal muscles. Only liver glycogen is readily available for immediate utilization. In 24 hours of continuous fasting, the liver is virtually depleted of glycogen, but the muscles still possess about 80% of their glycogen. With longer periods of starvation, the rate and ratio of glycogen depletion does not change either in the liver or muscles.

Proteins are not stored in the body in the usual sense since every known protein has a specific physiological role (enzymes, functional proteins as actin or myosin, structural as collagen and bone proteins). Every protein which is broken down and utilized for energy may affect some important physiological function. The major body proteins are collagen (25%) and actomyosin (20%) which, under conditions of increased demand, undergo degradation. Such degradation is more pronounced in myosin than in collagen. Loss of more than 10% of body proteins is known to cause major impairments of physiological functions, while a 30–50% loss is lethal.

Fat is a readily stored substrate. Not only does it have twice the caloric value of carbohydrates and proteins, but it is also unhydrated while the other two fuels are hydrated with about 4 times their weight of water. Therefore, 1 kg of fat yields the same amount of energy as 10 kg of carbohydrates or protein. Thus, storage of fat has a clearly evolutionary advantage over carbohydrates. Fat cannot supply the entire energy needs for the organism since the brain and some other tissues (red blood cells and the renal cortex) cannot utilize it. Such needs are supplied by the stored glycogen.

The average weight gain during pregnancy is about 12 kg, with the conceptus accounting for 4.950 kg (fetus, 3.5 kg; placenta, 0.65; amniotic fluid, 0.8 kg). Maternal tissues directly affected by pregnancy (uterus and breasts) along with fluid gain account for about 4.3 kg, for a total of 9.250 kg (34). The rest (2.75 kg) is believed to be the net fuel storage increase. Although the exact composition of this fuel store is still undefined in the human, it is assumed to be mainly fat (32) (Fig. 6.1). Weight gain during gestation is inversely related to maternal weight before pregnancy, for obese women gain less than the lean ones (41). More detailed information is available in experimental animals. In the rat, total body weight increases during gestation by about 30%, fat is increased 50%, while proteins are increased 20% (73). The proteins accumulated are well distributed among the various organs (liver, 35%; heart, 30%; kidneys, 28%; gastrointestinal tract, 40–50%) (81). Protein metabolism in the rat appears to be biphasic, anabolic in the early stages of pregnancy and catabolic later on (53).

It is not clear what changes in total body protein occur in pregnancy. Johnstone et al. (35) performed a 12-day nitrogen balance test in 68 normal pregnant women in late gestation (30–34 weeks), no nitrogen retention or loss could be demonstrated. A total gain of about 1 kg protein equivalent to 5 kg lean body mass in human pregnancy was calculated by Hytten and Leitch (31) and almost all of it has been related to the fetus, placenta, and uterus. The remainder of protein accumulation occurs earlier in pregnancy and is generated to accommodate the increased metabolic needs, but not for storage. Proteins are utilized as fuel in cases of fuel shortage as in starvation or when excess proteins are ingested.

INTERCONVERSION OF FUELS

The most essential fuel is glucose, which must be continuously available, yet it is stored in relatively small amounts. About as much glycogen is stored in the liver as is used by the brain over a 24-hour period. In the rat, placental transfer of fat is poor, and the fetus mobilizes its energy and synthesizes fat from glucose and amino acids (42). In other animals and man there is a limited placental transfer of fatty acids, primarily amino acids and glucose, across the placenta.

Some metabolic interconversion of fuels does exist. Glucose can be converted to fat through acetylcoenzyme A, the main pathway for excess carbohydrates and amino acids. The reverse pathway, fatty acids to glucose, is trivial. About 5% of the triglyceride carbons (the glycerol moiety) can be converted to glucose. Glucose can also be

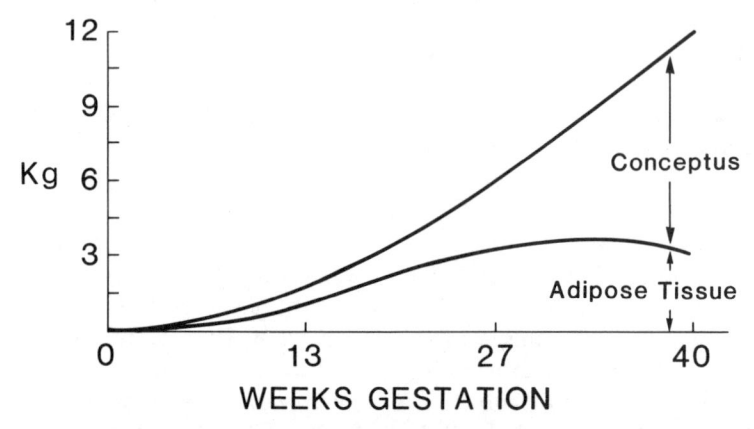

Figure 6.1. Constituents of maternal weight gain during pregnancy. Fat content is established from measurement of total body water. The conceptus consists of the fetus, placenta, uterus, amniotic fluid, and membranes. The conceptus plus fat could account for all maternal weight gain during pregnancy (31).

Fuel Metabolism in Pregnancy 85

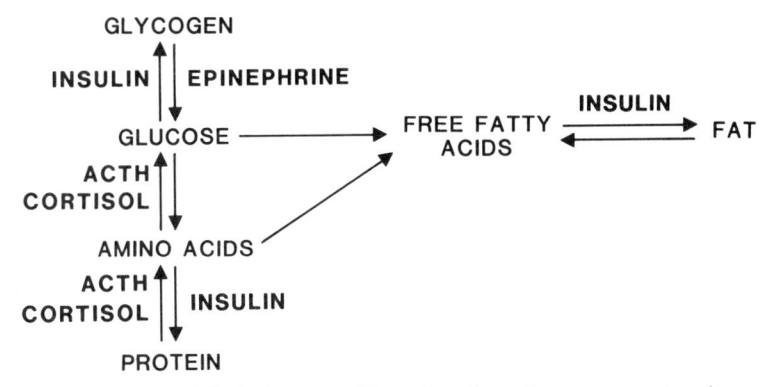

Figure 6.2. Interconversion of fuel elements. Note that there is no conversion from fatty acids to glucose. Epinephrine stimulates the breakdown of glycogen and fat. ACTH and cortisol stimulate breakdown of protein to amino acids and the transformation of these into glucose (gluconeogenesis). Insulin reverses the epinephrine and ACTH-cortisol effects.

utilized to form the carbon skeleton of almost all nonessential amino acids. Conversely, proteins can be converted to glucose, as mass, approximately 60 g of glucose for every 100 g of protein (Fig. 6.2).

THE CONTROLLED STRESS CONCEPT

Bessman and his group have recently proposed the "controlled stress" hypothesis to explain the biochemical effects caused by the interplay among the catabolic stress hormones and anabolic insulin (84). They postulated that all types of stress, including trauma, infection, psychologic, constitute an emergency survival mechanism in which the organism is rapidly supplied with large amounts of fuels, glucose for the brain and free fatty acids (FFA) for the muscle, to enable them to cope with the fight and flight requirements. Epinephrine, the most primitive stress hormone (18), is responsible for the primary stress reaction. Its mechanism of action is rapid, activating preexisting inactive enzymes through the cAMP-adenyl cyclase system (60, 75). Both glycogenolysis and lipolysis are markedly increased. By and large, the epinephrine effect is uncontrolled and results in excess supply of these fuels, exceeding the capacity of the cell to metabolize. This results in hyperglycemia, hyperlipidemia, ketonemia, and lactic acidemia from incomplete oxidation of FFA and glucose and those acids cause a decrease in blood bicarbonate and pH (Table 6.1). All these changes can be observed clinically in diabetic ketoacidosis. In the process, the epinephrine effect causes excessive expenditure of the limited glycogen depots. This is phase I of stress.

Table 6.1. Epinephrine Effects on Blood Chemistry

1. Glucose	↑
2. Free fatty acids	↑
3. Lactate	↑
4. Ketone acids	↑
5. Bicarbonate	↓
6. pH	↓

Table 6.2. Insulin Effects

Metabolism		Blood	
Glycogen synthesis	↑	Glucose	↓
Protein synthesis	↑	Amino acids	↓
Glucose transport	↑	Glucose	↓
Fatty acid synthesis	↑	Ketones	↓
Fat synthesis	↑	Free fatty acids	↓

Insulin is known to elicit anabolic reactions and, as such, can be regarded as the true growth hormone (6). Insulin counteracts the action of epinephrine (Table 6.2) by its stimulation of protein, fat and glycogen synthesis. Insulin limits the supply of all fuels by reference to the blood glucose level, for it is most important to conserve glucose for the brain. Insulin is secreted when the blood level of glucose rises higher than 100 mg which is the optimum level for brain metabolism. It acts by increasing the resynthesis of fat and glycogen without affecting their breakdown rate.

If stress continues for several hours, the effects of cortisol, ACTH, and growth hormone (phase II of stress) became manifest (Table 6.3). They are secreted along with epinephrine, but since their mechanism of action is slow, their effects are delayed (e.g., induction of enzymes). All these phase II hormones cause an increased breakdown of proteins to amino acids, thereby stimulating gluconeogenesis, so that an adequate supply of glucose for the brain continues even after the liver glycogen reserves are exhausted. Insulin controls phase II by increasing the opposite reaction, protein synthesis from amino acids, therefore, depriving gluconeogenesis of substrate when the blood level of glucose exceeds the optimum 150 mg/100 ml. Protein breakdown is not affected by insulin (46, 50). Since the fuel to be conserved is glucose, it represents the signal for pancreatic beta cell secretion of insulin.

When the stress is over, both epinephrine and the phase II hormones are no longer secreted. Epinephrine effects cease immediately, while phase II effects continue for hours or even days since their decline depends on the half-life of the newly synthesized enzymes evoked by the phase II hormones (cortisol, ACTH, GH) (Fig. 6.3).

Pregnancy appeared late in evolution. It exists only among vertebrates and, mainly, mammals. Gestation-related hormones, estrogen, progesterone, human placental lactogen, and prolactin, play a secondary role, as modifiers, in the main scheme of fuel metabolism discussed above. Their major metabolic role is to ensure adequate substrate supply to the fetus through an enhanced catabolism of maternal fuel stores. Moreover, they are secreted independently of the day to day metabolic variations so that the fine tuning of fuel metabolism is regulated by the major stress hormones and insulin.

HORMONES AFFECTING FUEL SUPPLY IN PREGNANCY

In nonstressful conditions, epinephrine levels do not change in pregnancy (85).

ACTH and cortisol do increase during pregnancy (36). Progressive increasing cortisol levels are accompanied by higher circulating cortisone-binding globulin under the influence of estrogen in pregnancy (13, 16). ACTH blood levels rise in late pregnancy. It was postulated (16) that the hypothalamus demonstrates a reduced sensitivity to cortisol due to high maternal concentrations of cortisone antagonists such as progesterone and 17-hydroxyprogesterone (12). A direct positive effect of estrogen on ACTH secretion was also suggested (53). The pregnant woman, therefore, can be considered to be continually in phase II of stress augmented by the catabolic effect of those hormones particularly associated with pregnancy.

Fasting growth hormone (hGH) is essentially unchanged throughout pregnancy. Pituitary hGH secretion in response to stimuli (as hypoglycemia) is increased during the first 24 weeks and depressed thereafter. The change may be due to the higher cortisone and/or human placental lactogen (hPL) at that period (79, 83).

In reviewing the current literature, it appears that glucagon plays only a minor role in modifying the pregnancy-related changes of fuel metabolism (41).

Estrogen secretion rises from below 100 μg/day to 33 mg/day near term gestation (55). This hormone increases lipolysis and gluconeogenesis via protein breakdown, the

Table 6.3. Steroid-Peptide Hormone Effects

Metabolism		Blood	
Protease	↑	Amino acids, ketones and lactate	↑
Glucose-6-phosphatase			
Fructose-1,6-diphosphatase		Glucose	↑
Pyruvate carboxylase			
Phosphoenolpyruvate carboxykinase			

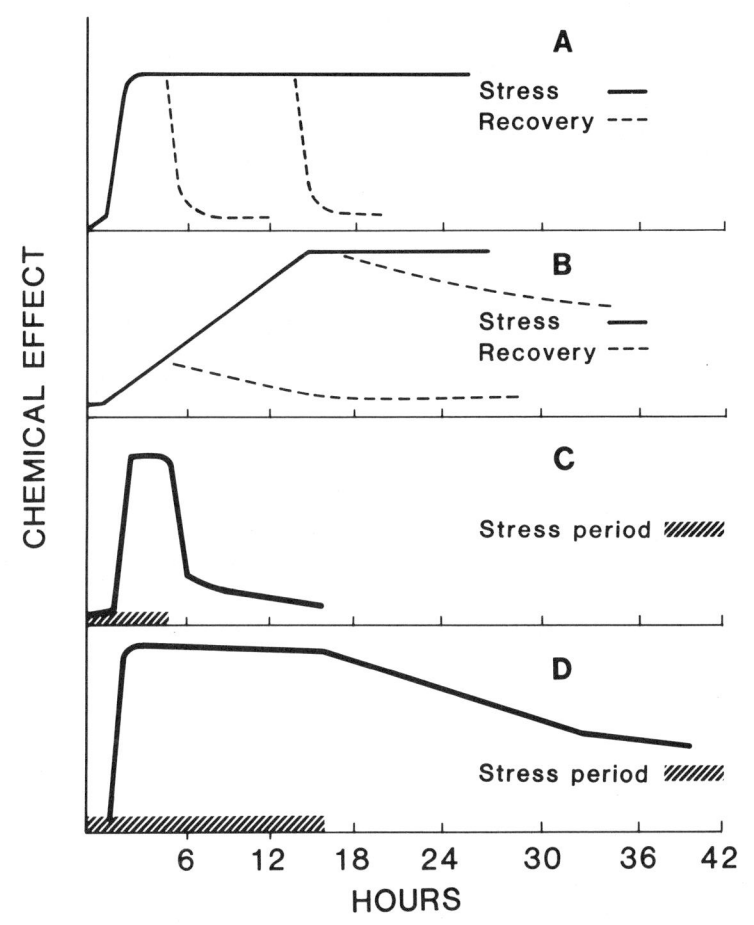

Figure 6.3. Schematic relationship between chemical effects of stress hormones of phase I and II stress and duration of actual stress. (*A*) Phase I of stress—epinephrine. (*B*) Phase II of stress—steroid-peptide hormones. (*C*) Actual manifestations of short-term stress—combined effect of phase I and II hormones. (*D*) Actual manifestation of long-term stress—combined effect of phase I and II hormones (84).

latter effect is assumed to be facilitated by ACTH secretion. Conversely, natural estrogen improves glucose tolerance, both in laboratory animals and in human subjects (36), probably through a positive effect on insulin secretion, for it also causes hypertrophy of pancreatic islets, which has been shown to occur in pregnancy (1). This process may explain the increased basal levels of insulin in late pregnancy in spite of lower fasting blood glucose.

Progesterone has limited effect, in the human, on glucose tolerance, but does increase basal plasma insulin (15, 37). Progesterone was also found to diminish insulin receptor response (43). Its secretion rises progressively, reaching a level of 250 mg/day at term.

hPL is a single chain, placenta-secreted polypeptide. Immunologically, it is closely related to hGH. hPL causes mobilization of FFA from maternal depots. It has a diabetogenic effect and its administration provokes glucose intolerance in women who have had impaired glucose tolerance tests in previous pregnancies (27). Blood levels at term are 5–8 μg/ml (23). It has been suggested that hPL is modulated by glucose and/or FFA (78).

Prolactin has actions similar to those of hGH. Its levels in pregnancy are steadily increasing (33, 62). Prolactin is secreted both in the pituitary and placenta. The "anti-insulin" effect of prolactin is well established. Its administration causes an elevation of blood FFA level in the human (5), and a delayed increase (5 hours) of blood glucose and glucose turnover in the dog (61). In hyperprolactinemic nonpregnant women, the glucose tolerance curve, basal insulin levels, and post-challenge plasma insulin responses are significantly higher than in normal women, mimicking the metabolic responses of late gestation (29). These phenomena can be explained through the "controlled stress" concept, since prolactin increases gluconeogenesis exactly the same as the other peptide hormones and an increase in glucose synthesis could appear clinically as diminution in insulin sensitivity. The delayed changes in glucose metabolism are similar to those seen in phase II of the stress mechanism, reflecting the effects caused by stimulated catabolic enzyme synthesis.

METABOLIC ADAPTATION TO PREGNANCY

Fat accumulation and increased protein synthesis start to occur early in pregnancy. These changes are partly explained by enhanced maternal appetite. Pregnancy is characterized by increased levels of circulating insulin and insulin resistance (45, 72). In response to excess fuel supply, fat is accumulated. Early in pregnancy, hPL, prolactin, and cortisone levels are low so that glucose tolerance is generally unaltered and may even improve in the diabetic (68), probably due to enhanced insulin secretion.

A major metabolic change occurs in the second half of pregnancy. Fat accumulation ceases; and, in many cases, there is an actual drop in fat depots. Some investigators report a reduction in lean body mass in laboratory animals. During this period cortisol, growth hormone, and insulin levels continue to rise. Fasting blood levels of glucose, amino acids, FFA and ketones do not significantly change through pregnancy (Fig. 6.4A). A further fast of 4–6 hours results in lower blood glucose and amino acids while FFA and ketones increase markedly (Fig. 6.5) (47, 49). The metabolic changes mimic those seen during prolonged starvation and, indeed, Freinkel termed them as a state of "accelerated starvation" (22).

The above metabolic shift is partly due to the fetal requirements. The fetus triples its weight in the last trimester of gestation. Although the fetus' metabolic expenditure per kg body weight, expressed in calories, is not much different from that of the mother, the composition of the substrates used is different. Since very limited amounts of fatty acids cross the placenta, fat and protein synthesis are derived solely from glucose and amino acids. The continuous transplacental drainage of glucose and amino acids does not affect maternal blood levels of these nutrients during the day. However, after overnight fasting, plasma glucose and amino acid levels are lower in late pregnancy. With exhaustion of liver glycogen stores, protein becomes the only source for glucose and amino acids. Under these conditions, lipolysis occurs. However, since glucose is drained, the organism does not respond with insulin secretion (19) to control the excess breakdown as in the normal compensated stress reaction. If the starvation persists, FFA formation exceeds its complete oxidation rate and ketones are produced (Fig. 6.4B). This simulates the sequence of events occurring during starvation in the nonpregnant individual. The process of starvation is faster during gestation and during exercise because the catabolic hormones are initially higher and glucose utilization is enhanced. An increased lipolytic activity was found in vitro in fat tissues of pregnant animals (40). The above tissues had been exposed to cortison and hPL. Once the lipolytic enzymes are hypertrophied, a decrease of lipolysis depends not on the hormone's presence, but on the decreasing of the enzymes, which is a function of their half-life.

The decreased glucose tolerance seen in late pregnancy is explained by the above mechanism. During glucose load, insulin

Fuel Metabolism in Pregnancy

A NORMAL (WITH OR W/O STRESS)

Conditions	Mother	Placenta	Fetus
Stress Hormones	Normal or High		
Insulin	Normal or High	FFA, Glucose, Lactate, Amino Acids	Amino Acids = ↑ Glucose =
Blood Levels	Normal Normal Normal		

Fat Glycogen Protein (↓↑ ↑ ↑)

B STARVATION

Conditions	Mother	Placenta	Fetus
Stress Hormones	Normal		
Insulin	Low	FFA, Glucose, Amino Acids, Ketones	Amino Acids = ↓ Glucose = ↓ Ketones ↑
Blood Levels	High Low Low		

Fat Glycogen Protein (↓ ↓ ↓)

C DIABETES (STRESS)

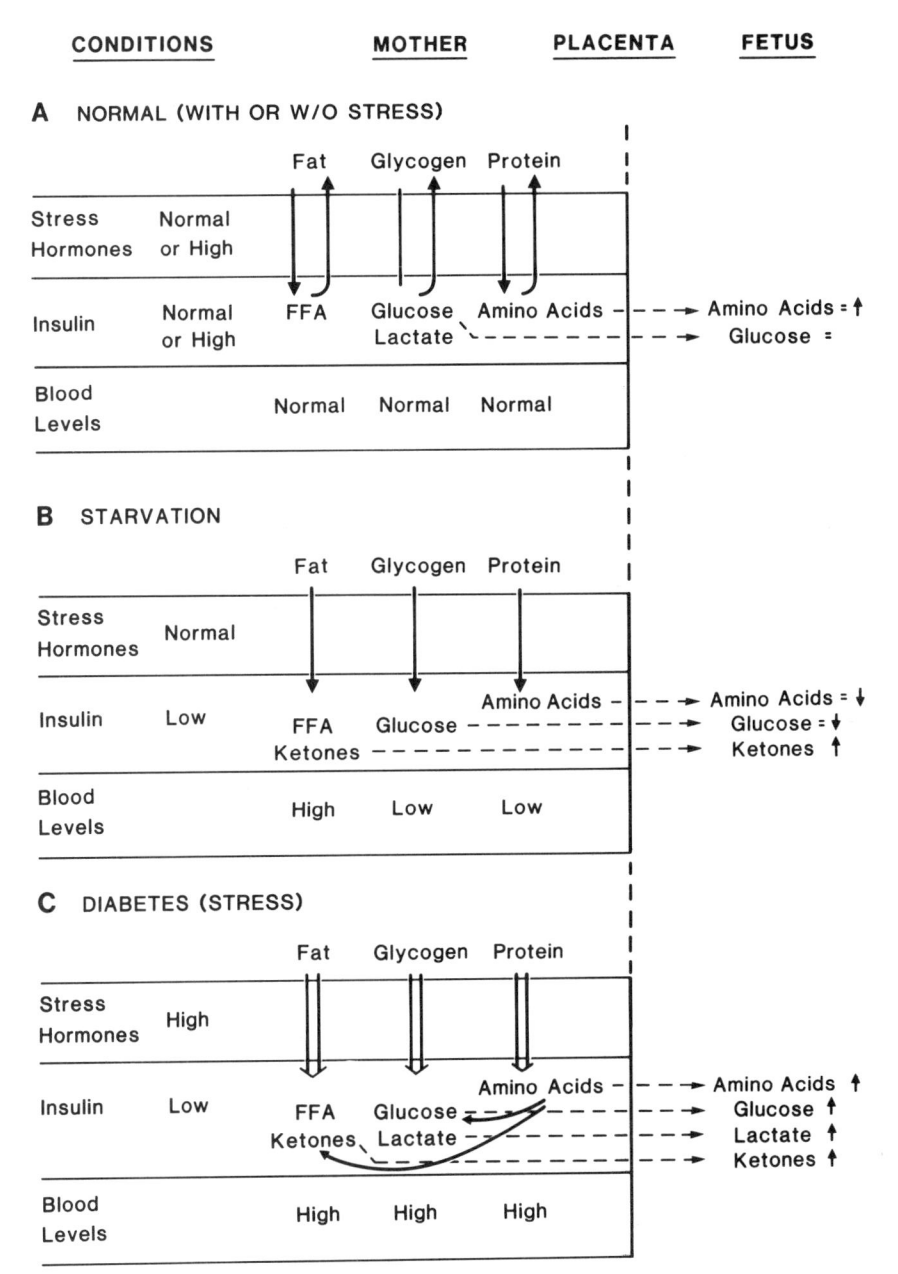

Conditions	Mother	Placenta	Fetus
Stress Hormones	High		
Insulin	Low	FFA, Ketones, Glucose, Lactate, Amino Acids	Amino Acids ↑ Glucose ↑ Lactate ↑ Ketones ↑
Blood Levels	High High High		

Fat Glycogen Protein (⇓ ⇓ ⇓)

Figure 6.4. Hormonal effects on fuel supply and availability in pregnancy. (*A*) *Normal*: A balance exists between breakdown and synthesis of fuels due to the mutual effects of stress hormones and insulin. Blood levels of fuels and their products are normal. No change is observed during stress since insulin secretion increases to counteract stress hormone activity. (*B*) *Starvation*: Due to glucose drainage from the maternal system, insulin activity is low. As fat breakdown continues without activation of fat synthesis by insulin, FFA and ketones rise, resulting in ketonemia in the mother and fetus. (*C*) *Diabetes with stress*: Both phase I and II of stress are activated and are not controlled by insulin. FFA, ketones, glucose, lactate, and amino acids are elevated in maternal blood (diabetic ketoacidosis). All of them except FFA are elevated also in the fetus. The fetus reacts with hyperinsulinemia and transforms these substrates to fat and proteins, resulting in the typical macrosomic baby seen in diabetic pregnancies.

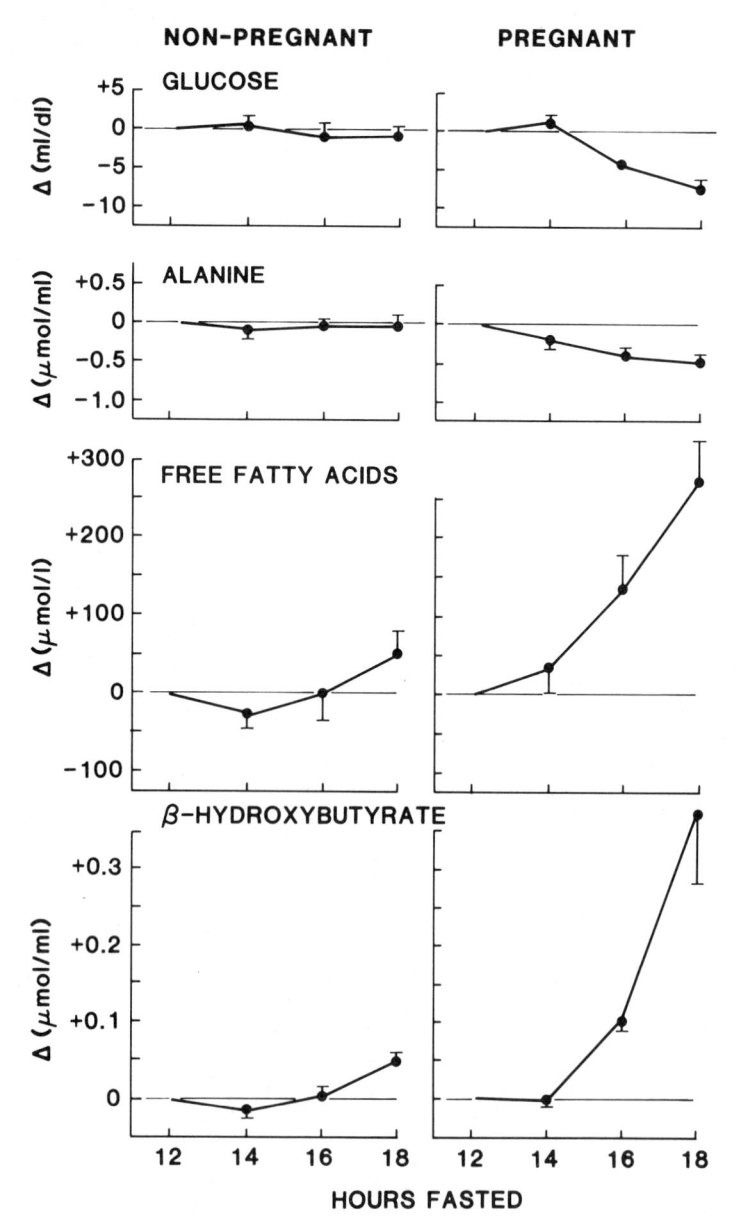

Figure 6.5. Changes in plasma concentrations of glucose, alanine, free fatty acids, and β-hydroxybutyrate in nonpregnant and pregnant women between 12 and 18 hours' fast. Values are shown as absolute increments or decrements from base values. (Modified from Metzger et al. (49).)

also has to counteract the increased gluconeogenesis effects of pregnancy hormones and cortisol by diverting glucose to fat and glycogen. Many other theories have been advanced to explain glucose intolerance in pregnancy despite elevated insulin secretion (45). They include: reduced binding affinity of insulin receptors (56), decreased postreceptor effect, faster removal of insulin from the circulation (28) by special binding protein (inactive receptors) or enhanced insulin catabolism by higher insulinase activity and/or concentration. The rat and human do have high insulinase activity in the placenta. While the rat has increased insulin clearance (21), the human placenta does not (4). The combined effect of these processes was termed "insulin insensitivity." It was calculated that insulin sensitivity in pregnancy is about one fifth of that found in the nonpregnant woman (20). At this point, it is not clear what are the major factors in determining this insulin insensitivity, e.g., hormone, enzyme, or receptor related. In general, the "insulin insensitivity" factors themselves can be explained by the "controlled stress" mechanism. Puavilai and co-workers (59) found, in late pregnancy, during glucose load, increased insulin binding to peripheral monocytes together with high plasma glucose to insulin ratio. They theorized that this is caused by a "post-receptor" defect in insulin action. The same data can be interpreted as an intact insulin action in the face of a high gluconeogenesis rate caused by ACTH, cortisol, and hPL, whose blood levels are elevated during late gestation without need to postulate unknown postreceptor effects.

CONSEQUENCES OF GESTATIONAL KETOSIS

As discussed above, gestational ketosis is common and should probably be regarded as a physiological rather than a pathological state. Unlike fatty acids, ketones readily cross the placenta (65). Whether this poses risks for the fetus is still under debate. Part of the debate lies in the fact that gestational ketosis in normal women is often considered to have the same pathological significance as diabetic ketoacidosis. The latter is a totally different metabolic situation in which there is no countervailing anabolic effect of insulin. Ketosis is accompanied by metabolic acidosis and glucose levels are usually highly elevated. Metabolic acidosis per se may harm the fetus by decreasing uterine blood flow (11).

The collaborative perinatal project of the National Institute of Neurological and Communicative Disorders and Stroke consists of an 8-year prospective follow-up of 53,518 pregnancies in 12 United States hospitals between 1959 and 1966 (77). Some studies were based upon the diabetic mothers' subgroup of this data base. Churchill et al. (14) found lower IQ scores (mean of 83) in infants of diabetic mothers who had had episodes of ketonuria within 24 hours of delivery as compared with those of diabetics who had not had such episodes (mean 101) or those of normal, nondiabetic mothers (mean 102). Analyzing the same data, Naeye (52) found no difference among either of these groups in the IQ scores. Stevens and co-workers (74) followed, prospectively, 80 children of diabetic mothers born at or transferred to the University of Iowa hospital shortly after birth. By the age of 5 years, they found a lower IQ score among those children whose mothers had had ketonuric episodes during pregnancy.

All these studies do not differentiate between patients with and without acidemia; the exact occurrence of ketoacidosis vs. ketosis only is unknown. Moreover, the results cannot be extrapolated to normal women with physiological ketosis of pregnancy. Naeye and Chez (51), analyzing the Collaborative Perinatal project data base, did not find any psychoneurological impairment among children of normal mothers who had had ketosis during starvation. It was also claimed that, in certain conditions, the fetus can even benefit from ketones since it can utilize them for energy (30) and for cerebral lipid synthesis (80).

The consensus is that ketosis should be avoided whenever possible. This can be easily accomplished by avoiding lengthy intervals between meals and having some snack prior to sleep. Skipping breakfast is another common habit which must be avoided in late pregnancy, since it prolongs the overnight fast to 16–18 hours, and it also should be avoided prior to exercise.

METABOLIC FATE OF GLUCOSE

On the average, pregnant women who do not limit their food intake consume approximately 2300–2800 kcal (39). Since very little net maternal weight gain (excluding pregnancy products and fluids) is observed during late gestation, all fuels are used for maternal and fetal energy needs. Assuming an average daily intake of 2500 kcal with 40% carbohydrates, the maximum available glucose to them will amount to 1000 kcal or 250 g. Maternal inflexible requirements are about 150 g/day (120 g for the brain and 30 g for other glucose dependent tissues).

Fetal oxygen consumption near term is about 5 ml/kg/hour (69). Based on the assumption that the primary fuel for the fetus is glucose, Widdowson (81) calculated that the fetal energy requirement per kg of body weight is the same as that of the mother. A full term fetus contains protein and fat equivalent to 8000 kcal, and during the last 4 weeks of gestation, fetal fat and protein accumulates at the rate of 126 kcal daily. The energy required for this synthesis is 32 kcal/day. The total energy requirement of the fetus is 110 kcal/day (28 g glucose). Fat is synthesized by the fetus from glucose at a daily rate of 38 g glucose. Total fetal glucose utilization is, therefore, 66 g and the combined fetal maternal inflexible glucose need is 216 g/day (81). In this type of situation, only 35 g of glucose are left for other metabolic purposes. The above is consistent with the common belief that, in late pregnancy, glucose is "reserved" for fetal needs.

In early pregnancy, fetal metabolic needs are practically nil. Glucose disappears from the blood after meals faster than it can be oxidized. When 50 g glucose are injected intravenously, blood glucose will return to the preload level within 1 hour. At the same time, only about 70 kcal are utilized for energy. Even if all of the energy were produced from glucose (which is probably an overestimation), it accounts for only 35% of the administered glucose. Most of the glucose is diverted into fat and a smaller amount into glycogen. Each molecule of glucose transformed into fat is lost for the maternal glucose dependent tissues and for the fetus later in pregnancy.

Glucose utilization by the resting muscle is insulin dependent. Glucose uptake by the tissues is increased in the presence of higher circulating glucose levels in the presence or absence of insulin (71). Glucose utilization for energy is higher in the absorptive period since both glucose and insulin are elevated at that time, and significantly diminished thereafter. In late pregnancy, muscle glucose oxydation is relatively higher since the absorptive period is prolonged (reduced glucose tolerance) and basal insulin levels are higher.

Exercising muscles increase energy production independently of insulin. In the diabetic, exercise lowers blood glucose, an insulin-like effect. The mechanism of this phenomenon was worked out by Bessman and his group (7, 8, 82). He suggested a creatine-phosphocreatine shuttle for energy transfer from the mitochondria to the myofibrils. When the muscle is exercised, more phosphocreatine is consumed by the myofibrils. The free creatine liberated diffuses to the mitochondrial membrane where phosphocreatine is regenerated. The latter reaction is ATP dependent and the net effect, in this mitochondrial compartment, is a depletion of ATP and an increased ADP. Since ADP controls energy generation, its greater availability results in a higher rate of energy production. It has been demonstrated by Artal et al. (3) that, during exercise in pregnancy, glucose is reduced similarly in the healthy and diabetic patients.

METABOLIC CONSIDERATIONS ON DIABETES IN PREGNANCY

Viewing insulin as the only antistress hormone, diabetes can be considered a disease of "uncontrolled stress." The organism is fully capable of producing the epinephrine and peptide hormone phases of stress, but unable to modulate them with pancreatic insulin and prevent the ill effects of the full blown stress reaction. Practically, a diabetic balanced with a certain dose of insulin can cope with normal life quite well. However, as soon as any kind of stress intervenes: infection, surgery or emotional stress, the diabetic patient is driven out of balance and goes into an excessive catabolic state that requires a higher dose of insulin.

Pregnancy may be considered a state of chronic stress, not only the original hormones related with phase II of stress are elevated, but also some pregnancy related stress hormones, i.e., hPL and prolactin.

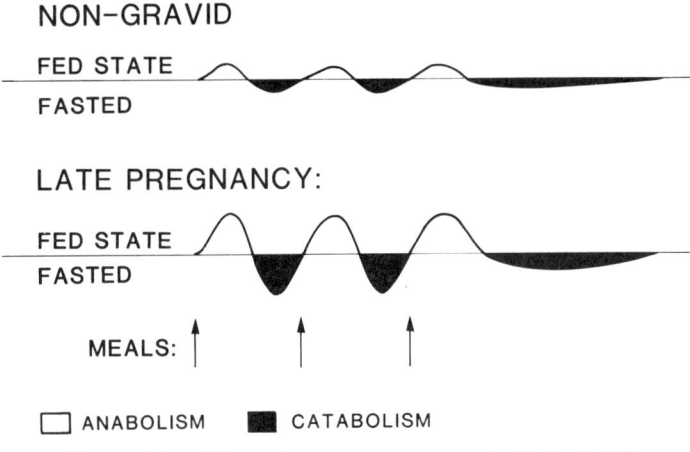

Figure 6.6. Effect of pregnancy on metabolic fuels (48).

Glucose levels fluctuate in normal late gestation more than in any other period and, with them, also insulin levels. Metzger and Freinkel (48) conclude that the effect of pregnancy on maternal fuel metabolism is to amplify the magnitude of the oscillation during transitions between the fed and fasted states (Fig. 6.6). Insulin oscillates in parallel with glucose. In gestational diabetes, the organism is incapable of secreting the required amount of insulin to glucose stimulation. Therefore, it is expected that fuel levels will have even higher oscillations than in normal pregnancy. The experimental data support the above theoretical consideration. Glucose levels are elevated in the fed state, although not reduced to normal at the fasting state due to increased gluconeogenesis (26). The same trend is observed for amino acids (48). Circulating FFA and ketones are higher in gestational diabetes than in normal pregnancy, both in the fed and in the fasted states (57). The increase is most pronounced after an overnight fast (25).

In insulin-dependent diabetes, the physician and the patient take the place of the pancreas in monitoring the metabolic state and controlling stress. The better the control, the closer the patient to normal. Any metabolic study of diabetes reflects only the success or the failure of a certain treatment scheme in a certain group of patients (2).

Normally, insulin secretion is adjusted many times a day to control the correct supply and storage of the main fuels as reflected by glucose blood levels. A diabetic, given 2-3 doses of insulin a day, may get his average requirement of the hormone, but certainly not his immediate needs. Most of the time, the diabetic has either too much or too little circulating insulin. The organism oscillates enormously between anabolic and catabolic states. This constant shift between synthesis and breakdown, especially of proteins, may be responsible for the late complications of the disease. For the short run, the body can accommodate to such fluctuations unless a rapid increase in insulin levels is needed as in the case of severe stress. Pregnancy is a period of rapid daily metabolic changes requiring a better adjustment of insulin administration. Moreover, for reasons beyond the scope of this paper, fetal outcome appears best when maternal glucose levels are constantly stabilized around 80-100 mg/100 ml (2, 17, 24, 38, 76). Accomplishing better metabolic control necessitates strict dietary (66, 67) and activity control as well as regular monitoring of blood glucose (2, 70), a better distribution of insulin dosage and avoidance of prolonged fasting and any possible stress.

Several open loop insulin pumps have been introduced (58, 63). They administer insulin continously and may take into account the changes in insulin requirements during meals, and be programmable for ac-

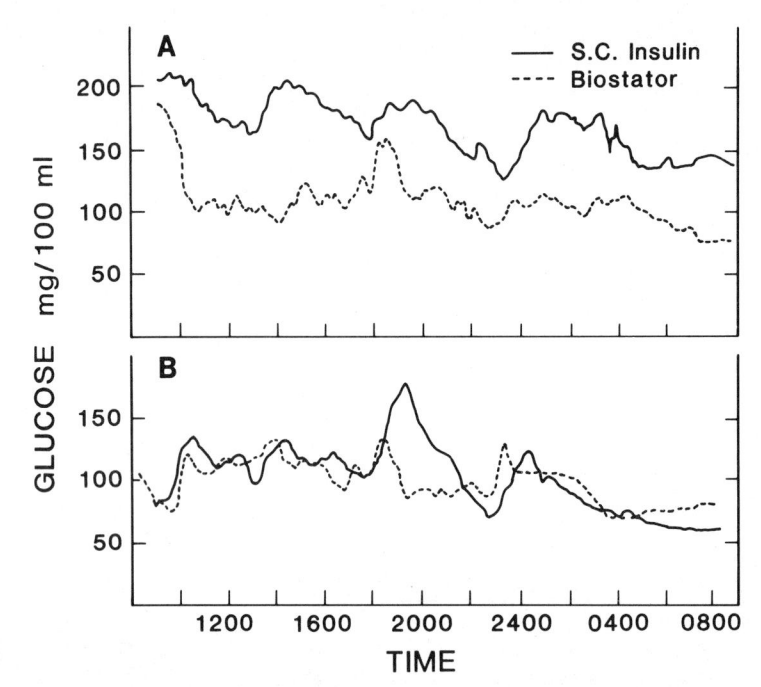

Figure 6.7. Blood glucose levels obtained with a closed loop insulin delivery system (Biostator, Miles Laboratories, Elkhart, Ind.) and optimal conventional therapy with diet and multiple injections of subcutaneous insulin. (*A*) Juvenile diabetes. (*B*) Mature onset diabetes. The closed loop system not only brings mean blood glucose done to a predetermined level, but also reduces the catabolic and anabolic fluctuations represented by glucose levels.

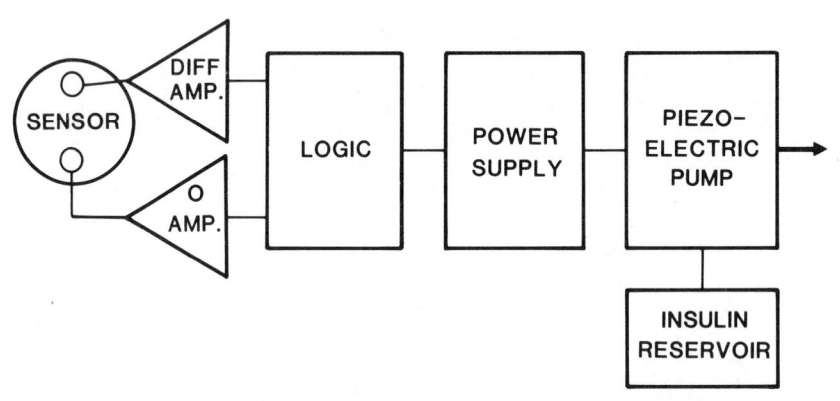

Figure 6.8. Schematic representation of the implantable artifical beta cell. The glucose oxidase electrode senses *tissue* glucose and activates the piezoelectric pump when glucose levels are above predetermined value. Insulin is delivered either subcutaneously or intraperitoneally. Note that the vascular system is not involved to avoid coagulation problems.

tivity and overnight fasting. However, since they are preprogrammed, strict dietary and activity control must be retained, and no factor which cannot be predetermined is taken into account. These periods of increased insulin requirement due to stress are, we believe, most destructive. The optimal solution is a closed loop system which will monitor blood glucose and deliver the exact amount of insulin needed as does the normal pancreas. A large, relatively immobile unit is available and has proved efficient for short-term treatment such as delivery, cesarean section or ketoacidotic events (Fig. 6.7) (54, 64). An implantable long-term device was developed by Bessman and his group. This "artificial pancreas" is based on a glucose oxidase sensor measuring directly tissue glucose and activating a piezoelectric pump to deliver minute amounts of insulin as needed (Fig. 6.8). Experimental models for human use are now being manufactured (9, 10, 44). Such a system may prove to be essential in the individual with juvenile diabetes who wishes to engage in regular physical activities.

REFERENCES

1. Aerts L, Van Asshe FA: Ultrastructural changes of the endocrine pancreas in pregnant rats. *Diabetologia* 11:285–289, 1975.
2. Artal R, Golde SH, Dorey F, McClellan SN, Gratacos J, Lirette T, Montoro M, Wu PYK, Anderson B, Mestman J: The effect of plasma glucose variability on neonatal outcome in the pregnant diabetic. *Am J Obstet Gynecol* 147:537–541, 1983.
3. Artal R, Wiswell R, Romem Y, Kammula RK, Sperling M: Hormonal responses to exercise in pregnant diabetic and non-diabetic patients. In Proceedings of the Society for Gynecologic Investigation 1983, p 225.
4. Bellman O, Hartmann E: Influence of pregnancy on the kinetics of insulin. *Am J Obstet Gynecol* 122:829–833, 1975.
5. Berle P, Finsterwalder E, Apostolakis M: Comparative studies on the effect of human growth hormone, human prolactin and human placental lactogen on lipid metabolism. *Horm Metab Res* 6:847–350, 1974.
6. Bessman SP: Diabetes mellitus: Observations, theoretical and practical. *J Pediatr* 56:191–203, 1960.
7. Bessman SP: Interrelations of various food materials. In Ghadim H (ed): *Total Parenteral Nutrition.* New York, John Wiley & Sons, 1975, pp 335–342.
8. Bessman SP, Fonio A: The possible role of the mitochondria bound creatine kinase in regulation of mitochondrial respiration. *Biochem Biophys Res Commun* 22:597–602, 1966.
9. Bessman SP, Geiger PG: Transport of energy in muscle: the phosphorylcreatine shuttle. *Science* 211:448–452, 1981.
10. Bessman SP, Schultz RD: Progress toward a glucose sensor for the artificial pancreas. In *Ion Selective Microelectrodes.* New York, Plenum Press, 1974, pp 184–197.
11. Blechner JN, Stenger VG, Prystowski H: Blood flow to the human uterus during maternal metabolic acidosis. *Am J Obstet Gynecol* 121:789–794, 1975.
12. Burden J, Harrison DJ, Hillhouse EW, Ironmonger MR, Jones MT: Effect of chlorpromazine, pentabarbitone, vasopressin, angiotensin II, bradykinin and ACTH on secretion of CRF from hypothalamus in vitro. *J Endocrinol* 67:45p, 1975.
13. Burke CW, Roulet F: Increased exposure of tissues to cortisol in late pregnancy. *Br Med J* 1:657–659, 1970.
14. Churchill JA, Berendes HW, Nemore J: Neuropsychological deficits in children of diabetic mothers. A report from the collaborative study of cerebral palsy. *Am J Obstet Gynecol* 105:257–268, 1969.
15. Costrini NV, Kalkhoff RK: Relative effects of pregnancy estradiol and progesterone on plasma insulin and pancreatic islet insulin secretion. *J Clin Invest* 50:992, 1971.
16. Demey-Ponsart E, Foidart JM, Sulon J, Sodoyez JC: Serum CBG, free and total cortisol and circadian patterns of adrenal function in normal pregnancy. *J Steroid Biochem* 16:165–169, 1982.
17. Fadel HE, Hammond SD: Diabetes mellitus and pregnancy. *J Reprod Med* 27:56–66, 1982.
18. Falkmar S, Wilson S: Comparative aspects of the immunology and biology of insulin. *Diabetologia* 3:519–528, 1967.
19. Felig P, Lynch V: Starvation in human pregnancy: Hypoglycemia, hypoinsulinemia and hyperketonuria. *Science* 170:990–992, 1970.
20. Fisher PM, Sutherland HW, Bewsher PD: The insulin response to glucose infusion in gestational diabetes. *Diabetologia* 19:10, 1980.
21. Freinkel N: Effect of the conceptus on maternal metabolism during pregnancy. In Liebel GS, Wrenshall CA (eds): *On the Nature and Treatment of Diabetes.* Amsterdam, Excerpta Medica Foundation, 1965.
22. Freinkel N, Metzger BE, Nitzan M, Daniel R, Surmaczynska BZ, Nagel TC: Facilitated anabolism in late pregnancy: some novel maternal compensation for accelerated starvation. In Malaisse WJ, Pirart J (eds): *Proceedings of the Eight Congress of the International Diabetes Federation.* Amsterdam, Excerpta Medica, 1975.
23. Genazani AR, Pocolar F, Neri P, Fioretti P: Human chorionic somatomammotropin (HCS): plasma levels in normal and pathological pregnancies and their correlation with placental function. *Acta Endocrinol* 167(suppl):1–39, 1972.
24. Gillmer MDG, Beard RW, Brooke FM, Oakley NW: Carbohydrate metabolism in pregnancy; Part I. Durnal plasma glucose profile in normal and diabetic women. *Br Med J* 3:399–401, 1975.
25. Gillmer MDG, Beard RW, Oakley NW, Brooke FM, Elphick MC, Hall D: Durnal plasma free fatty acid profile in normal and diabetic pregnancies. *Br Med J* 2:670–673, 1977.
26. Gillmer MDG, Persson B: Metabolism during normal and diabetic pregnancy and its effect on neonatal outcome. In *Pregnancy Metabolism, Diabetes and the Fetus.* Ciba Foundation Symposium No. 63, 1979, pp 93–121.
27. Goebelsmann U: Protein and steroid hormones in pregnancy. *J Reprod Med* 23:166–177, 1979.
28. Goodner CJ, Frienkel N: Carbohydrate metabolism in pregnancy: The turnover of I^{131}-insulin in the pregnant rat. *Endocrinology* 67:862–872, 1960.
29. Gustafson AB, Banasiak MF, Kalkhoff RK, Hagen

TC, Kim HK: Correlation of hyperprolactinemia with altered insulin and glucagon: similarity of effects of late human pregnancy. *J Clin Endocrinol Metab* 51:242–246, 1980.
30. Hawkins RA, Williamson DH, Krebs HA: Ketone body utilization by adult and suckling rat brain in vivo. *Biochem J* 122:13–18, 1971.
31. Hytten FE, Leitch I: *The Physiology of Human Pregnancy*, ed 2. Oxford, Blackwell, 1971, pp 333–369.
32. Hytten FE, Thompson AM, Taggart N: Total body water in normal pregnancy. *Obstet Gynaecol Br Commonw* 73:553–561, 1966.
33. Jacobs LS, Daughaday WH: Physiologic regulation of prolactin secretion in man. In Josimovich JB, Reynolds M, Cobo E (eds): *Lactogenic Hormones, Fetal Nutrition and Lactation*. New York, John Wiley & Sons, 1974, pp 351–377.
34. Jacobson HN: Nutrition and pregnancy. In Wallace H, Gold EM, Lis EF (eds): *Maternal and Child Health Practices*. Springfield, Ill., Charles C Thomas, 1973.
35. Johnstone FD, Campbell DM, MacGillivaray I: Nitrogen balance studies in human pregnancy. *J Nutr* 111:1884–1893, 1981.
36. Kalkhoff RH, Kissebah AH, Kim HG: Carbohydrates and lipid metabolism in pregnancy: relationship to gestational hormone action. *Semin Perinatol* 2:291–307, 1978.
37. Kalkhoff RK, Jacobson M, Lember D: Progesterone pregnancy and the augmented plasma insulin response. *J Clin Endocrinol Metab* 31:24–28, 1970.
38. Karlsson K, Kjellmer I: The outcome of diabetic pregnancies in relation to the mother's blood sugar level. *Am J Obstet Gynecol* 112:213–220, 1972.
39. King JC: Protein metabolism during pregnancy. *Clin Perinatol* 2:243–254, 1975.
40. Knopp RH, Herrera E, Freinkel N: Carbohydrate metabolism in pregnancy; VIII. Metabolism of adipose tissue isolated from fed and fasted pregnant rats during late gestation. *J Clin Invest* 49:1438–1446, 1970.
41. Knopp RH, Montes A, Childs M, Job RL, Hirushi M: Metabolic adjustments in normal and diabetic pregnancy. *Clin Obstet Gynecol* 24:21–49, 1981.
42. Koren Z, Shafrir E: Placental transfer of free fatty acids in the pregnant rat. *Proc Soc Exp Biol Med* 116:411–414, 1964.
43. Krauth MC, Schillinger E: Changes in insulin receptor concentration in rat fat cells following treatment with the gestagens clomegestone acetate and cyproterone acetate. *Acta Endocrinol (Copenh)* 86:667–672, 1977.
44. Layne EC, Schiltz RD, Thomas LJ, Slama G, Sayler DF, Bessman SP: Continuous extracorporeal monitoring of animal blood using the glucose electrode. *Diabetes* 25:81–89, 1976.
45. Lind T, Billewicz WZ, Browh G: A serial study of changes occurring in the oral glucose tolerance test in pregnancy. *J Obstet Gynaecol Br Commonw* 80:1033–1039, 1973.
46. Londholm K, Edstrom S, Ekman L, Karlberg I, Walker P, Schersten T: Protein degradation in human skeletal muscle tissue: the effect of insulin, leucine, amino acids and ions. *Clin Sci* 60:391–326, 1981.
47. McDonald-Gibson RG, Young M, Hytten FE: Changes in plasma nonesterified fatty acids and serum glycerol in pregnancy. *Br J Obstet Gynaecol* 82:460–466, 1975.
48. Metzger BE, Freinkel N: Effects of diabetes mellitus in the endocrinologic and the metabolic adaptation of gestation. *Semin Perinatol* 2:309–318, 1978.
49. Metzger BE, Ravnikar V, Vileisis RA, Freinkel N: "Accelerated starvation" and the skipped breakfast in late normal pregnancy. *Lancet* 1:588–592, 1982.
50. Mohan C, Bessman SP: In vitro protein degradation measured by differential loss of methionine and 3-methylhistidine: The effect of insulin. *Anal Biochem* 118:11–22, 1981.
51. Naeye RL, Chez RA: Effects of maternal acetonuria and low pregnancy weight gain on childrens' psychomotor development. *Am J Obstet Gynecol* 139:189–193, 1981.
52. Naeye RL: *The Outcome of Diabetic Pregnancies: A Prospective Study*. Amsterdam, Ciba Foundation Symposium No. 63, Excerpta Medica, 1979, pp 227–241.
53. Naismith DJ: The fetus as a parasite. *Proc Nutr Soc* 28:25–31, 1969.
54. Nattras M, Alberti KGMM, Dennis KJ, Gillbrand PN, Letchworth AT, Buckle ALJ: A glucose-controlled insulin infusion system for diabetic women during labour. *Br Med J* 2:599–601, 1978.
55. Oakey RE: The progressive increase in estrogen production in human pregnancy: an appraisal of factors responsible. *Vitam Horm* 1:36, 1970.
56. Pagano G, Cassoder M, Massobri M, Bozzon C, Tossare GF, Menato G, Lenti G: Insulin binding in human adipocytes during late pregnancy in healthy, obese and diabetic states. *Horm Metab Res* 12:177–181, 1980.
57. Persson B, Lunell NO: Metabolic control in diabetic pregnancy. *Am J Obstet Gynecol* 122:737–745, 1975.
58. Potter JM, Reckless JPD, Cullen DR: The effect of continuous subcutaneous insulin infusion and conventional insulin regimes on 24-hour variations of glucose and intermediary metabolites in the third trimester of pregnancy. *Diabetologia* 21:534–539, 1981.
59. Puavilai G, Drobny EC, Domont LA, Baumann G: Insulin receptors and insulin resistance in human pregnancy: evidence for a post-receptor defect in insulin action. *J Clin Endocrinol Metab* 54:247–253, 1982.
60. Rall TW, Sutherland EW: Formation of cyclic adenine ribonucleotide by tissue particles. *J Biol Chem* 232:1065–1076, 1958.
61. Rathgeb I, Winkler B, Steel R, Alszuler N: Effect of ovine prolactin adminstration on glucose metab-

olism and insulin levels in the dog. *Endocrinology* 88:718–722, 1971.
62. Rigg LA, Lein A, Yen SSC: Pattern of increase in circulating prolactin levels during human gestation. *Am J Obstet Gynecol* 129:454–456, 1977.
63. Rudolf MCJ, Coustan DR, Sherwin RS, Bates SE, Felig P: Efficacy of insulin pump in the home treatment of pregnant diabetics. *Diabetes* 30:891–895, 1981.
64. Santiago JV, Clarke WL, Arias F: Studies with a pancreatic beta cell simulator in the third trimester of pregnancy complicated by diabetes. *Am J Obstet Gynecol* 132:455–463, 1978.
65. Schade DS, Perkins RP, Drumm DA: Interpreting Ketosis warning in pregnancy. *Contemp Obstet Gynecol* 21(6):91–109, 1983.
66. Schulman PK, Gyves MT, Merkatz IR: Role of nutrition in the management of the pregnant diabetic patient. In Merkatz IR, Adams PAJ (eds): *The Diabetic Pregnancy: A Perinatal Perspective.* New York, Grune & Stratton, 1979, pp 35–44.
67. Seeds AE, Knowles HC: Metabolic control of diabetic pregnancy. *Clin Obstet Gynecol* 24:51–62, 1981.
68. Silverstone FA, Solomon E, Rubricius J: The rapid intravenous glucose tolerance test in pregnancy. *J Clin Invest* 40:2180–2189, 1961.
69. Sinclair JC: Metabolic rate and temperature control. In Smith CA, Nelson NM (eds): *The Physiology of the Human Infant,* Ed 4. Springfield, Ill., Charles C Thomas, 1976, p 354.
70. Sonksen PH: Home monitoring of blood glucose by diabetic patients. *Acta Endocrinol* 94(238):145–155, 1980.
71. Soskin S: *The Endocrines in Diabetes.* Springfield, Ill., Charles C Thomas, 1948.
72. Spellacy WN, Goetz FC: Plasma insulin in normal late pregnancy. *N Engl J Med* 268:988–991, 1963.
73. Spray CM. A study of some aspects of reproduction by means of chemical analysis. *Br J Nutr* 4:354–360, 1950.
74. Stehbens JA, Baker GL, Kitchell M: Outcome at age 1, 3 and 5 years of age of children born to diabetic women. *Am J Obstet Gynecol* 127:408–413, 1977.
75. Sutherland EW, Rall TW: The relation of adenosin 3′,5′-phosphate and phosphorylase to the action of catecholamines and other hormones. *Pharmacol Rev* 12:265–299, 1960.
76. Tevaarwerk GJM, Harding PGR, Milne KJ, Jaco NT, Rodger NW, Hurst C: Pregnancy in diabetic women: Outcome with a program aimed to normal glycemia before meals. *Can Med Assoc J* 125:435–441, 1982.
77. The Collaborative Study on Cerebral Palsy: Mental retardation and other neurological and sensory disorders of infancy and childhood manual. Bethesda, Md., U.S. Department of Health, Education and Welfare, 1966.
78. Tyson JE, Austin K, Farinholt J, Fiedler J: Endocrine-metabolic response to acute starvation in human gestation. *Am J Obstet Gynecol* 125:1073–1084, 1976.
79. Tyson JE, Jones GS, Huth J, Thomas P: Patterns of insulin, growth hormone, and placental lactogen release after protein and glucose protein ingestion in pregnancy. *Am J Obstet Gynecol* 110:934, 1971.
80. Webber RJ, Edmond M: The in vivo utiliation of acetoacetate, D-(−)-3-hydroxybutyrate, and glucose for lipid synthesis in brain of 18-day-old rat. Evidence for an acetyl-CoA bypass to sterol synthesis. *J Biol Chem* 254:3912–3920, 1979.
81. Widdowson EM: The demands of the fetal and maternal tissues for nutrients, and the bearing of these on the need of the mother to "eat for two." In Dobbing J (ed): *Maternal Nutrition in Pregnancy—Eating for Two?* London, Academic Press, 1981, pp 1–17.
82. Yang WCT, Geiger PJ, Bessman SP, Borrebaek B: Formation of creatine phosphate from creatine and 32P-labeled ATP by isolated rabbit heart mitochondria. *Biochem Biophys Res Commun* 76:882–887, 1977.
83. Yen SSC, Samaan N, Pearson OH: Growth hormone levels in pregnancy. *J Clin Endocrinol Metab* 27:1341–1347, 1967.
84. Zaidise I, Bessman SP: The diabetic syndrome—uncontrolled stress. In Belfiore F, Galton DJ, Reaven GM (eds): *Frontiers in Diabetes.* Basil, Karger, 1984, vol 4, pp 77–92.
85. Zuspan SP: Urinary excretion of epinephrine and norepinephrine during pregnancy. *J Clin Endocrinol* 30:357–360, 1970.

7
Nutritional Needs of Physically Active Pregnant Women

During pregnancy, the mother's diet supplies the nutrients needed by the fetus for development. If the nutrient supply from the diet is deficient, fetal growth may slow and an infant with a high risk of morbidity and mortality may be born (4). The dramatic detrimental effect of severe maternal food restriction on fetal growth was demonstrated in western Holland during the winter months of 1944–1945 when, as a result of a food embargo, the population had its average daily food ration reduced from 1800 to 600 kcal per day (50). The famine lasted 28 weeks, and some women were affected during the last two trimesters of pregnancy. In these women, the average birth weight fell 327 g, or 9%, compared to the prefamine mean value. Also, the incidence of stillbirths and neonatal mortality increased.

Today, situations still exist where a poor maternal diet reduces fetal growth. Among low income women in developing countries, the food supply is limited, and infants born to these underfed women weigh an average of 300 g less at birth than infants born to well-fed mothers. However, maternal malnutrition also exists among more affluent women who either are advised to or choose to limit their food intake. For example, the average birth weight of all infants born in Motherwell, Scotland, between 1938 and 1977 was 400 g less than in Aberdeen, Scotland, because all pregnant women in Motherwell at that time were advised to restrict their food intake (35). Fetal growth retardation is very likely if the maternal food supply and, therefore, dietary energy supply is restricted.

Heavy maternal physical activity can expend the available maternal energy and possibly deprive the fetus of needed energy for growth. For example, the birth weights of infants born to women in developing countries during the months of heavy agricultural labor are lower than those born at other times of the year (47). Due to a poor food supply, these women are also consuming low calorie diets. In more affluent societies, recreational physical activity has become quite popular, and it is frequently continued throughout pregnancy. It is unlikely that this physical activity will restrict fetal growth because the total energy expenditure of these women is not as great as that of women agricultural workers in developing countries and their food supply is not limited. But, these physically active women may have some nutritional needs which differ from those of sedentary pregnant women.

At this time, the nutritional needs of physically active pregnant women are undefined. Therefore, inferences must be drawn from knowledge of the nutritional requirements of pregnant, sedentary women and of nonpregnant, active women. Before discussing the nutritional needs of active pregnant women in this chapter, we will first review those of pregnant sedentary women and those of active nonpregnant women.

NUTRIENT REQUIREMENTS OF PREGNANT SEDENTARY WOMEN

Nutritional advice given to pregnant women varies between and within cultures. Some cultures recommend nutritious foods for the pregnant woman, such as leafy greens, fruits, and milk. Others forbid foods that clearly make an important nutrient contribution to the diet. For example, one African tribe forbids eggs and milk during pregnancy (49). Within Westernized cultures, nutritional advice seems to change with generations. Presently, pregnant women are advised to eat to appetite, gain approximately 25 lb, salt their food to taste, and breast-feed their infants. This prescription is exactly the opposite of what their mothers were told.

It is becoming evident from a historical and cultural review of food practices during pregnancy that there are many different, acceptable ways of providing the nutrients needed for fetal growth. This diversity of practice is an important issue to keep in mind when counseling pregnant women about their dietary habits. It is not necessary that all women consume meat, milk, vegetables, and bread. But, it is important that they select carefully from a wide variety of foods to provide the calories and nutrients needed for the fetus and themselves.

Energy

Total caloric intake appears to be the most important nutritional factor affecting infant birth weight. It has been estimated that a typical pregnancy requires about 80,000 additional calories, or approximately 300 extra calories per day above that needed in the nonpregnant state (34). About one-third of these calories are accounted for by maternal fat gain. The remainder is primarily the energy needed for metabolism by the new tissue gained.

If energy intake is sufficient, the total weight gain during pregnancy averages between 10 and 12 kg (34). However, individual energy intakes and weight gains vary widely. Maternal pregravid weight and daily energy expenditure are two factors which influence appetite, energy intake, and weight gain.

Women who begin pregnancy weighing 15% or more below the suggested weight for their height deliver low birth weight infants more frequently and have a greater risk of developing preeclampsia and preterm labor (33). Intensive nutritional counseling and provision of supplemental calories in the form of high quality foods has been successful in improving their weight gain and in increasing infant birth weight (48). Therefore, underweight women should be encouraged to increase their energy intake and to gain between 12 and 15 kg.

Obese women (greater than 20% above standard weight for height) more frequently deliver large infants (greater than 4.0 kg). These women also are prone to develop glucose intolerance or hypertension during gestation. Food restriction and weight reduction are not recommended during pregnancy, however. Past studies of food restriction in obese pregnant women indicate that maternal fat losses are very low. For example, a 500-kcal restriction daily during the last 10 weeks of pregnancy caused less than a 0.5-kg maternal fat loss (16). This small fat loss does not warrant the discomfort of a restricted food intake during pregnancy when appetite is increased and the woman is prone to hypoglycemia.

A gradual, progressive weight gain of 9–11 kg is ideal for obese pregnant women. This goal is best attained through individual diet assessment and counseling with emphasis on foods rich in nutrients but low in fat. Breast-feeding should be encouraged, and, following weaning, a comprehensive program of exercise and diet for weight reduction suggested. Occasionally, a very obese woman loses weight during pregnancy without conscious dieting. The mechanism for this weight loss is unknown, but infant birth weight is not affected negatively.

In all pregnant women, a weight gain of less than 1.0 kg per month during the last two trimesters is considered to be insufficient (44). A low rate of weight gain may lead to delivery of a low birth weight infant. In obese women, a low weight gain does not seem to be as detrimental as in an underweight woman (26). Possibly, lower weight gains are better tolerated by obese women because some of the energy needed for pregnancy can be provided by maternal stores. Or, the metabolic adjustments associated with obesity may alter the use of energy for fetal growth.

Identification of excessive weight gain can be difficult in pregnant women. Individual variability leads to a wide range of weight gains compatible with appropriate birthweights. What is excessive for one woman may not be for another. Also, in pregnancy, excessive weight gain may result from accumulation of body water as well as body fat, and it is difficult to distinguish the two types of tissue gain. Sometimes the pattern of weight gain is helpful in assessing the composition of tissue gain. Water may be accumulated more rapidly than fat.

Excessive fat gain during pregnancy does not appear to cause preeclampsia, as thought previously. But, unless the woman is underweight or carrying twins or triplets, gaining more than 16–18 kg can lead to postpartum obesity and a source of anxiety for some women. If weight gain is high, food restriction should not be initiated in the third trimester when fetal growth is maximal and most sensitive to growth retardation. Instead, reduced intakes of fats and sweets and increased exercise can help normalize the rate of weight gain until term.

It is insufficient to consider only the total energy intake when counseling pregnant women; the source of calories should also be reviewed. Nutrient density, the quantity of protein, vitamins and minerals per 100 calories, is a measure of diet quality. The recommended additional calories for pregnancy, 300 kcal per day, can easily be provided by many different foods. Depending on the food choice, additional nutrients may also be provided or the food may only provide "empty calories." A pint of low fat milk or a peanut butter sandwich on whole grain bread each provide about 300 kcal, as do six small cookies or a 12-oz can of soda and 10 french-fried potatoes. The milk or sandwich have a much higher nutrient density than the cookies or soda with french fries. The iron density of common foods is compared in Table 7.1. This information may be helpful in counseling pregnant women to select foods with a high iron density.

Protein

An additional 30 g protein, or a total of 76 g, is recommended for pregnancy (41). But, protein-rich foods are plentiful in the United States, and *nonpregnant* women often select diets which provide more than the amount recommended for pregnancy. If this is true, no further increase in protein is needed for pregnancy. Protein-containing foods are excellent sources of many vitamins and minerals essential for fetal growth and development, such as iron, vitamin B_6, and zinc. There is, however, no evidence that high protein diets, greater than 100 g per day, are beneficial during prgnancy, and at least one study has suggested that "excessive amounts" may be harmful (51). An intake of 75–100 g protein per day, or 12% of the calories as protein calories, should be appropriate for pregnancy. Some animal protein sources, such as red meat, whole milk, and cheese are high in saturated fats. These foods should be limited and consumption of chicken, fish, nonfat milk, and vegetable protein sources, such as beans, encouraged.

Vegetarian Diets

Within the past 10 years, diets which exclude some or all animal protein sources have become quite popular. These diets can provide adequate nutrition for pregnant women, but more care in food selection is needed. Diets that include dairy products and/or eggs easily provide the nutrients needed for pregnancy. But, if all animal protein sources are avoided, vitamin B_{12} intakes will be inadequate and zinc, iron, calcium, vitamin D, and riboflavin intakes may

Table 7.1. Iron Density of Some Foods

Food	Serving Size	Iron mg/serving	Iron mg/100 kcal
Dairy products			
Milk			
Whole	1 cup	0.1	0.1
Nonfat	1 cup	0.1	0.1
Yogurt, plain	8 oz	0.2	0.1
Cheese, cheddar	1 oz	0.2	0.2
Meat and meat alternatives			
Hamburger	3 oz	2.6	1.1
Beef stew	1 cup	2.9	1.3
Chili	1 cup	4.3	1.3
Chicken			
Thigh	1 medium	1.2	1.0
Breast	½	1.3	0.8
Eggs	1 whole	1.0	1.2
Fish sticks	4 sticks	0.4	0.2
Salmon	1 average steak	1.5	0.7
Sardines	3 oz	2.4	1.4
Tuna, in water	3 oz	1.6	1.2
Lamb, leg	3 oz	1.9	1.2
Lentils, cooked	½ cup	2.1	1.9
Liver, calf	3 oz	12.1	5.5
Macaroni and cheese	1 cup	1.8	0.4
Oysters	6	8.6	7.8
Peanut butter	1 tbsp	0.3	0.3
Pork chop	1 medium	1.6	1.5
Frankfurter	1 average	0.7	0.5
Liverwurst	1 oz	1.5	1.8
Tofu	1 2-inch cube	2.3	2.7
Turkey			
Dark	3 oz	2.0	1.2
Light	3 oz	1.0	0.7
Vitamin C-rich fruits and vegetables			
Grapefruit	½ raw	0.4	1.0
Lemonade	1 cup	0.1	0.1
Cantaloupe	½ melon	0.6	1.2
Orange juice	¾ cup	0.4	0.5
Green peppers	½ cup	0.5	3.3
Dark leafy green vegetables			
Broccoli	½ cup	0.6	3.0
Romaine lettuce	1 cup	0.8	8.0
Spinach	½ cup cooked	2.0	10.0
Swiss chard	½ cup cooked	1.3	8.7
Other fruits and vegetables			
Apricots, canned	4 halves	0.4	0.4
Banana	1 medium	0.8	0.8
Cabbage, cooked	½ cup	0.2	1.3
Carrots, boiled	½ cup	0.4	2.0
Corn, sweet	½ cup	0.4	0.6
Peas, canned	½ cup	1.6	2.1
Potatoes			
Baked	1 large	1.1	0.8
French-fried	20 each	0.8	0.4
Sprouts, alfalfa	1 cup	1.4	3.5
Raisins	½ cup	1.3	1.3

Table 7.1.—*Continued*

Food	Serving Size	Iron mg/serving	Iron mg/100 kcal
Breads and cereals			
Whole wheat bread	1 slice	0.8	1.2
White			
Enriched	1 slice	0.6	0.9
Unenriched	1 slice	0.2	0.3
Cereals			
Bran flakes	1 cup	12.4	12.4
Corn flakes	1 cup	0.6	0.6
Puffed rice	1 cup	0.3	0.5
Oatmeal	½ cup	0.7	1.1
Grits	½ cup	0.2	0.3
Other foods			
Cracker, graham	1 cracker	0.2	0.4
Doughnut, cake	1 average	0.6	0.4
Noodles, enriched	⅔ cup cooked	0.9	0.9
Popcorn	1 cup w/oil	0.2	0.5
Wheat germ	1 oz	2.5	2.1

be low. Also, due to the low fat and high bulk of vegetarian food sources, pregnant women may have difficulty consuming sufficient energy. Vitamin and mineral supplements may be recommended when the dietary assessment shows that intakes are inadequate. Use of vegetable oils and fats should be encouraged if the rate of weight gain is low as a result of insufficient energy intakes. Vegetable protein foods should be combined to ensure adequate protein quality at each meal. Guidelines for patient education have been prepared (14).

Iron

Additional iron is needed during pregnancy for expansion of maternal red blood cell volume and for fetal erythropoiesis and tissue gain. About 800 mg iron are gained during the last half of pregnancy; this is about 5–6 mg daily (39). Since most women cannot provide this iron without depletion of their own stores, a daily oral supplement providing 30–60 mg elemental iron is recommended (41) for all pregnant women. A reduction in mean corpuscular volume along with a fall in hemoglobin and hematocrit is indicative of iron depletion during pregnancy. Women with such iron depletion should be given therapeutic doses of iron.

Food selection not only influences the amount of iron ingested (Table 7.1), but it also influences the amount of iron which will be absorbed. Some foods enhance iron absorption in the gut, whereas others inhibit it. Animal protein, or the "meat factor," and ascorbic acid enhance iron absorption (41). Tea binds iron in the gut and reduces its absorption. Tea should be avoided at meals when good iron sources are consumed. Also, iron absorption will be reduced if iron pills are taken with tea or milk. Cast iron pans may provide significant amounts of iron, particularly if acidic foods, such as spaghetti sauce, are cooked in the pans.

Calcium

A daily allowance of 1200 mg calcium is recommended to provide the 30 g of calcium gained during pregnancy without maternal skeletal demineralization (41). Although rare, neonatal hypocalcemia has been reported when maternal calcium and/or vitamin D intakes were inadequate (45).

A quart of cow's milk would provide most of the calcium and vitamin D recommended for pregnancy and a signifciant amount of protein. But, many ethnic groups, including people of Asian, Black, and Middle Eastern descent, are lactase deficient and are unable to digest the lactose in milk. These people may experience abdominal cramping, bloating, flatulence, and diarrhea when milk is consumed. Low lactose dairy products are cheese and yogurt. These foods may be substituted for milk. Other calcium-rich foods include salmon or sardines, fortified soymilk, ground sesame seeds, and leafy green vegetables.

Sodium

The increase in total body water by pregnant women also causes an increase in total body sodium. The net gain is about 22 g sodium (34). This gain occurs even though there is an increase in the glomerular filtration rate and in natriuretic hormones.

In the past, salt was forbidden to pregnant women, and diuretics were used whenever edema occurred. It was then thought that high sodium intakes caused toxemia and that the condition could be treated effectively with sodium restriction and diuretics (18). Now it appears that sodium restriction does not prevent toxemia, nor is it an effective way to treat toxemia. Diuretics are discouraged during pregnancy because they can cause electrolyte imbalances, hyperglycemia, hyperuricemia and other problems, and women are told to "salt to taste." High salt diets are not condoned, however, because they may precipitate hypertension in susceptible individuals. A diet composed primarily of natural foods can be safely salted "to taste"; processed foods are already seasoned with salt and should be used in moderation without further salting.

Other Nutrients

The dietary need for folic acid is increased during pregnancy for support of tissue synthesis. A 200–400-μg supplement may be needed to meet the 800 μg suggested intake (41). Foods rich in folic acid include eggs, leafy vegetables, oranges, legumes, whole grain cereals, and wheat germ.

Refinement of grains removes many nutrients in the germ and bran. Of particular concern are zinc, vitamin B_6, magnesium, and vitamin E because these nutrients are not replaced during the enrichment process. To assure an adequate intake of these nutrients for increased metabolic needs of pregnancy, whole grain cereals should be used. Whole grains also are excellent sources of fiber.

WOMEN AT NUTRITIONAL RISK DURING PREGNANCY

Women who may be at risk for nutritional problems are listed in Table 7.2. In general, women at risk are those who have economic, social, or medical problems that may lead to nutritional problems. Women with these problems often develop malnutrition because they do not consume enough food or because they make poor food choices. Asking a woman what she usually eats and then estimating her intake during the previous 24 hours will identify nutritional problems due to insufficient amounts of food or poor food choices. Presence of a poor weight gain pattern, obesity or under-

Table 7.2. Nutritional Risks during Pregnancy

1. Pregravid weight 15% below or 20% above suggested weight for height
2. Insufficient or excessive rate of weight gain
3. Age of less than 15 years or more than 35 years
4. Presence of social, cultural, religious, psychological or economic factors that limit or affect adequacy of nutrition
5. History of a low birth weight baby or other obstetric problems
6. Chronic disease, such as diabetes, thyroid disorders, or sickle cell disease
7. Presence of twins or triplets
8. Pica
9. Abnormal laboratory values, such as low hemoglobin level, abnormal blood glucose level, albuminuria, and ketonuria

weight, or anemia is documentation of poor dietary habits and malnutrition. These women need in-depth nutritional counseling and follow-up.

NUTRITIONAL ADVICE FOR PREGNANT WOMEN

Nutritional counseling for pregnant women should emphasize the use of a wide variety of foods. A low fat diet composed of lean animal foods, nonfat dairy products, and limited amounts of added fat is recommended for the average women. Soft drinks, alcoholic beverages, pastries, and candy have a low nutrient density and should be limited in the diet along with high fat, salty snacks such as potato chips. Total food intake should be increased to provide about 300 additional calories daily. A supplement providing 30–60 mg iron and 200–400 µg folic acid is suggested as is the use of iodized salt. A prenatal vitamin-mineral supplement may be provided, but probably is not necessary if nutrient dense foods are routinely selected.

NUTRIENT REQUIREMENTS OF ACTIVE NONPREGNANT WOMEN

At present, there is little specific information regarding nutrient needs of active women; most studies of nutrient needs of athletes have been done on men. In general, however, the needs of the athlete differ little from those of the sedentary individual, with the exception of those nutrients lost during an exercise bout (energy, water, and electrolytes) and those nutrients necessary for release of the energy expended. The general dietary advice for the physically active woman is similar to that of the nonactive pregnant women, i.e., to eat to appetite from a wide variety of foods, and to give special attention to those foods which replace the components lost during a training event.

Energy

As with the pregnant woman, energy is the most important nutrient for the athlete. Without adequate energy intake to cover that expended in all daily activities, both training and routine maintenance, lean tissue mass, the predominant component of which is muscle, is lost (15). In addition, fat stores cannot be maintained. Recommendations for energy intakes, as set by the National Research Council (41) assume only a small proportion of light activity daily in addition to sedentary maintenance activities. To estimate total energy needs for the woman who participates in significant strenuous activity, an amount of energy equivalent to that expended during the strenuous activities must be added to the maintenance need (see Table 7.3 for list of energy expenditures for nonpregnant women performing various strenuous activities). In addition, exercise may increase the basal energy needs (9) and/or the energy expended in response to a meal (22), contributing further to an increased energy requirement.

Table 7.3. Approximate Energy Expenditure at Various Strenuous Activities[a]

Activity	Energy Expended (kcal/min)
Walking, on level, without load	
2 mph	2.5
2.5 mph	2.9
3 mph	4
4 mph	6
Walking, uphill, 2 mph	
10% grade	5
20% grade	6.5
Running	
Cross country (3–4 mph)	10
Track (10 mph)	20
Cycling	
5.5 mph	4
10 mph	6.5
13 mph	9
Dancing	
Waltz	5
Square	8
Swimming	
Leisurely	4.5
Breast or back stroke	9
Crawl	13

[a] Adapted from G. M. Briggs and D. H. Calloway: *Nutrition and Physical Fitness*, ed. 11, Philadelphia, W. B. Saunders Co., 1984; and P. Astrand and K. Rodahl: *Textbook of Work Physiology*, ed. 2, New York, McGraw-Hill, 1977.

Actual energy intakes of many active women seem to fall far short of the theoretical totals derived from their maintenance and activity requirements. In some cases, such as ballet dancers (42) and gymnasts (38), these low energy intakes are designed to maintain body weight (and body fat) well below the mean for age and height. In other cases, such as runners, these lower than expected intakes are associated with maintenance of normal body weight (12). In women running less than 25 miles per week (considered moderately active), energy intakes were similar to those reported by sedentary women. Maintenance of body weight on lower than expected energy intakes has been reported for individuals in underdeveloped countries, but the adaptive mechanism has not been identified. Both a decrease in time spent at other high energy expending activities, as found in individuals placed on an energy restricted diet (30), and an increase in the efficiency of energy utilization, as implicated in some obese individuals (46), are feasible mechanisms.

Composition of the food used to replace energy utilized in activities is also important. Complex carbohydrates are recommended in amounts to cover the energy expended at the activity because a high carbohydrate diet best replaces the critical fuel (muscle glycogen) lost during the exercise bout (20). Complex carbohydrates, such as whole grains, breads, pastas, and whole grain pastries, have the added benefit of providing matching amounts of the vitamins, niacin, and thiamin, required for energy release. The recommendation for these vitamins is proportional to energy intake (41). Fat, although providing energy in a very concentrated form, is ineffective at replacing the glycogen stores, and as such is discouraged as a major fuel replacement source.

Protein

There is evidence that protein is used both as a muscle fuel and as a substrate for gluconeogenesis at rest and during exercise. This utilization of protein may increase with training (54). However, the effect of these uses of protein on long-term total body protein (after days or weeks of exercise) in the athlete is not clear. Some investigators suggest 1.5–2 g dietary protein/kg body weight to maximize protein accumulation and to avoid the transient signs of protein insufficiency that may accompany initiation of an exercise program (i.e., decreased hemoglobin levels (53), or transient negative nitrogen balance (29). However, others have found accumulation of body protein in individuals initiating a moderate exercise program on protein intakes as low as 0.57 g/kg body weight provided energy intake was adequate for the added exercise (10). In any event, as stated above, the average protein intake in the United States is high and generally exceeds 1.5 g/kg body weight in women who have increased their overall food intake to accommodate an exercise program. There appears to be no increased need for protein with exercise which would warrant an increase in protein intake over that usually consumed.

In fact, a further increase in protein intake may have deleterious effects. Increased dietary protein has been shown to increase calcium and water excretion. Over the long-term, urinary calcium losses may contribute to bone demineralization and the development of osteoporosis (2). More immediately, the increase in water loss necessary to remove the by-products of protein degradation could contribute to an already potential dehydration state. In addition, high protein intakes have recently been implicated in the deterioration of kidney function in chronic renal failure (28).

Iron

Iron is a functional component of several of the elements necessary for oxygen transport (hemoglobin, myoglobin) and energy release (cytochromes). As these elements increase with training, one might expect the requirement for iron to increase. Such thinking, as well as reports of significant decreases in hemoglobin levels with repeated, strenuous activity (23), has led many coaches to recommend iron supplements to their athletes, both male and female. However, reports in the literature of anemia in athletes, as defined either by hemoglobin levels or iron binding capacity, indicate the condition to be no more prevalent in the athletes than in the general population (8). Evaluation of the effects of iron supplementation in active women with previously adequate hemoglobin levels have shown no consistent improvement in parameters of iron status or performance after supplementation (32). Assessment of iron store in a group of active women suggested that, as with the pregnant women, iron status is related more to dietary intake than to activity level (27). The effect of exercise on iron absorption is unknown.

Calcium

Exercise has a beneficial effect on bone density in men (55) and women (43), both young and old. The greater bone density of active individuals implies that calcium retention is higher in the active individual than it is in the inactive and that, perhaps, calcium utilization is improved by activity. There are also reports of increased bone density in postmenopausal women who have initiated an exercise program while consuming their usual intake of calcium (43). Thus, the need for calcium in the athlete is probably not greater than that of a sedentary individual. However, the high protein diets of many athletes, may, as indicated above, counteract any improvement in calcium utilization by increasing calcium excretion. Calcium intakes as high as 2 g/day were inadequate to maintain calcium balance in a group of male runners consuming 2 g protein/kg body weight (11).

Water

For every 580 kcal of energy used during an exercise bout, 1 liter of water may be lost in removing that heat from the body. This loss of body water leads to a decrease in circulating blood volume, which in turn, decreases the ability to further remove heat. Over a training session, as much as 3 or 4% of the body water may be lost, equivalent to about 6 lb in a 150-lb person. Such a decrease may hamper performance. Replacement of the water lost during an exercise bout as well as that required for removal of the waste products of protein degradation is necessary to ensure continued ability to train and perform. Unfortunately, in the chronically exercising individual, the thirst mechanism alone does not seem to be sufficient to insure complete rehydration; rather, only about 50% of that water lost over the day will be replaced, leaving the athlete chronically dehydrated, and with diminished blood volume (31). Maintenance of a preexercise weight log, with return to the previous day's pre-exercise weight as goal is a useful tool in insuring appropriate rehydration (7). A daily intake of 10–12 glasses of water or other fluids is not unreasonable for the training athlete.

A number of electrolytes are lost in association with water. (See Table 7.4 for primary components of sweat.) Of primary concern are sodium and potassium. Replenishing these electrolytes is mandatory for continued performance, and can be accomplished primarily by careful dietary choices.

Sodium

Although the loss of sodium in sweat is significant, several factors in the active individual compensate for that loss so that sodium is not an important concern for most athletes. First, with training, sweat sodium content decreases slightly, from 1.0 g/liter to around 0.8 g/liter, decreasing slightly the overall losses. In addition, the kidney conserves sodium when extracellular levels start

Table 7.4. Electrolyte Composition of Sweat (g/liter)[a]

Sodium	0.8–1.4
Chloride	1.0–1.75
Potassium	0.25–1.0
Magnesium	0.0004–0.004
Calcium	0.02–0.16

[a] Adapted from: C. F. Consolazio, R. E. Johnson, and L. J. Pecora: *Physiological Measurements of Metabolic Function in Man.* New York, McGraw-Hill, 1963.

to drop; this adaptive mechanism compensates for the loss of sodium in sweat. Many common foods naturally contain a significant amount of sodium so that the average intake may be as high as 5 or 6 g/day. With such high intakes and the ability to conserve body sodium, losses in sweat seldom become critical. Salt intake should only be monitored when exercising in the heat for extended periods of time (more than 2 hours). Under such circumstances, salting food to taste and eating salty foods should be adequate to replace the increased losses (24). Salt tablets are unnecessary.

Potassium

The question of potassium replacement is controversial. Potassium content of sweat (0.25–1 g/liter) is low in comparison to usual intakes (6–8 g), and highly variable. However, potassium losses in sweat during exercise in the heat may be as high as 6 g/day (13). Overt signs of potassium deficiency in athletes have not been reported, although the possibility of a subclinical deficiency leading to muscle necrosis has been suggested (36). Potassium is normally an intracellular cation; when extracellular potassium increases above a threshold level, the kidney excretes it. Because potassium is stored with glycogen, it is released when glycogen is burned, increasing the blood potassium levels during and immediately following an exercise bout. This transient increase may trigger the kidney's excretory mechanisms. Thus, significant amounts of potassium may be excreted post-exercise, with replenishment required to accompany replacement of the glycogen stores. Negative potassium balances have been reported in active individuals given 2–4 g of potassium per day (37). However, tissue potassium levels have been maintained in individuals exercising repeatedly for 4 days while consuming less than 1 g of potassium/day (19). In any event, thoughtful inclusions in the diet of high potassium foods such as citrus, cantaloupe, bananas and nuts may help to avoid any potential depletion.

Other Nutrients of Concern

Nutrient supplements often recommended for athletes include riboflavin, vitamin C, and vitamin E. Because riboflavin is necessary for the release of energy from foods, as are niacin and thiamin, one might expect the increased energy release which accompanies physical activity to create a need for riboflavin. Recent work on riboflavin requirements show an increased need in women *initiating* a moderate exercise program (3), but no improvement in riboflavin status or performance in trained swimmers given a 60-mg riboflavin/day supplement (52). In any event, the magnitude of any increased need is small and could be easily provided by the increased food intake accompanying exercise provided foods rich in riboflavin such as milk, yogurt, and whole wheat breads are included.

The answer to the question of need for the vitamins C and E is not so clear. Both of these vitamins act as antioxidants; in association with the increased flow of oxygen through the tissues with physical activity, there is an increase in tissue oxidative damage (21). It is not known if this increased need for detoxification of oxygen radicals increases the need for the antioxidant nutrients, vitamins C and E. In rats fed a vitamin E-deficient diet, red blood cell hemolysis, a sign of vitamin E deficiency, appeared more slowly in exercising animals than in sedentary ones (1). The need for vitamin C is even more controversial. Scientific evidence suggests there is no increase in need with exercise but lay publications continue to suggest supplementation. Studies of the effect of vitamin C supplementation on performance suggest that supplementation has little effect in individuals previously ingesting adequate amounts of vitamin C. In a group of individuals consuming a diet containing only that vitamin C found in foods (about 350 mg/day), serum levels of the vitamin were consistently higher in the active individuals than in the sedentary ones (25). In general, any increased need of athletes for these nutrients can probably be fulfilled by consuming a diet of a variety of foods from all of the food groups.

NUTRIENT RECOMMENDATIONS FOR ACTIVE PREGNANT WOMEN

As stated above, nutritional needs of the physically active pregnant woman have not been studied. However, based on our knowledge of the nutritional needs for pregnancy and for heavy activity, some general recommendations can be made.

Energy

The recommended additional energy for pregnancy, 300 calories per day, provides for only the increased basal metabolic needs. Energy needs for physical activity are greater in the pregnant than nonpregnant state because of the increased body weight; more energy is required to move the heavier body. At present, recommendations for energy intake during pregnancy include no addition for the increased energy cost of activity because it is assumed that pregnant women decrease their level of activity during pregnancy (41).

However, surveys of the activity patterns of pregnant women do not show that they become more sedentary (6). Instead, they tend to maintain the same pattern of activity throughout pregnancy, and the energy required for activities involving movement of the body, i.e., walking, is greater late in pregnancy than in mid-pregnancy (40). These data suggest that physically active pregnant women need more than 300 additional calories per day.

The energy needs of the physically active pregnant woman will vary with the amount of activity she performs. Therefore, it is impossible to make a general recommendation. As a beginning, however, 500 additional calories may be recommended for women who are maintaining a 30-min daily exercise program during pregnancy. (It is not advisable to initiate an exercise program during pregnancy.) More might be needed by those women who exercise more. If the rate of weight gain begins to fall below normal at any stage of pregnancy (Fig. 7.1), additional calories should be recommended. At all times, the physically active pregnant woman should be encouraged to eat to appetite since mankind has some ability to adjust energy intake to the physiological need. A physically active pregnant woman may be able to unconsciously adjust her intake to her level of expenditure. A diet high in complex carbohydrates is advised since carbohydrate best replaces muscle glycogen lost during exercise (See above).

Protein

Pregnancy increases the need for protein and, some feel that physical activity may do so as well. However, the usual dietary intake of protein in the United States is above the requirement for pregnancy and probably provides the additional needs for both pregnancy and exercise. It may be useful to base the protein recommendation for physically active pregnant women on energy intakes to assure that a high energy, high carbohydrate, low protein diet is not consumed. As stated previously, a diet providing 12% of the energy as protein should be adequate. This means that a woman consuming 2300 kcal/day should ingest 69 g protein, whereas a woman consuming 3000 kcal/day should ingest 90 g protein.

Iron

The iron needs of the trained pregnant woman maintaining her level of physical fitness are similar to those of sedentary pregnant women since additional iron does not appear to be required by the trained woman. Both sedentary and physically active pregnant women need to accumulate about 800 mg iron in the last half of pregnancy (39). To prevent depletion of maternal iron stores, this need is best provided by a 30–60-mg iron supplement. A pregnant woman initiating a training program would have greater iron needs since additional iron would be needed for blood volume expansion associated with training. Initiation of a training program during pregnancy is not recommended, however.

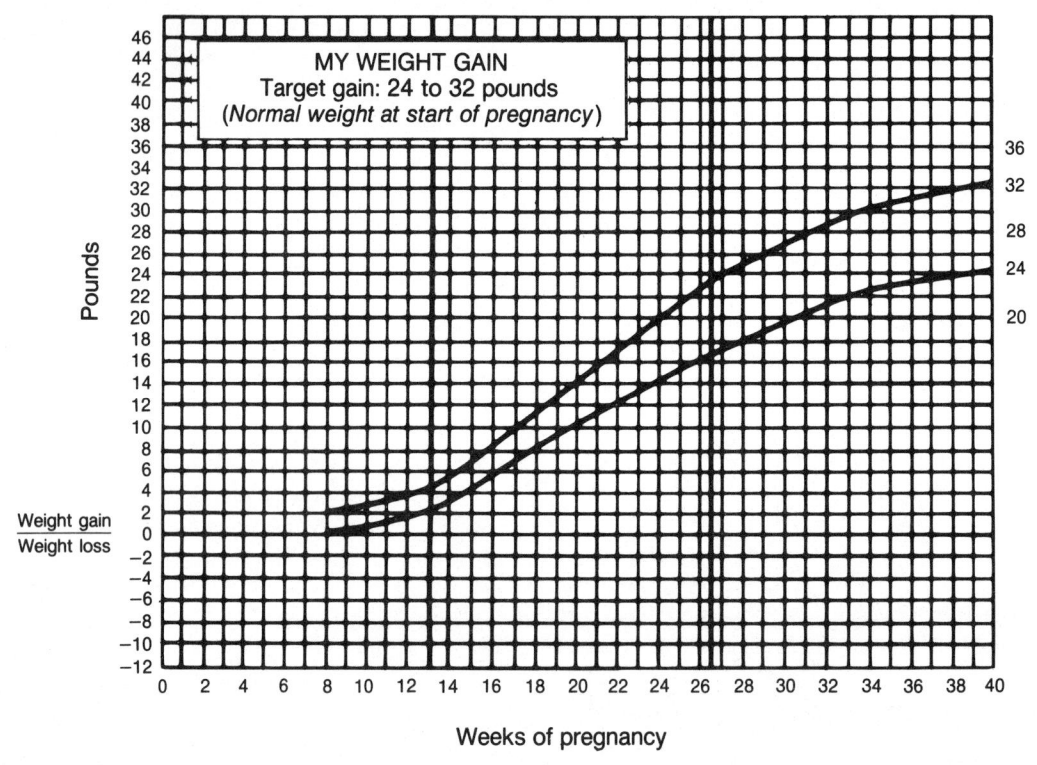

Figure 7.1. Weight gain chart for pregnant women. (From J. E. Brown: *Nutrition for Your Pregnancy*, Minneapolis, Minn., University of Minnesota Press, 1983.)

Water

Water retention is normal during pregnancy, but the amount retained varies from 7 to 12 liters (34). Administration of diuretics is associated with a reduction in birth weight (17). This expansion of the total body water is an important determinate of pregnancy outcome, and it should not be impaired.

The physically active pregnant woman probably has an increased need for water to support expansion of total body water and to maintain normal body temperature (see above). Consumption of 8–12 cups of water daily is probably prudent to maintain normal hydration and expansion of total body water under circumstances of exercise.

Sodium

Additional sodium is needed for expansion of the extracellular fluid volume in the sedentary pregnant woman (34). This additional need coupled with increased sodium losses during exercise may place the physically active pregnant woman at risk for sodium depletion if her exercise is vigorous and if her sodium intake is low. Most pregnant women in the United States consume at least twice as much sodium as is needed. Thus, it is quite unlikely that sodium depletion will develop in the physically active pregnant woman. Pregnant, as well as nonpregnant, women participating in prolonged exercise in the heat should be advised to consume salty foods and to salt their foods to taste following the exercise bout.

SUMMARY

Based on current knowledge, energy seems to be the major nutritional concern for physically active pregnant women. If energy needs are met, it seems likely that the other nutritional needs will be satisfied as long as a wide variety of foods are consumed. Maternal appetite may be the best indicator of total energy needs, and all women should be urged to eat to appetite. This advice, however, does not mean that food intake should not be controlled. The rate of maternal weight gain is the best clinical measure of the adequacy of maternal energy intake. Weight gain of physically active pregnant women should be monitored monthly throughout pregnancy. If the rate of gain deviates from the ranges around the normal curve (Fig. 7.1) at any time, daily energy intakes should be estimated using a 24-hour recall of all food eaten, and the intake adjusted appropriately.

REFERENCES

1. Aikawa K, Quintanilha AT, DeLumen BO, Brooks GA, Packer L: Exercise endurance training alters vitamin E levels and red blood cell hemolysis in rodents (submitted for publication), 1984.
2. Anonymous: High protein diets and bone homeostasis. Nutr Rev 39:11, 1981.
3. Belko AZ, Ovarzanek E, Kalkway HJ, Rotler MA, Bogusy DA, Miller D, Hass JD, Roe DA: Effects of exercise on riboflavin requirements of young women. Am J Clin Nutr 39:509, 1983.
4. Bergner L, Susser MW: Low birthweight and prenatal nutrition: an interpretive review. Pediatrics 46:946, 1970.
5. Bielinski R, Schutz Y, Jequier E: Energy metabolism during the postexercise recovery in man. Int J Vitam Nutr Res 53:226, 1983.
6. Blackburn MW, Calloway DH: Energy expenditure and consumption of mature, pregnant and lactating women. J Am Dietet Assoc 69:29, 1976.
7. Block, A, Ikeda J: Eat to Compete, a Workbook on Proper Eating Habits for Teenage Athletes, Cooperative Extension, University of California, Berkeley, 1982.
8. Brotherhood J, Brozovic B, Pugh LGC: Haematological status of middle- and long-distance runners. Clin Sci Mol Med 48:139, 1975.
9. Butterfield G: Utilization of protein and energy by young men under two conditions of energy balance and work. Doctoral dissertation, University of California, Berkeley, 1980.
10. Butterfield GE, Calloway DH: Physical activity improves protein utilization in young men. Br J Nutr 51:171, 1984.
11. Butterfield GE, Deshaies Y, Shattuck S: Calcium balance in male runners given a high protein diet (in preparation), 1984.
12. Butterfield GE, Gates J, Hamilton S, Kotula K, Nerad J: Energy intake in women runners (manuscript in preparation), 1984.
13. Cade TR, Spooner GR, Schlien EM, Pickering MJ, Dean RC: Effect of fluid, electrolyte and glucose replacement during exercise on performance, body temperature, rate of sweat loss, and compositional changes of extracullular fluid. J Sports Med Phys Fitness 12:150, 1972.
14. California Department of Health: Nutritional during Pregnancy and Lactation: For Professional Use. Sacramento, Calif., 1975.
15. Calloway DH, Spector H: Nitrogen balance as related to caloric and protein intake in active young men. Am J Clin Nutr 2:405, 1954.
16. Campbell DM: Dietary restriction in obesity and its effects on neonatal outcome. In Campbell DM, Gillmer MDG (eds): Nutrition in Pregnancy. London, Royal College of Obstetrics and Gynaecologists, 1982, pp 243.
17. Campbell DM, MacGillivray I: The effect of a low calorie diet or a thiazide diuretic on the incidence of pre-ecalmpsia and on birth weight. Br J Obstet Gynaecol 82:572, 1975.
18. Committee on Maternal Nutrition, Food and Nutrition Board, National Research Council: Maternal Nutrition and the Course of Pregnancy. Washington, D.C., National Academy of Sciences, 1970.
19. Costill DL, Cate R, Fink WJ: Dietary potassium and heavy exercise: effects on muscle water and electrolytes. Am J Clin Nutr 36:266, 1982.
20. Costill DL, Miller JM: Nutrition for endurance sport: carbohydrate and fluid balance. Int J Sports Med 1:2–14, 1980.
21. Davies KJA, Quintanilha AT, Brooks GA, Packer L: Free radicals and tissue damage produced by exercise. Biochem Biophys Res Commun 107:1198, 1982.
22. Davis JR, Tagliaferro AR, Kertzer R, Gerardo T, Nichols J, Wheeler J: Variations in dietary-induced thermogenesis and body fatness with aerobic capacity. Eur J Appl Physiol 50:319, 1983.
23. Dressendorfer RH, Wade CE, Amsterdam EA: Development of pseudoanemia in marathon runners during a 20-day road race. JAMA 246:1215, 1981.
24. Fink WJ: Fluid intake for maximizing athletic performance. In Haskell W, Scala T, Whittam J (eds): Nutrition and Athletic Performance. Palo Alto, Calif., Bull Publishing, 1982, pp 52–63.
25. Fishbaine B, Butterfield G: Ascorbic acid status of running and sedentary men. Int J Vitam Nutr Res (in press), 1984.
26. Garrow JS: Treat Obesity Seriously. A Clinical Manual. Edinburgh, Churchill Livingstone, 1981, pp 174–177.
27. Gates J, Hamilton S, Butterfield G: Iron and ascorbic acid status in women runners. Fed Proc 42:803, 1983.
28. Giordana C: Early diet to slow the course of chronic renal failure. In Proceedings of the 8th International Congress Nephrology, Athens, 1981, pp 71–78.
29. Gontzea I, Sutrescu P, Dumitreche S: The influence of adaptation to physical effort on nitrogen balance in men. Nutr Rep Int 11:231, 1975.

30. Gorsky RD, Calloway DH: Activity pattern changes with decreases in food energy intake. *Hum Biol* 55:;577, 1983.
31. Greenleaf JE: The body's need for fluids, In Haskell W, Scala J, Whittam J (eds): *Nutrition and Athletic Performance.* Palo Alto, Calif., Bull Publishing, 1982, pp 34–50.
32. Hegenauer G, Strause L, Saltman P, Dann D, White J, Green R: Transitory hematological effects of moderate exercise are not influenced by nonsupplementation. *Eur J Appl Physiol* 52:57, 1983.
33. Hunscher HA, Tompkins WT: The influence of maternal nutrition on the immediate and long-term outcome of pregnancy. *Clin Obstet Gynecol* 13:130, 1970.
34. Hytten FE, Chamberlain G (eds): *Clinical Physiology in Obstetrics.* Oxford, Blackwell, 1980.
35. Kerr JF, Campbell-Brown BM, Johnstone FD: Dieting in pregnancy. A study of the effect of a high protein, low carbohydrate diet on birthweight in an obstetric population. In Sutherland HW, Stowers JM (eds): *Carbohydrate Metabolism in Pregnancy and the Newborn.* New York, Springer-Verlag, 1978, pp 518–534.
36. Knochel JP: Rhabdomyolysis and effects of potassium deficiency on muscle structure and function. *Cardiovasc Med* 3:247, 1978.
37. Lane HW, Roessler GS, Nelson EW, Cerda JJ: Effect of physical activity on human potassium metabolism in a hot and humid environment. *Am J Clin Nutr* 31:838, 1978.
38. Ledoux M, Brisson G, Peronnet F: Nutritional status of adolescent female gymnasts. *Med Sci Sports Exerc* 14;145, 1982.
39. Lind T: Iron supplementation during pregnancy. In Campbell DM, Gillmer MDG (ed): *Nutrition in Pregnancy.* London, Royal College of Obstetricians and Gynaecologists, 1982, pp 181.
40. Nagy L, King JC: Energy expenditure of pregnant women at rest or walking self-paced. *Am J Clin Nutr* 38:369, 1983.
41. National Research Council: *Recommended Dietary Allowances*, ed 9. Washington, D.C., National Academy of Sciences, 1980.
42. Novak LP, Magill LA, Schultz JE: Maximal oxygen intake and body composition of female dancers. *Eur J Appl Physiol* 39:277, 1978.
43. Oyster N, Morton M, Linnell S: Physical activity and osteoporosis in post-menopausal women. *Med Sci Sports Exerc* 16:44, 1984.
44. Pitkin RM: Obstetrics and gynecology. In: Schneider HA, Anderson CE, Coursin DB (eds): *Nutritional Support of Medical Practice.* Hagerstown, Md.: Harper & Row, 1977, pp 407–421.
45. Pitkin RM: Calcium metabolism in pregnancy: a review. *Am J Obstet Gynecol* 121:724, 1975.
46. Pittet PH, Chappuis PH, Acheson K, De Techtermann F, Jéquier E: Thermic effect of glucose in obese studied by direct and indirect calorimetry. *Br J Nutr* 35:281, 1976.
47. Prentice AW, Whitehead RG, Roberts SB, Paul AA: Long-term energy balance in child-bearing Gambian women. *Am J Clin Nutr* 34:2790, 1981.
48. Primrose T, Higgens A: A study of human antepartum nutrition. *J Reprod Med* 7:257, 1971.
49. Root BA, King JS: Maternal nutrition. In Creasy RK, Resnik R (eds): *Maternal-Fetal Medicine.* Philadelphia, W.B. Saunders, 1984, p 181.
50. Rosso O, Cramoy C: Nutrition and pregnancy. In Winick M (ed): *Human Nutrition. A Comprehensive Treatise.* New York, Plenum Press, 1979, vol 1.
51. Rush D, Stein Z, Susser M: A randomized controlled trial of prenatal nutritional supplementation in New York City. *Pediatrics* 65:683, 1980.
52. Tremblay A, Boilard F, Breton, M-F, Bessette H, Roberge AG: The effects of riboflavin supplementation on the nutritional status and performance of elite swimmers. *Nutr Res* 4:201, 1984.
53. Yoshimura H, Inoue T, Yamada T, Shiraki K: Anemia during hard physical training (sports anemia) and its causal mechanism with special reference to protein nutrition. *World Rev Nutr Diet* 35:1, 1980.
54. Young VR, Torun B: Physical activity. Impact of protein and amino acid metabolism and implications for nutritional requirements. Nutrition in Health and Disease and International Development. In Symposia from XIIth International Congress of Nutrition 1981, pp 59–85.
55. Williams JA, Wagner J, Wasnick R, Heilbrun L: The effect of long-distance running upon appendicular bone mineral content. *Med Sci Sports Exerc* 16:223, 1984.

8
Changes in Maternal Hemodynamics during Pregnancy

CARDIAC OUTPUT

Maternal cardiac output increases during mammalian pregnancy; however, a quantitative description of that generalization is difficult for humans. The following statements appear tenable at this time. First, cardiac output increases before and in excess of the increment in uterine blood flow. Second, the increase in cardiac output can be attributed mainly to cardiac enlargement, rather than to changes in loading or contractility. Third, posture dominates the control of cardiac output late in pregnancy because of its influence on venous return. Finally, exercise capacity is reduced in pregnancy because a portion of cardiac output is committed to nonmuscular tissue and because venous return may be impaired.

Maternal Hemodynamics at Rest

TIME COURSE, MAGNITUDE AND EFFECTS OF POSTURE

The clinician who examines a young, healthy woman in the second trimester of pregnancy receives many clues to the presence of a hyperkinetic circulation. The rosy cheeks, warm skin, active precordium, ejection murmur, and bounding peripheral pulses support this impression. It is not surprising, therefore, that most values for resting cardiac output are 30–50% greater during mid-pregnancy (1–5) than postpartum. Cardiac output is increased and probably does not increase further after the second trimester. This time course has clinical relevance when considering the interaction between pregnancy and cardiac pathophysiology: the maximal stress on the cardiovascular system probably occurs by the second trimester. The fact that cardiac output reaches maximum values by mid-pregnancy also suggests that mechanisms other than increased uterine blood flow are responsible.

Early measurements of cardiac output during human pregnancy were made in supine subjects and showed a reduction of output to near postpartum levels in the third trimester (1–3). Following the demonstration that the inferior vena cava is occluded in the supine position during late pregnancy (6), it was realized that posture played a crucial role in the hemodynamics at that time. Nevertheless, two studies (4, 7) have taken posture into account and have yielded different results, although reliable indicator-dilution techniques were used in both. Lees et al. (7) concluded from a serial study of five subjects that cardiac output did not decline in the third trimester when subjects were studied in lateral recumbency. In contrast, a serial study of 11 subjects by Ueland et al. (4) showed that cardiac output peaked in the second trimester, then fell toward postpartum levels. The fall from the second to the third trimester was greatest when women were studied supine, but also occurred in lateral recumbency and in seated subjects. In the absence of additional serial measurements of cardiac output, using invasive methods, inferential corroboration from noninvasive techniques is enlightening. A serial study of 27 women before, during, and after pregnancy by Atkins et al. (5) confirmed the findings of Ueland et al. Impedance cardiography, a less accepted technique, was used, but the study was well controlled. Left ventricular size has been measured by echocardiography in two published serial studies (9, 10). In both, calculated stroke volume was increased above nonpregnant levels by about 30% in the third trimester. A similar unpublished study from our institution showed that stroke volume peaked in the first and second trimesters, then fell almost to nonpregnant values during the third trimester.

This persistent conflict in findings suggests that a better understanding of the maternal circulation in the third trimester is needed. As Lees et al. (7) pointed out, "cardiac output measurements...are valid only for the experimental conditions under which they are made and have no universal applicability." It appears to us that the absolute value of cardiac output in the third trimester of human pregnancy is less important than the persuasive evidence that resting cardiac output is substantially increased by the second trimester and becomes highly variable in the third trimester. Assumption of a sitting or supine position causes output to fall below values measured in lateral recumbency (4). Supine recumbency may lead to symptomatic reductions of cardiac output in about 5% of pregnancies (11), the "supine hypotensive syndrome."

Determinants of Cardiac Output Changes

HEART RATE

Cardiac output is the product of heart rate and stroke volume. Of the two, heart rate is more variable, ranging on average from resting values of 60/min to almost 200/min during maximal exercise in women of childbearing age. Because of this great range, heart rate is a powerful protector of circulatory stability. Heart rate per se may be affected by pregnancy or altered reflexly to maintain blood pressure in the face of altered vascular resistance or stroke volume. (A review of cardiac and circulatory control can be found in Braunwald et al. (12).)

The *intrinsic* heart rate of healthy human adults averages approximately 110 beats/min. It is normally suppressed by vagal tone and minimally supported at rest by adrenergic drive. Vagal suppression of the sinus node originates in the carotid sinus baroreceptors. Vagal release with resultant tachycardia acts to defend blood pressure; however, tachycardia alone does not increase cardiac output: for that to happen, an increase in venous return must accompany the increase in heart rate.

In human pregnancy, maternal heart rate is elevated over postpartum values in all three trimesters. Whether the mechanism is an increase in intrinsic rate, a decrease in vagal tone, or an increase in adrenergic drive (or a combination of these) is unknown. Most measurements show that heart rate increases progressively throughout pregnancy (4, 8–10). From our preceding discussion of cardiac output, it should be evident that heart rate will be quite sensitive to maternal posture in the third trimester. Accordingly, investigations that show a decline of cardiac output in the third trimester also show in general that heart rate rises simultaneously.

The importance of the relative tachycardia lies in two areas. First, increased heart rate elevates myocardial oxygen requirements. This is probably not important in normal women but it may become so in the presence of important cardiovascular pathology. Second, an increased resting heart rate diminishes the increment in output that can occur with maximal exercise; maximal work capacity falls. For example, if the maximal heart rate is 200/min and basal heart rate increases from 60 to 80 beats/min during pregnancy, then the maximal increment in heart rate will fall from 3.3-fold to 2.5-fold.

STROKE VOLUME

Stroke volume increases progressively during the first and second trimesters of human pregnancy, to a peak value 30% above postpartum (4). Thereafter, stroke volume becomes quite unstable and may remain the same or fall to postpartum levels, especially with changes in body position.

Left ventricular stroke volume is accomplished by the shortening and thickening of left ventricular muscle against a closed mitral valve. The determinants of muscle shortening are muscle length before shortening (*preload*), average muscle stress during shortening (*afterload*), and the intrinsic strength of the muscle (*contractility*). These three variables affect stroke volume on a beat-to-beat basis. Preload and contractility are regulated by the circulatory system to meet instantaneous demands. On a long-term basis, stroke volume is most affected by altering *heart size*. For example, stroke volume increases about 10-fold in the years from birth to adulthood, with unimportant changes in contractility and preload. This increment is not achieved entirely by increasing cell size (*hypertrophy*): rather, the conformation of the ventricle is continually remodeled: as a result, the size of the lumen increases progresively without a change in filling pressure.

PRELOAD

At the ultrastructural level, Starling's law of the heart is based upon the fact that extension of the filaments of the sarcomere during diastole increases the extent of their shortening during the subsequent systole. However, humans, when supine, are very near the "top of their Starling curve" (13); further lengthening of the sarcomere filaments evokes only minor increases in shortening. The evidence for this statement rests upon the observation that acute increases in filling pressure produce little or no change in left ventricular stroke volume of human subjects in supine recumbency. Certainly the 30% increase in stroke volume that occurs during pregnancy could not come entirely from an increased end-diastolic pressure in the ventricle. Additionally, there is no evidence that ventricular filling pressure increases during pregnancy (1). Blood volume is elevated by 40% (14), but the substantial increase in venous capacitance (15) and the enlargement of the pelvic vascular bed appear to accommodate the expanded blood volume without altering cardiac filling pressures.

A definitive statement regarding the importance of changes in preload as a mechanism for increasing stroke volume during pregnancy must await measurements of sarcomere length. From the available evidence, we doubt that increases in preload are important: in late gestation, however, *reduced* preload probably is important in restricting stroke volume.

AFTERLOAD

Accurate and simultaneous measurements of ventricular dimensions and pressures during systole are required to calculate muscle stress; they have not been made in pregnancy. However, we can examine several factors that affect afterload and assess the performance of the ventricle by techniques that are sensitive to changes in afterload. Extrapolation from these data suggests that reduced afterload is not responsible for the 30% increase in stroke volume during pregnancy.

Left ventricular muscle stress during systole is determined largely by the product of its radius:wall thickness ratio (r/h) and the simultaneous intraventricular pressure. In pregnancy, the r/h ratio is increased. Pressure during systole is determined by the volume of blood in the ventricle, its rate of ejection, and the impedance of the vascular system. The intraventricular volume and the rate of ejection are increased in pregnancy (9), but the effect of these upon afterload appears to be offset by a diminished systemic vascular resistance. Additionally, and not previously recognized, aortic capacitance (the other component of impedance besides peripheral resistance) increases during pregnancy, leading to a further fall in afterload. In the study of Katz et al. (9), aortic diastolic dimension increased progressively throughout gestation, but the change did not reach statistical significance; however, aortic diastolic pressure was significantly lower in the second and third trimesters, so aortic dimension increased despite a lower distending pressure.

The three reported echocardiographic studies show no important changes in fractional shortening, ejection fraction, or normalized velocity of shortening during pregnancy (9, 10, 16). These ejection-phase indices of ventricular function are sensitive to changes in both contractility and afterload; they are less sensitive to changes in preload. Accordingly, reduced afterload is unlikely to be important in explaining the 30% increase in stroke volume that occurs in pregnancy. Ejection fraction would need to exceed 90% in order for either reduced afterload or increased contractility to accomplish an increase in stroke volume of this magnitude.

During pregnancy a large, relatively thin left ventricle delivers a larger stroke volume to a compliant, low-resistance arterial circuit. Myocardial mechanics and vascular impedance are nicely matched to provide an increased cardiac output at a normal or slightly reduced arterial pressure.

CONTRACTILITY

Direct measurements of the intrinsic strength of contraction in pregnant human subjects are not available. The ejection-phase indices of function discussed above do not show important changes in contractility. Two studies that used measurements of systolic time intervals have been reported (8, 17); both suggest that small increases in contractility occur early in pregnancy. However, the changes were small and interpretations of their significance were based on repeated applications of the *t*-test. If the statistical significance of these findings is in doubt, their functional importance is clear: changes in contractility that do not increase ejection fraction cannot, by themselves, increase stroke volume.

HEART SIZE

The important cardiac change during pregnancy, then, is an increase in heart size. Circumstantial evidence for this assertion comes from echocardiographic studies showing that the internal diameter of the left ventricle enlarges during pregnancy (9, 10, 16). From our knowledge of filling pressure and the relationship between left ventricular pressure and volume, an increased filling pressure can be excluded as the mechanism causing left ventricular end-diastolic volume to increase by 30%. Investigation of pregnancy in a laboratory animal was necessary to evaluate this phenomenon further. In guinea pigs, pregnancy is associated with a "rightward shift" of the left ventricular pressure-volume relationship; at a constant filling pressure, left ventricular volume is increased about 25% at term, compared with weight-matched controls (18); hypertrophy was not present. We concluded that the ventricle was remodeled during pregnancy. Although the human left ventricle also appears to enlarge during pregnancy, some hypertrophy may be present, on the order of 10–15% (9, 10, 19).

Mechanisms

Having acknowledged that the changes in the circulation during pregnancy are still incompletely defined, we can only speculate on the mechanisms that bring them about. One point seems clear; the cardiovascular changes of pregnancy cannot be attributed entirely to increased maternal blood flow to the uterus. Reductions in peripheral vascular resistance and increases in cardiac output and blood volume all antedate important changes in uterine blood flow. It has been demonstrated that hormonal factors are implicated in the cardiovascular adaptions to pregnancy. The hemodynamic changes that occur early in pregnancy appear to establish a circulatory reserve that can be drawn upon later in gestation to satisfy the needs of the developing fetus in the uterus.

A crucial step toward understanding cardiocirculatory physiology during pregnancy will be taken when we learn whether the generalized enlargement of the system results from plethora or is a parallel rather than a cause-and-effect phenomenon. Conventional physiologic dogma would favor the former: mean systemic pressure increases in pregnancy (20); increased venous return and cardiac output follow from well-developed mechanisms (21). We are not convinced that parameters which function as powerful short-term regulators of the cardiovascular system are responsible for the major long-term adaptations of pregnancy. We support the thesis that hormonal changes early in pregnancy evoke a decrease in vascular resistance and increases in venous and arterial capacitance: simultaneously, blood volume rises.

In the third trimester, resting cardiac output is variable, depending upon body position. The enlarged uterus, and the distensible large veins that must drain past it, encourage venous pooling: as a result, cardiac output may fall below postpartum levels. The implications of this observation are clear. When cardiac output falls, the maternal organism is forced to choose between maintaining uterine blood flow at the expense of maternal tissue, or placing fetal health in jeopardy. Since women spend the majority of their time, even in the third trimester, in positions other than lateral recumbency, the maternal blood supply to the uterus probably becomes increasingly variable towards term, as venous return becomes more vulnerable.

Exercise

Women in our society are increasingly entering the work force and participating in exercise programs or sports. It is important to consider the health consequences of these activities during gestation.

The enlarged heart of pregnancy might be ideally suited for exercise. Distance athletes also show significant cardiac enlargement (although with more hypertrophy) in response to training (22). Bicycle exercise, when performed in the supine position during pregnancy, produces changes in cardiac output which parallel those observed at rest; the level of cardiac output achieved during standard exercise falls in the third trimester. Even with the active muscle pump and elevated legs, cardiac output during exercise achieves a value similar to that recorded in resting subjects early in the second trimester. This observation suggests two possible explanations: either the dilated heart of pregnancy is poorly suited to perform work at the higher arterial pressures characteristic of exercise, or venous return is so impeded in the supine position that the heart is continually "running dry," even during leg exercise.

Subsequent studies made during upright bicycle exercise suggest a better cardiac reserve. Guzman and Caplan (23) showed that maternal cardiac output at work loads of 150, 250, and 350 kpm was increased throughout gestation. It is of interest that stroke volume at the highest work load was 77 ml near term compared with a nonpregnant value of 74 ml. Heart rate was higher throughout gestation at all work loads than corresponding control values. Ueland and colleagues (4) studied subjects at 100 and 200 kpm during upright bicycle exercise. At both work loads, cardiac output increased with excercise and was minimally increased or unchanged with respect to postpartum values: in agreement with Guzman and Caplan's findings, stroke volume fell progressively at both work loads as gestation advanced. Near-term values could not be distinguished from postpartum levels. To summarize, cardiac output increased during upright bicycle exercise to values that exceeded or equaled postpartum values; however, stroke volume fell progressively as gestation advanced, reaching values near term similar to those found postpartum.

We have recently begun to measure maternal cardiac output before, during, and after exercise using impedance cardiography and echocardiography. Our preliminary data strongly suggest that impaired venous return restricts cardiac performance during upright bicycle exercise near term. The ability of the left ventricle to increase contractility during exercise appears to be normal

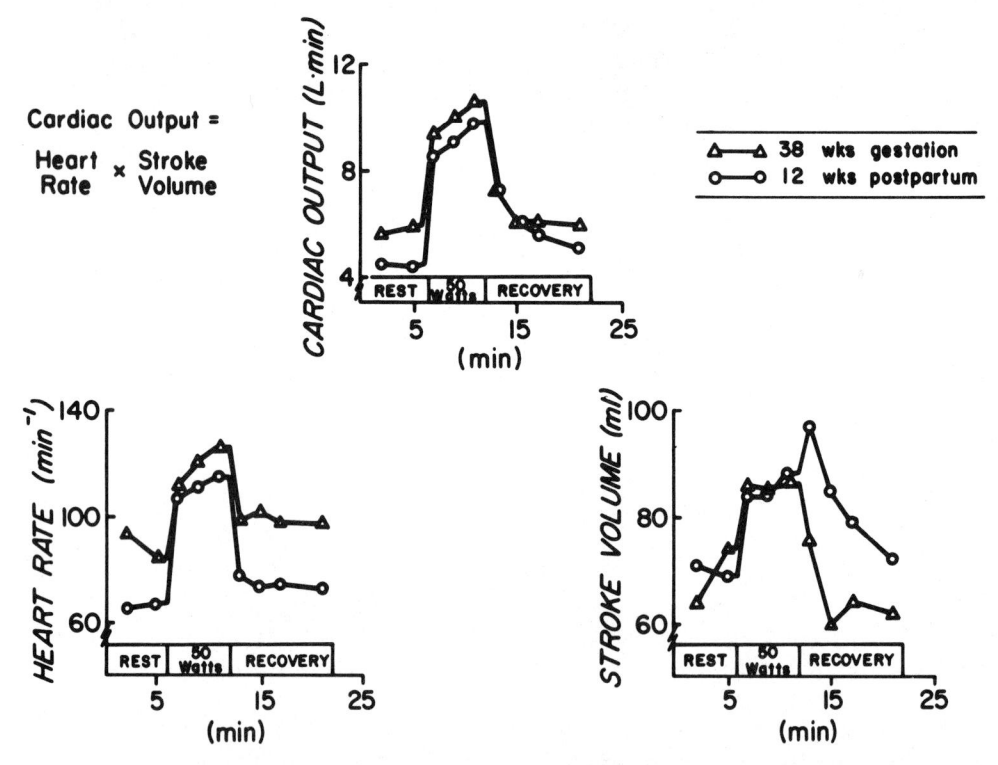

Figure 8.1. Exercise hemodynamics at 38 weeks of gestation ($N = 9$). Cardiac output, heart rate, and stroke volume are shown in late gestation and postpartum during an upright bicycle exercise protocol. Stroke volume was determined by impedance cardiography.

in late gestation. Figure 8.1 shows cardiac output, heart rate, and stroke volume before, during, and after 6 min of upright bicycle exercise at 50 watts (300 kpm) intensity. Nine women were studied at 38 weeks of gestation and again 12 weeks postpartum. Steady-state values, both at rest and during exercise, are similar to those of Guzman and Caplan (23) and Ueland et al. (4). In late gestation, stroke volume during exercise is not significantly different from the postpartum value. The most striking finding is a precipitous drop in stroke volume when exercise stops in late gestation. We interpret this to mean that the leg muscle pump is crucial for maintenance of venous return during upright exercise in late gestation. Even with active pedaling, however, stroke volume in late gestation does not exceed postpartum levels. This is difficult to reconcile with the finding of a larger heart unless venous return is impeded, even during exercise.

We do not believe that these findings can be attributed to a reduced contractile response to exercise. We are studying this problem with M-mode echocardiography (Fig. 8.2). Figure 8.3 shows left ventricular dimension and normalized dimension shortening ($\Delta D/D$) obtained by echocardiography performed on one woman serially before and during pregnancy. A small increase in end-diastolic dimension is noted early in exercise except in the first trimester. The increase of fractional shortening in response to exercise remains stable throughout gestation. When exercise stops, end-diastolic dimension falls sharply, especially in the third trimester. These findings support the concept that a restriction of venous return causes the reduction in stroke volume after exercise. The fact that the response of fractional shortening to exercise is normal throughout pregnancy is strong evidence that contractility is maintained during gestation.

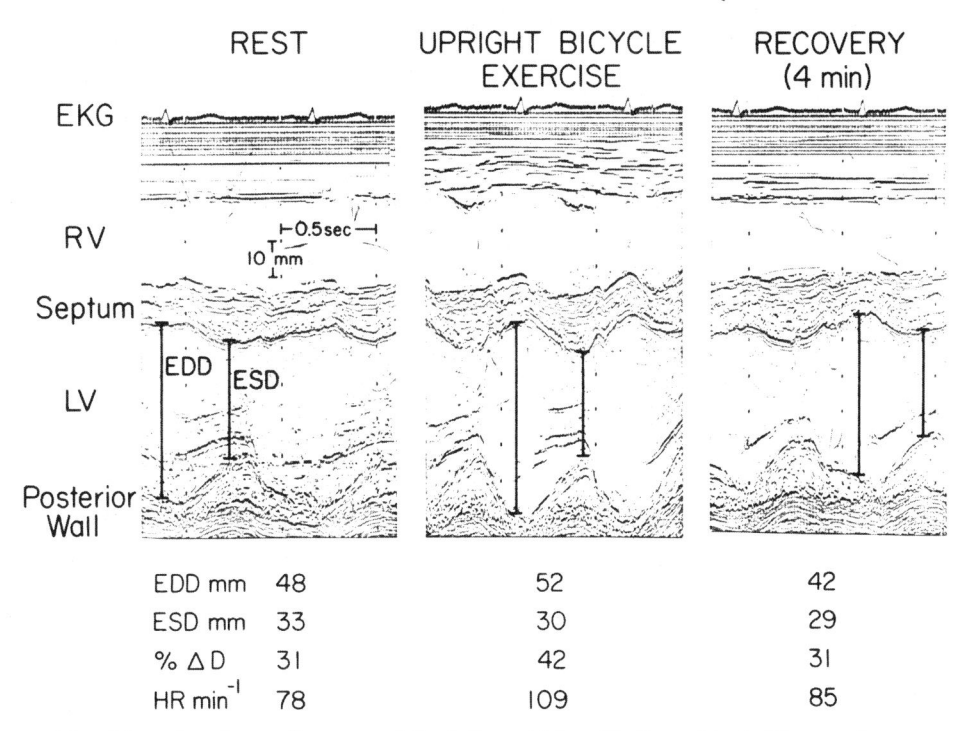

Figure 8.2. M-mode echocardiograms of the left ventricle with the subject sitting on the ergometer at rest, during upright bicycle exercise, and during recovery. Measurements of end-diastolic (*EDD*) and end-systolic dimension (*ESD*) are indicated. Cardiac output is increased during exercise by increases in both EDD and percent shortening (%ΔD). During recovery in this subject in late gestation, impaired venous return results in a marked reduction in EDD. This appears to be the mechanism for the reduced stroke volume after exercise that is shown in Figure 8.1.

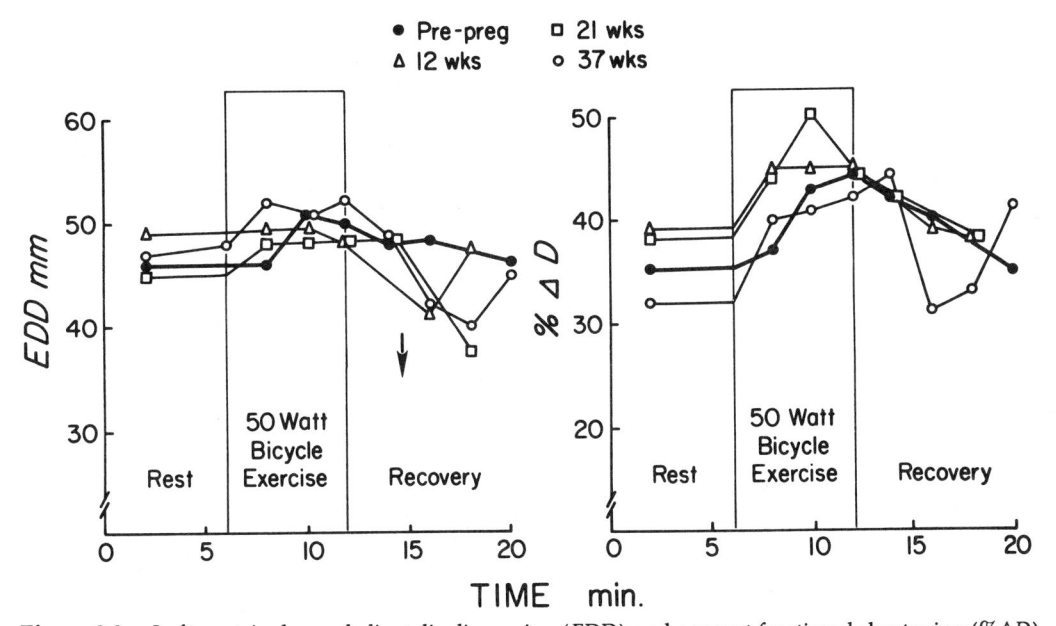

Figure 8.3. Left ventricular end-diastolic dimension (*EDD*) and percent fractional shortening (%Δ*D*) are shown before and throughout gestation in one subject. The decrease in EDD that occurs after exercise during pregnancy is evident; so is the falling %Δ*D* that occurs after exercise in the 37th week of pregnancy.

119

The importance of venous return may not be confined to maintenance of cardiac output. We have suggested (24) that the volume of venous return at the onset of exercise plays an important role in the ventilatory response.

UTERINE BLOOD FLOW

The extra cardiac output furnished to the periphery by the maternal heart during pregnancy does not go entirely to reproductive tissues. Early in gestation the kidneys receive the major share of the increment. As pregnancy proceeds some of the extra blood flow goes to the maternal skin, presumably to provide for the increased loss of heat that is required by the actively metabolizing and growing tissues of the fetus. Measurements of mammary blood flow have not been made in humans, but estimates based upon plethysmography and thermometry indicate that breast blood flow increases progressively during pregnancy, reaching its highest levels postpartum (25). The uterine circulation is an essential link in the chain of transport that supplies nutrients and oxygen to the placenta and removes waste products, including heat.

Resting Values for Uterine Blood Flow

Early estimates of uterine blood flow were made using nitrous oxide. Equilibration of the foreign gas between maternal blood and the tissues of the uterus and its contents was either assumed (26) or estimates of tissue nitrous oxide concentrations were made, based upon analyses of fetal blood samples and samples of amniotic fluid (27). Sampling of uterine vein blood was accomplished either by retrograde catheterization or by venipuncture under direct vision at term cesarean section.

MAGNITUDE, TIME COURSE AND EFFECTS OF POSTURE

These studies yielded estimates of approximately 500 ml/min at term (27). Measurements made with electromagnetic flowmeters implanted acutely at surgical interruption of pregnancy gave values of approximately 50 ml/min at the 10th week of pregnancy and 200 ml/min at the 28th week (28). More recent estimates, based upon placental scintigraphy of indium-113m, produced values of approximately 1200 ml/min at 37 weeks of pregnancy when the subjects were lying in the left lateral position (29): calculated values were 30% lower when normal subjects were studied supine, the position in which the original nitrous oxide estimates were all made. It seems appropriate to consider that the early estimates, especially those made during term cesarean section, gave low values that reflected vena caval obstruction by the term uterus. Accordingly, we now consider that uterine blood flow at term approximates 1 liter/min in the resting woman lying in the left lateral position.

MECHANISMS CONTROLLING UTERINE BLOOD FLOW

Studies of the control of uterine blood flow have not been performed in humans. Early observers (30) postulated that the fall in uterine vascular resistance that is responsible for the increase in uterine blood flow during pregnancy was due to erosion of vessels in the maternal endometrium by trophoblastic invasion. Since that time, work with other species has shown that the resistance to blood flow falls strikingly even in those animals, like sheep and goats, where no erosion of the uterine vessels occurs (31–33).

ESTROGENS AND PROGESTERONE

Evidence drawn from work with animals supports the concept that many of the changes in vascular resistance that occur within the pregnant uterus are mediated by steroid hormones produced by the ovaries and placenta. The administration of estrogens to nonpregnant sheep evokes a fall in peripheral vascular resistance (34), and contraceptives that contain estrogenic compounds cause cardiac output to rise by an augmentation of stroke volume (35). Furthermore, estrogen infused directly into the uterine artery of nonpregnant sheep produces a major fall in uterine vascular resistance after a latent period that is attributed to the time required to synthesize a mediator protein (36). Exogenous progesterone, on the other hand, appears to exert an action antagonistic to estrogen, evoking a decrease in the rate of uterine blood flow when administered to sheep in early pregnancy (37). This body of evidence leads to the concept that the long-term regulation of uterine blood flow during pregnancy, at least in sheep, depends upon a balance between the vasodilator action of estrogens from either the ovary or the chorion and an antagonistic action of progesterone.

RENIN, ANGIOTENSIN AND PROSTAGLANDINS

Against this background, several other hormones apparently act in the short-term regulation of blood flow to the pregnant uterus, modulating from minute to minute the long-term effects of the steroid hormones. Renin-like substances have been isolated from the pregnant uterus of several animal species. The intravenous infusion of angiotensin II in subpressor doses evokes an increase in blood flow to the uterus of nephrectomized rabbits near term (38) and larger doses produce the same effect in pregnant sheep (39). It has been suggested that the vasodilating action of angiotensin is mediated through the local release of prostaglandin E (40).

CATECHOLAMINES

The uterine vasculature of sheep is very sensitive to norepinephrine and epinephrine; infusion of either of these agents causes a decrease in uterine blood flow and a redistribution of the maternal circulation within the pregnant uterus (39, 41–43).

Exercise

Plasma catecholamine levels increase during exercise, by an amount that depends upon the intensity and the duration of exercise (44). Psychological stress also evokes the release of catecholamines: in contrast with exercise, which is characterized by the release of norepinephrine, emotional stress elevates the circulating level of epinephrine (45). From these considerations one would predict that exercise during pregnancy would be associated with a decrement in uterine blood flow, the amount of decrease depending upon exercise intensity, exercise duration and the psychological components of the exercise.

ANIMALS STUDIES

Studies made in experimental animals support these predictions (46), and raise doubts about whether experience derived from the study of women who are forced to work by economic necessity (47, 48) can be applied to women who exercise "for the fun of it."

Physical training diminishes the magnitude of the increase in plasma catecholamines associated with a standard exercise task (49, 50). Accordingly, one would predict that with the same intensity and duration of exercise, well-trained women will show a lesser decrement in uterine blood flow than untrained women. Since training also lessens the degree of ketosis and of hypoglycemia (50) protection might be afforded the fetus during maternal exercise by prior physical training of the mother.

HUMAN STUDIES

Against this theoretical background and data from the study of experimental animals showing that uterine blood flow diminishes during exercise, evidence from the study of humans is fragmentary and indirect. When radiolabeled sodium is injected into the muscle of the uterus, its rate of removal (monitored by an external counter) is considered to reflect the rate of blood flow. Using this technique, Morris et al. (51) demonstrated that when normal women exercised late in pregnancy, the time required for "clearance" of the radiosodium increased. These data were originally interpreted as indicating that uterine blood flow decreased during maternal exercise (51) but the interpretation and its implications require modification because, as shown by animal studies (46) nonplacental uterine blood flow may behave differently than placental blood flow during maternal exercise. We would now interpret the radiosodium studies as suggesting that nonplacental uterine blood flow falls during maternal exercise in humans as it does in experimental animals (46). In addition, the studies using radioactive sodium (51) were apparently performed using subjects in the supine position, raising concern about obstruction of the inferior vena cava by the pregnant uterus (11).

The hypothesis that uterine blood flow falls during maternal exercise is consistent with a large literature concerning the redistribution of blood flow that occurs during exercise in nonpregnant human subjects (52). This visceral vasoconstriction is proportional to the severity of the exercise and is thought to be mediated by the sympathetic nervous system except at exhausting levels of exertion (52). Several pieces of evidence suggest that pregnancy, perhaps acting via the steroid hormones, blunts the action of the autonomic nervous system on blood vessels. As early as 1862, Raynaud (53) reported that a woman suffering from attacks of severe, painful, and inappropriate peripheral vasoconstriction (Raynaud's syndrome) found relief during each of her pregnancies. Sjöberg (54) reported that norepinephrine in the uterine vasculature is depleted during pregnancy in rabbits. Ford et al. (55) found that the response of the sheep uterine artery to sympathetic nerve stimulation was lessened during pregnancy. Other inferential evidence comes from a report by Doležal and Figar (56) who measured blood flow to the finger in nonpregnant and pregnant women: several different stimuli were presented with the general vascular response being constriction in nonpregnant subjects and dilation in women in the first and second trimester of pregnancy: near term, the vasoconstrictor response returned. Accordingly, we are hesitant about transposing data on sympathetic response to exercise from nonpregnant to pregnant subjects.

MATERNAL EXERCISE AND FETAL HEALTH

The effects of exercise upon uterine blood flow and fetal oxygenation have been inferred from measurements of fetal heart rate. Hon and Wohlgemuth (57) demonstrated abnormal fetal heart rate patterns following maternal exercise close to term and other workers have confirmed this finding (58, 59). Pommerance et al. (60) measured the fetal heart rate response to maternal exercise in 54 normal women: 5 fetuses had an increase in heart rate greater than 16 beats/min following maternal exercise and 4 of these subsequently showed signs of fetal distress during labor: the fetal tachycardia following maternal exercise was considered to indicate uteroplacental insufficiency and its occurrence in 5 out of 54 women to suggest that about 10% of clinically healthy women are unable to maintain an "adequate" uterine blood flow during muscular exercise. Pernoll et al. (61) confirmed the occurrence of fetal tachycardia after healthy women completed 6 min of mild bicycle exercise near term. However, the mechanism that evokes fetal tachycardia following maternal exercise is not clear. Although it may indicate a significant decrement in uterine blood flow, the evidence is certainly not conclusive.

Another line of evidence suggesting that maternal exercise may jeopardize uterine blood flow arises from data showing that fetal growth is handicapped by maternal exercise. In animals, exercise of severe intensity is associated with several undesirable effects upon the fetus, including increased mortality, decreased weight gain, and delayed bone ossification (62). Naeye and Peters (47) have presented evidence that women who work in the third trimester of pregnancy deliver infants weighing significantly less (at term) than newborn infants of mothers who remain at home. Because "work" has different psychological implications than "exercise" in our society, the relevance of data obtained from working women to women who exercise by choice and for relatively short periods of time can be questioned. Nevertheless, it seems likely that exercise of unaccustomed severity or duration should be regarded as potentially threatening the maintenance of uterine blood flow. Until convincing evidence to the contrary is presented, we believe that the appropriate advice for healthy pregnant women who are accustomed to exercise is to limit the intensity of their exercise to that which causes their heart rate to rise to levels less than 70% of the age-predicted maximum, for durations of half an hour or less, and with a frequency of three times weekly. Even this restrained exercise program should be interrupted if vaginal bleeding occurs or if there is evidence of fetal growth retardation. Furthermore, because excessive heat is recognized to have harmful effects on the fetus and leads to vasodilatation that further encourages venous pooling, exercise should probably not be performed in a hot environment.

REFERENCES

1. Bader RA, Bader ME, Rose DJ, Braunwald E: Hemodynamics at rest and during exercise in normal pregnancy as studied by cardiac catheterization. *J Clin Invest* 34:1524–1536, 1955.
2. Roy SB, Malkani PK, Virik R, Bhatia ML: Circulatory effects of pregnancy. *Am J Obstet Gynecol* 96:221–225, 1966.
3. Walters WAW, MacGregor WG, Hills M: Cardiac output at rest during pregnancy and the puerperium. *Clin Sci* 30:1–11, 1966.
4. Ueland K, Novy MJ, Peterson EN, Metcalfe J: Maternal cardiovascular dynamics; IV. The influence of gestational age on the maternal cardiovascular response to posture and exercise. *Am J Obstet Gynecol* 104:856–864, 1969.
5. Atkins AFJ, Watt JM, Milan P, Davies P, Crawford JS: A longitudinal study of cardiovascular dynamic changes throughout pregnancy. *Eur J Obstet Gynaecol Reprod Biol* 12:215–224, 1981.
6. Kerr MG, Scott DB, Samuel E: Studies of the inferior vena cava in late pregnancy. *Br Med J* 1:532–533, 1964.
7. Lees MM, Taylor SH, Scott DB, Kerr MG: A study of cardiac output at rest throughout pregnancy. *J Obstet Gynaecol Br Commonw* 74:319–328, 1967.
8. Burg JR, Dodek A, Kloster FE, Metcalfe J: Alterations of systolic time intervals during pregnancy. *Circulation* 49:560–564, 1974.
9. Katz R, Karliner JS, Resnik R: Effects of a natural volume overload state (pregnancy) on left ventricular performance in normal human subjects. *Circulation* 58:434–441, 1978.
10. Laird-Meeter K, van de Ley G, Bom TH, Wladimiroff JW, Roelandt J: Cardiocirculatory adjustments during pregnancy: an echocardiographic study. *Clin Cardiol* 2:328–332, 1979.
11. Kerr MG: The mechanical effects of the gravid uterus in late pregnancy. *J Obstet Gynaecol Br Commonw* 72:513–529, 1965.
12. Braunwald E, Ross J, Jr, Sonnenblick EH (eds): *Mechanisms of Contraction of the Normal and Failing Heart*, ed 2. Boston, Little, Brown, 1976.
13. Parker JO, Case RB: Normal left ventricular function. *Circulation* 60:4–11, 1979.
14. Hytten FE, Paintin DB: Increase in plasma volume during normal pregnancy. *J Obstet Gynaecol Br Commonw* 70:402–407, 1963.
15. Fawer R, Dettling A, Weihs D, Welti H, Schelling JL: Effect of the menstrual cycle, oral contraception and pregnancy on forearm blood flow, venous distensibility and clotting factors. *Eur J Clin Pharmacol* 13:251–257, 1978.
16. Rubler S, Damani PM, Pinto ER: Cardiac size and performance during pregnancy estimated with echocardiography. *Am J Cardiol* 40:534–540, 1977.
17. Rubler S, Hammer N, Schneebaum R: Systolic time intervals in pregnancy and the postpartum period. *Am Heart J* 86:182–188, 1973.
18. Morton MJ, Tsang H, Hohimer AR, Ross D, Thornburg K, Faber J, Metcalfe J: Left ventricular size, output and structure during guinea pig pregnancy. *Am J Physiol* 246:R40–R48, 1984.
19. Larcher D: De l'hypertrophie normale du coeur pendant la grossesse, et de son importance pathogénique. *Arch Gen Med* 13:291–306, 1859.
20. Douglas BH, Harlan JC, Lanford HG, Richardson TQ: Effect of hypervolemia and elevated arterial pressure on circulatory dynamics of pregnant animals. *Am J Obstet Gynecol* 98:889–894, 1967.
21. Guyton AC, Coleman TG, Granger HJ: Circulation: Overall regulation. *Annu Rev Physiol* 34:13–46, 1972.
22. Morganroth J, Maron BJ, Henry WL, Epstein SE: Comparative left ventricular dimensions in trained athletes. *Ann Intern Med* 82:521–524, 1975.
23. Guzman CA, Caplan R: Cardiorespiratory response to exercise during pregnancy. *Am J Obstet Gynecol* 108:600–605, 1970.
24. Edwards MJ, Metcalfe J, Dunham MJ, Paul MS: Accelerated respiratory response to moderate exercise in late pregnancy. *Respir Physiol* 45:229–241, 1981.
25. Pickles VR: Blood flow estimations as indices of mammary activity. *J Obstet Gynaecol Br Emp* 60:301–311, 1953.
26. Assali NS, Douglass RA Jr, Baird WW, Nicholson DB, Suyemoto R: Measurement of uterine blood flow and uterine metabolism; IV. Results in normal pregnancy. *Am J Obstet Gynecol* 66:248–253, 1953.
27. Metcalfe J, Romney SL, Ramsey LH, Reid DE,

Burwell CS: Estimation of uterine blood flow in normal human pregnancy at term. *J Clin Invest* 34:1632–1638, 1955.
28. Assali NS, Rauramo L, Peltonen T: Measurement of uterine blood flow and uterine metabolism; VIII. Uterine and fetal blood flow and oxygen consumption in early human pregnancy. *Am J Obstet Gynecol* 79:86–98,1960.
29. Lunell NO, Nylund LE, Lewander R, Sarby B: Uteroplacental blood flow in pre-eclampsia measurements with indium-113m and a computer-linked gamma camera. *Clin Exp Hypertens (B)* 1:105–117, 1982.
30. Burwell CS: The placenta as a modified arteriovenous fistula, considered in relation to the circulatory adjustments to pregnancy. *Am J Med Sci* 195:1–7, 1938.
31. Hoversland AS, Metcalfe J, Parer JT: Adjustments in maternal blood gases, acid-base balance, and oxygen consumption in the pregnant pygmy goat. *Biol Reprod* 10:589–595, 1974.
32. Hoversland AS, Parer JT, Metcalfe J: Hemodynamic adjustments in the pygmy goat during pregnancy and early postpartum. *Biol Reprod* 10:578–588, 1974.
33. Metcalfe J, Parer JT: Cardiovascular changes during pregnancy in ewes. *Am J Physiol* 210:821–825, 1966.
34. Ueland K, Parer JT: Effects of estrogen on the cardiovascular system of the ewe. *Am J Obstet Gynecol* 96:400–406, 1966.
35. Walters WAW, Lim YL: Cardiovascular dynamics in women receiving oral contraceptive therapy. *Lancet* 2:879–881, 1969.
36. Resnik R, Battaglia FC, Makowski EL, Meschia G: The effect of actinomycin-D on estrogen-induced uterine blood flow. *Gynecol Obstet Invest* 5:24, 1974.
37. Caton D, Abrams RM, Lackore LK, James G, Barron DH: Effect of exogenous progesterone on the rates of uterine blood flow and oxygen consumption of sheep in early pregnancy. *Q J Exp Physiol* 59:233–239, 1974.
38. Ferris TF, Stein JH, Kauffman J: Uterine blood flow and uterine renin secretion. *J Clin Invest* 51:2827–2833,1972.
39. Assali NS, Holm LW, Sehgal N: Regional blood flow and vascular resistance of the fetus in utero: Action of vasoactive drugs. *Am J Obstet Gynecol* 83:809–817, 1962.
40. Venuto RC, O'Dorisio T, Stein JH, Ferris TF: Uterine prostaglandin E secretion and uterine blood flow in the pregnant rabbit. *J Clin Invest* 55:193–197, 1975.
41. Barton MD, Killam AP, Meschia G: Response of ovine uterine blood flow to epinephrine and norepinephrine. *Proc Soc Exp Biol Med* 145:996–1003, 1974.
42. Anderson SG, Still JG, Griess FC Jr: Differential reactivity of the gravid uterine vasculatures: Effects of norepinephrine. *Am J Obstet Gynecol* 129:293–297, 1977.
43. Clapp JF III: Effect of epinephrine infusion on maternal and uterine oxygen uptake in the pregnant ewe. *Am J Obstet Gynecol* 133:208–212, 1979.
44. Manhem P, Lecerof H, Hökfelt B: Plasma catecholamine levels in the coronary sinus, the left renal vein and peripheral vessels in healthy males at rest and during exercise. *Acta Physiol Scand* 104:364–369, 1978.
45. Dimsdale JE, Moss J: Plasma catecholamines in stress and exercise. *JAMA* 243:340–342, 1980.
46. Hohimer AR, Bissonnette JM, Metcalfe J, McKean TA: Effect of exercise on uterine blood flow in the pregnant pygmy goat. *Am J Physiol* 246:H207–H212, 1984.
47. Naeye RL, Peters EC: Working during pregnancy: Effects on the fetus. *Pediatrics* 69:724–727, 1982.
48. Briend A: Maternal physical activity, birth weight and perinatal mortality. *Med Hypotheses* 6:1157–1170,1980.
49. Winder WW, Hagberg JM, Hickson RC, Ehsani AA, McLane JA: Time course of sympathoadrenal adaptation to endurance exercise training in man. *J Appl Physiol* 45:R370–R374, 1978.
50. Winder WW, Hickson RC, Hagberg JM, Ehsani AA, McLane JA: Training-induced changes in hormonal and metabolic responses to submaximal exercise. *J Appl Physiol* 46:R766–R771, 1979.
51. Morris N, Osborn SB, Wright HP: Effective uterine blood-flow during exercise in normal and pre-eclamptic pregnancies. *Lancet* 2:481–484, 1956.
52. Rowell LB: Human cardiovascular adjustments to exercise and thermal stress. *Physiol Rev* 54:75–159, 1974.
53. Raynaud AGM: De l'asphyxie locale et de la gangrène symétrique des extrémités. Paris, 1862.
54. Sjöberg N-O: Considerations on the cause of disappearance of the adrenergic transmitter in uterine nerves during pregnancy. *Acta Physiol Scand* 72:510–517, 1968.
55. Ford SP, Weber LJ, Stormshak F: Response of ovine uterine arteries to nerve stimulation after perfusions of prostaglandin-F$_{2\alpha}$, norepinephrine or neurotransmitter antagonists. *Endocrinology* 101:659–665, 1977.
56. Doležal A, Figar Š: The phenomenon of reactive vasodilation in pregnancy. *Am J Obstet Gynecol* 93:1137–1143, 1965.
57. Hon EH, Wohlgemuth R: The electronic evaluation of fetal heart rate; IV. The effect of maternal exercise. *Am J Obstet Gynecol* 81:361–371, 1961.
58. Štembera ZK, Hodr J: The "exercise test" as an early diagnostic aid for foetal distress. In Horský J, Štembera ZK (eds): *Intra-uterine Dangers to the Foetus*. Amsterdam, Excerpta Medica Foundation, 1967, pp 349–353.
59. Pokorný, Rouš J: The effect of mother's work on

foetal heart sounds. In Horský J, Stembera ZK (eds): *Intra-uterine Dangers to the Foetus.* Amsterdam, Excerpta Medica Foundation, 1967, pp 354–357.
60. Pommerance JJ, Gluck L, Lynch VA: Maternal exercise as a screening test for uteroplacental insufficiency. *Obstet Gynecol* 44:383–387, 1974.
61. Pernoll ML, Metcalfe J, Paul M: Fetal cardiac response to maternal exercise. In Longo LD, Reneau DD (eds): *Fetal and Newborn Cardiovascular Physiology, Vol. 2, Fetal and Newborn Circulation.* New York, Garland STPM Press, 1978, pp 389–398.
62. Terada M: Effect of physical activity before pregnancy on fetuses of mice exercised forcibly during pregnancy. *Teratology* 10:141–144, 1974.

9

Maternal Cardiovascular Response to Exercise during Pregnancy

Important questions frequently arise regarding the influence of maternal exercise on pregnancy and its outcome. Since the metabolic demands of pregnancy effect many changes in maternal resting physiological status, it is of particular relevance that we recognize whether the additional stress of exercise induces adjustments that might exceed the threshold of safety for mother and/or child. In this chapter, we will review the information published on the adaptations of the pregnant circulatory system to exercise stress.

In Chapter 8, Morton and Metcalfe provided information related to the changes occurring in the cardiovascular system as a result of pregnancy. Significant changes occur in the circulatory system such as increases in blood volume, heart rate, and cardiac output and a decrease in resting arterial blood pressure. Table 9.1 summarizes the most significant changes. There is no question that such changes could affect the women's ability to perform exercise.

Most of these changes arise from the need to compensate for the continuing normal alterations of pregnancy. In addition to the specific changes presented in Table 9.1, a general adaptation toward blood redistribution occurs. Blood flow to the kidney may increase up to 400 ml/min at rest while to the uterus a 500 ml/min increase occurs, in general there is a greater distribution of blood to the splanchnic organs (Fig. 9.1) (1).

The major shift in blood distribution to the various organs is part of the normal changes associated with pregnancy. The demands of exercise require a major redistribution of blood away from the splanchnic organs toward the working muscles (Fig. 9.2). The possible negative effect of the shunting of blood away from the reproductive organs is of major concern during exercise in pregnancy. While several studies have been conducted investigating this problem, there is no conclusive evidence as to whether or not the human fetus actually is affected as a result of this apparent deprivation.

This review focuses on the cardiovascular effects of acute exercise on the mother and the possible effect of physical conditioning on maternal function.

CARDIOVASCULAR RESPONSE TO MATERNAL EXERCISE

The earliest investigations of maternal cardiovascular response to exercise were performed using a variety of different step tests (3). During the exercise bout attempts were made to measure several noninvasive parameters, such as heart rate, blood pressure, oxygen uptake, and respiratory capacity. These measurements gave the researchers some insights as to what to expect during exercise, but because maximal work capacity is difficult to access using step testing procedures, the results were limited to inference about submaximal exercise response. Further, due to the fact that step

Exercise in Pregnancy

Table 9.1. Cardiovascular Changes That Influence Exercise Capacity during Normal Pregnancy

Function	Nonpregnant	Pregnant	Percentage Change
Blood volume (ml)	2500	3900	55
Heart volume (ml)			12
Heart rate (bpm)			
Rest	70	85	20
Exercise	190	170	15
Cardiac output (ml/min)	4500	6000	30[a]
Stroke volume (ml/beat)	60–70	85–90	30[b]
A-V oxygen difference (ml)	45	40	12
Arterial pressure			
Systolic	120	112	5
Diastolic	75	70	5
Systemic vascular resistance (dynes/sec/cm^{-5})	1700	1250	30

[a] Greatest during mid-pregnancy.
[b] Greatest by the end of the second trimester.

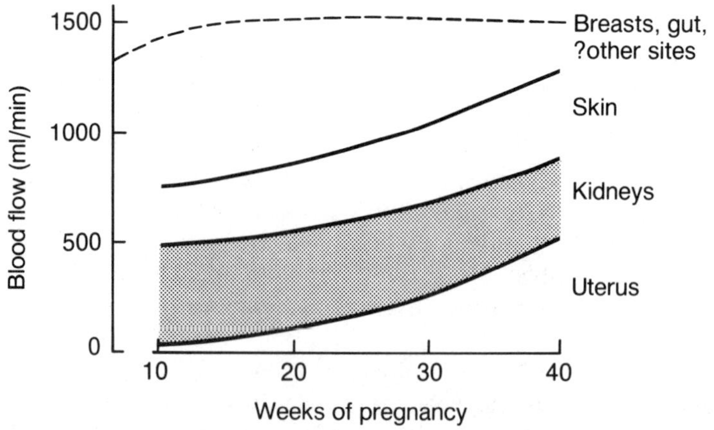

Figure 9.1. Distribution of increased cardiac output during pregnancy. (From M. deSwiet: In F. Hytten and G. Chamberlain (eds.), *Clinical Physiology in Obstetrics*, Oxford, Blackwell Scientific Publications, 1980, pp. 3–42 (1).)

testing is a weight-dependent exercise, interpretation of metabolic and circulatory response was very difficult. Widlund (3) found no significant differences in the metabolic cost or the oxygen debt incurred during low intensity exercise in his pregnant subjects. These results are surprising in view of the fact that the subjects were gaining weight. The possible implication is that pregnancy is associated with improved efficiency, at least during low intensity work. At the higher work intensity, Widlund reported a 10% increase in oxygen cost and a 15% higher oxygen debt.

It is of much relevance to analyze work efficiency in pregnancy in relation to the circulatory system. If the pregnant woman is more efficient in the use of oxygen, the circulatory demands associated with a given work load may be lessened. As a result, many physiological changes that might lead us to interpret submaximal response to exercise, as indicative of improved fitness, may prove incorrect or at least misleading.

Using bicycle ergometers, a non-weight-dependent exercise, several investigators have reported an increased oxygen cost of exercise in pregnancy and an increase in oxygen debt (4–6). As a result one must assume that the same amount of work in the pregnant woman represents a greater physiological stress than during nonpreg-

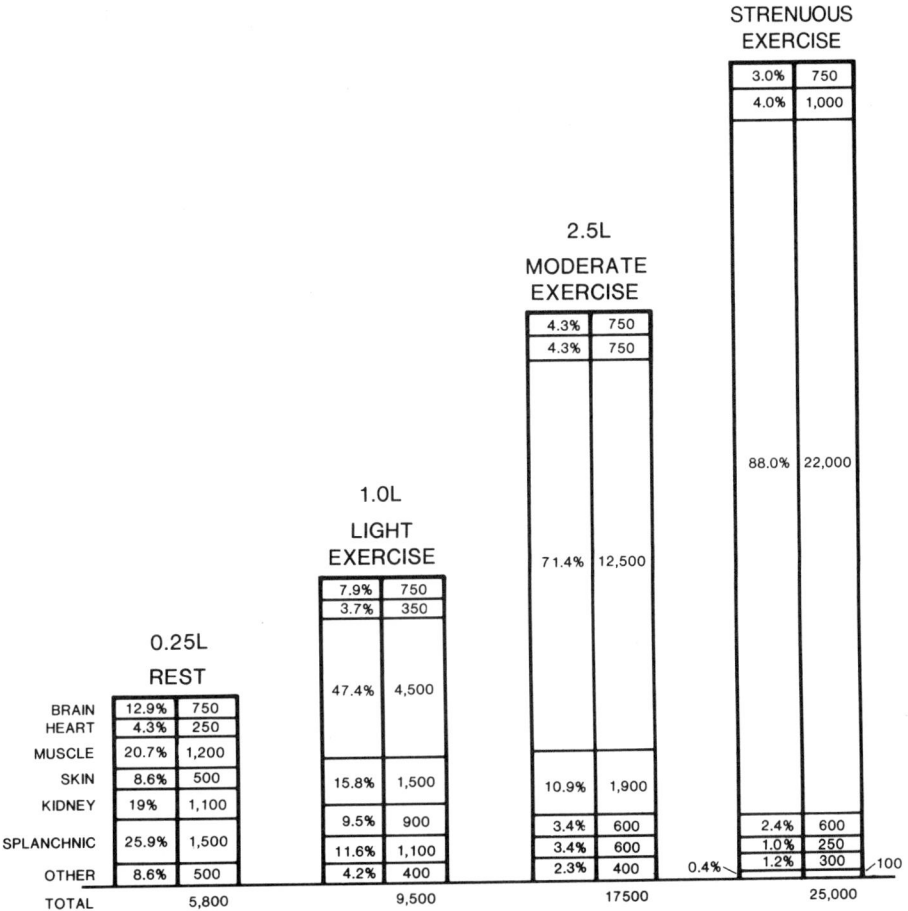

Figure 9.2. Effects of exercise at various intensities on distribution of cardiac output to organ systems. (Adapted from S. M. Horvath: *Diabetes*, 28 (suppl.):33–38, 1979 (2).)

nancy. Thus, we expect the circulatory system to adjust accordingly, that is, by increasing heart rate, blood pressure, and cardiac output for any given work task. However, the literature is not in universal agreement that this is the case.

Bader et al. (7) catheterized the right heart and pulmonary artery of 46 healthy pregnant women to observe hemodynamic changes during 10 min of supine exercise on a cycle ergometer. Intensity of exercise was not indicated, but the mean exercise heart rate of 108 beats/min (bpm) (rest = 94) suggested a rather light work intensity. The authors concluded that the decrease in total peripheral resistance and the increase in cardiac output, arterial blood pressure, heart rate, and arteriovenous oxygen difference were all within normal limits for exercise of such intensity in nonpregnant women. The difficulty in interpreting these results relates to the lack of appropriate controls and the fact that the exercise intensity was at such a low level. Again, the failure to show a significant effect in cross-sectional research of this nature may relate to the fact that the general circulatory effects of pregnancy, that is increased blood volume, reduced peripheral resistance, and arterial blood pressure, are effective at increasing the efficiency of the circulatory and metabolic response to exercise at low work loads. As the intensity of work increases, the response may lead to an entirely different interpretation.

Bader's investigation was subsequently

carried further by Rose et al. (8), who, employing the same subjects and exercise protocol, calculated left ventricular work using cardiac output and mean brachial arterial pressure. Left ventricular work increased during exercise, but in subjects near term the increase was somewhat smaller. The authors concluded that because the increase in cardiac output was proportional to the increase in $\dot{V}_{O_2}$ and that this relationship was normal, pregnancy effected no impairment of myocardial reserve during exercise. This was a cross-sectional study and did not attempt to extrapolate the observed effects to adaptations and requirements of pregnancy. While our own studies suffer from some of the same design weaknesses, by using maximal exercise rather that low intensity exercise, our data suggest that pregnancy may impose a major detriment to exercise tolerance (9).

More appropriate design strategies appeared in the late 1960s which employed longitudinal designs or, at least compared pregnancy to a postpartum condition. In a longitudinal study throughout the duration of pregnancy, Dahlstrom and Irhman (25) measured the cardiorespiratory response and predicted maximal work capacity of pregnant and nonpregnant women performing cycle ergometry. Exercise heart rates at the lower work intensity and heart rate recovery following all three exercise intensities increased as pregnancy progressed. Exercise heart rates at the higher work intensities did not change and were similar to controls. As a result, the predicted maximal work capacity, which was the same for both groups, remained constant throughout the study. Maximal exercise capacity was not assessed.

Ueland et al. (10) measured cardiac output, heart rate, stroke volume, and arterial blood pressure of pregnant women at rest, during exercise and recovery by catheterization of the brachial artery and the antecubital vein. Exercise was performed on a cycle ergometer at light and moderate intensities. Heart rate ranges were 116–128 bpm (rest = 92) for light work and 125–135 bpm (rest = 83) for moderate work, increasing through pregnancy. The exercise-induced increase in cardiac output for moderate work decreased progressively throughout pregnancy. These investigators concluded that the increase in cardiac output was well within the normal limits for nonpregnant women, indicating no impairment in myocardial reserve during pregnancy; yet because of the smaller rise in cardiac output later in pregnancy, there may be a progressive decline in circulatory reserve most likely due to peripheral pooling of the blood. These findings suggest that submaximal work does in fact require a greater cardiac output for the pregnant woman and that the requirement for enhanced cardiac output to meet the demands of the exercise may diminish in late pregnancy. This does not imply that the system responds better to stress in late pregnancy but that the process of homeostasis to adjust the maternal circulation to the needs of pregnancy has perhaps become more refined or permanent.

In another longitudinal study, Guzman and Caplan (11) measured heart rate, oxygen uptake, and cardiac output of healthy pregnant women exercising on a cycle ergometer (Fig. 9.3). Postpartum values were used as controls. Oxygen uptake remained essentially unchanged throughout pregnancy except for an increase at low intensity during 29–35 weeks of gestation. Heart rate responses were significantly higher during all stages of pregnancy with the most marked differences occurring at the lowest intensity. Stroke volume and cardiac output were also significantly higher throughout pregnancy. The arteriovenous oxygen difference remained constant throughout pregnancy but was lower than postpartum levels. It was concluded that the pregnant woman reaches her maximum work capacity at lower levels of work than in the nonpregnant state.

To summarize the literature regarding the acute response of the pregnant mother to

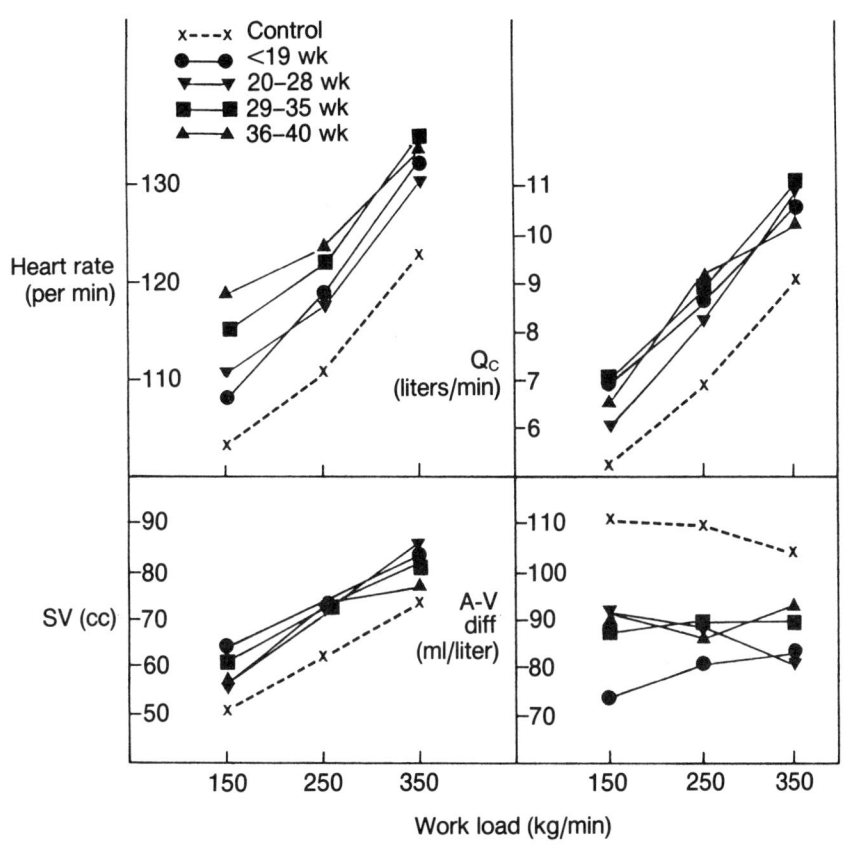

Figure 9.3. Effects of pregnancy on heart rate, cardiac output (Q_c), stroke volume (*SV*) and A-V difference at 3 work loads. *Dotted lines* represent measurements in the nonpregnant state; *solid lines*, values during various stages of pregnancy. (From C. Guzman and R. Caplan: *American Journal of Obstetrics & Gynecology*, 108:600–605, 1970 (11).)

exercise, we can conclude that:
1. There is a slight increase in cardiac output during mild and moderate exercise with a significant drop in maximal cardiac output.
2. There is an increase in stroke volume at any given work load.
3. There may be an increased heart rate at low intensity exercise, a normal heart rate at moderate intensity exercise, and a reduced maximal heart rate.
4. There is no difference in A-V oxygen difference during work in pregnancy.
5. There may be an error associated with the prediction of maximal work capacity from submaximal heart rate.

Table 9.2 summarizes studies investigating maternal response to acute exercise.

CARDIOVASCULAR CONDITIONING DURING PREGNANCY

Exercise training during pregnancy may be arbitrarily classified into three types: (*a*) psychoprophylactic preparation for childbirth, (*b*) cardiovascular or aerobic conditioning, and (*c*) sports or athletic training. Interest in decreasing duration of labor, facilitating delivery and improving probability of infant normalcy have been among the motivations prompting conditioning programs. Unfortunately, none of those effects could be demonstrated.

Several studies have attempted to relate physical fitness to the outcome of pregnancy (12–14). Physical fitness does not seem to have a significant effect on duration of labor

Table 9.2. Summary of the Studies of Exercise Response during Pregnancy[a]

Investigators	Date	Type of Study	Type of Subject Experimental	Type of Subject Control	Mode	Work Rate	Duration	Mets[b]	Variables Measured
Widlund (3)	1945	X-S	157 pg	60 n-pg	Step	22/min 40/min 52/min	82 s 45 s 52 s	4.8 8.7 11.3	HR, BP, $\dot{V}O_2$, VC, RR, O_2 debt
Bader (8)	1955	X-S	46 pg		Supine Bike		10 min		$\dot{Q}$, BP, HR, TPR
Rose (9)	1955	X-S	46 pg		Supine Bike		10 min		LVW
Gemzell (24)	1957	Long	20 pg		Bike	200 kg 400 kg 600 kg	6 min 6 min 6 min	3.3 5.2 7.1	PWC
Morris (36)	1956	X-S	19 pre	21 pg	Supine Bike		10 min		HR, BP, uterine flow
Dahlstrom (25)	1960	Long	46 pg	12 n-pg	Bike	200 kg 400 kg 600 kg	6 min 6 min 6 min	3.3 5.1 7.1	HR, BV, Hct, RR, PWC
Hon (37)	1961	X-S	26 pg		Dbl. Master				Fetal HR
Sovia (29)	1964	X-S	19 pg	11 hyp pg	Bike	200 kg 400 kg 700 kg	6 min 6 min 6 min	3.3 5.1 7.8	BP, HR, PWC
Seitchik (4)	1967	X-S	133 pg	28 post 34 n-pg	Bike	306 kg	10 min	4.2	$\dot{V}_{O_2}$, O_2 debt
Ueland (10)	1969	Long	11 pg	11 post	Bike	100 kg 200 kg	3 min 3 min	2.3 3.3	$\dot{Q}$, HR, BP, SV
Guzman (11)	1970	Long	8 pg	8 post	Bike	150 kg 250 kg 350 kg	4 min 4 min 4 min	2.8 3.7 4.6	HR, RR, $\dot{V}_e$, $\dot{V}_{O_2}$, $\dot{Q}$

Study	Year	Type	Subjects		Mode	Load	Duration	Response/RER	Measurements
Emmanouilides (38)	1972	Long	12 pg, ewe		Mill	2.5 mph	30–60 min		pH, P_{CO_2}, P_{O_2}, BP, HR
Orr (39)	1972	Long	2 pg, ewe	2 n-pg ewe	Mill	3 mph, 10%	34 min		P_{O_2}, pH, $\dot{Q}$, BP, HR, uterine flow
Blackburn (40)	1973	X-S	21 pg	16 post	Bike	300 kg	5 min	4.1	HR, $\dot{V}_{O_2}$
						400 kg	5 min	5.2	
					Mill	3 mph, 0%	5 min	3.3	
						3 mph, 5%	5 min	5.3	
						3 mph, 10%	5 min	7.4	
Knuttgen (27)	1974	Long	13 pg	13 post	Bike	367 kg	6 min	4.8	$\dot{V}_{O_2}$, HR, $\dot{V}_e$, RR, TV, R
					Mill	4 mph, 4%	6 min		
Sandström (22)	1974	X-S	10 pg		Bike	200 kg	6 min	3.3	PWC, HR, BP
						400 kg	6 min	5.2	
						600 kg	6 min	7.1	
Pomerance (41)	1974	X-S	54 pg		Bike				Fetal HR
Pernoll (6)	1975	Long	12 pg	12 post	Bike	300 kg	6 min	4.1	$\dot{V}_{O_2}$, HR, $\dot{V}_e$, RR, TV, $\dot{C}O_2$, P_{CO_2}, PWC
Erkkola (17)	1976	Long	62 pg		Bike	Max			PWC, Hct, Hb, BP, HR, Lactate
Curet (34)	1976	Long	5 pg, ewe	6 n-pg ewe	Mill	3 mph, 10%	45–60 min		$\dot{Q}$, SV, BP, TPR, uterine flow

[a] HR = heart rate, BP = blood pressure, SV = stroke volume, $\dot{Q}$ = cardiac output, RR = respiration rate, TV = tidal volume, PWC = physical work capacity, R = respiratory exchange ratio, TPR = total peripheral resistance, LVW = left ventricular work, Hct = hematocrit, HB = hemoglobin, BV = blood volume, pg = pregnant, n-pg = nonpregnant, post = postpartum, hyp = hypertensive, pre = pre-eclamptic, Long = longitudinal study, X-S = cross-sectional study, min = minute, s = second.

[b] Body weight = 62 kg.

except in multiparas in which labor appears to be shorter (12).

Studies correlating maternal maximal work capacity with maternal and fetal pH and lactate levels at delivery were carried out by Erkkola and Rauramo (15) on healthy pregnant women. Lactate levels of fit mothers were lower during work tests. All lactate concentrations after delivery were significantly higher than during the work tests, with the more fit women having values indicating that fit women work harder during labor and delivery. Blood lactate concentration after delivery exceeded work levels that would be elicited by an exercise intensity of 600 watts for 12 min. Erkkola attributed the differences in pH to the ability of more fit women with higher oxygen carrying capacity to compensate for metabolic acidosis.

Ihrman (16) used cardiovascular conditioning as a means of childbirth preparation during the 20–30th week of gestation. Conditioning involved aerobic exercise that elicited exercise heart rates of 170–180 bpm. As a result of conditioning, there were no differences in total hemoglobin, total blood volume, or in heart rate or blood pressure response to exercise between the two groups. Ihrman concluded that circulatory adjustments of pregnancy are not altered by heavy physical training during the 20–30th week of pregnancy. These results are in contrast to the study conducted by Erkkola (17, 18) who reported a 27.7% increase in maximal work capacity in mothers that actively exercised between the 10th and 38th week of gestation.

A summary of the exercise training studies during pregnancy are presented in Table 9.3.

SUMMARY AND CONCLUSIONS

This review examined how the circulatory system of pregnant women adapts to exercise. Some general conclusions can be drawn although the human studies cited are limited in number and depth. There is no consistency in exercise test protocol or in methods of training therefore the conclusions are not readily applicable to every day activities and several areas require further investigation. These findings support our position that exercise programs should not be undertaken in pregnancy by unfit women.

No significant increase in energy expenditure of executing simple daily activities under 4 METs was found during pregnancy. Thus, pregnant women continued to execute simple daily activities until term (19–21). However, since there is a decrease in physical work capacity during the first trimester (17, 22), the energy expenditure of the simple daily activities becomes a relatively greater percentage intensity of maximum capacity (23). Therefore, it is postulated that exercise during the first trimester should depend on the previous exercise habits of the mother and her physical work capacity. If the physical work capacity of the mother is high, she can probably tolerate greater daily activity and exercise. On the other hand, simple daily activities could most likely be at the upper limits of exercise tolerance for a mother with a low physical working capacity. Thus, the woman with a low physical work capacity may not be able to initiate an exercise program during the first trimester.

Most studies agree that energy expenditure throughout a wide range of cycle ergometer intensities, heart rate at high intensities, and oxygen debt at low intensities are no different for pregnant than for nonpregnant women (3, 4, 7, 10, 11, 24, 25, 27).

Weight-dependent exercise requires increasing oxygen uptake as pregnancy progresses (5, 19, 27). Oxygen debt is larger and recovery heart rates are higher for the pregnant woman exercising at higher weight-dependent intensities (3, 4, 19). Because the maximal work capacity remains unchanged or reduced during the second and third trimesters, yet the energy demand for weight-dependent exercise increases, the absolute intensity of weight-dependent exercise should be decreased as pregnancy progresses. There appears to be no reason to alter the relative intensity at which preg-

Table 9.3. Summary of the Exercise Training Studies during Pregnancy

Investigators	Date	Subjects Experimental	Subjects Control	Mode	Frequency	Intensity	Duration Workout	Duration Study
Read (30)	1949	516		Relaxation Breathing				Last 20 wk
Rodway (32)	1947	340	340	Relaxation Breathing Posture Muscle Tone	2/mo			
Thoms (31)	1951	1000		Relaxation Breathing Posture	4/preg			
Burnett (33)	1955	2675		Lamaze	2/wk			
Curet (34)	1976	5 ewe	6 ewe	Treadmill	2/wk	3 mph, 10%	45–60 min	3 wk
Ihrman (16)	1960	26		Cardiovasc. Relaxation		170–180 beat/min	35 min 10 min	20–30th wk of gestation
Erkkola (15)	1976	31	31	Individual preference	3/wk	HR 140/min onset sweat, dyspnea	60 min	Last 28 wk of gestation
Dressendorfer (14)	1978	1		Jogging Lamaze		170 m/min		Continuous
Kasch (35)	1976	1		Jogging Aerobic dancing Lamaze	5/wk	177 m/min	40 min	Continuous

nant women exercise, unless of course, there is a complication of pregnancy.

Cardiac output, arterial blood pressure, arteriovenous oxygen difference, left ventricular work and peripheral resistance adjust within normal limits during exercise (7, 8, 28). Thus, all forms and intensities of exercise presented in these studies appear to have no adverse effects on the pregnant woman.

Cardiovascular function is impaired in pregnancy induced hypertension and heart disease (26, 29), therefore, exercise for mothers with these conditions is contraindicated. More research is required on the pregnant diabetic, hypertensive and obese response to exercise.

Psychoprophylactic preparation for childbirth may show a slightly shorter duration of labor for the primipara and significantly shorter duration of labor for the multipara if participation is regular (30, 31). Other studies failed to indicate such conditioning-related improvements (32, 33). The success of such programs cannot be fully assessed until there is better control over participants' participation in the conditioning program.

Physical fitness as predicted through various physical work tests has shown no correlations with Apgar scores and as yet no convincing effect upon the duration of labor although the possibility of a decrease is suggested (12, 13). Since a prediction of maximal work capacity is often unreliable, perhaps the preceding information on pregnancy outcome is also unreliable.

Two studies utilizing cardiovascular conditioning during pregnancy demonstrated an improvement in cardiovascular function (17, 34), while one study did not (16). These training studies lacked adequate training duration (16, 34) and standardization of exercise mode and intensity (17). In the few case study reports available (14, 35) the regimen was well quantified, but more extensive investigations are needed before convincing conclusions can be drawn regarding the conditioning effects on pregnancy and its outcome.

Since 1915 basic work has been compiled to understand the pregnant woman's physiological alterations at rest and during exercise. Much of the knowledge on exercise is limited and some is contradictory. Thus, the impact of exercise on pregnancy is open for further investigation.

REFERENCES

1. deSweit M: The cardiovascular system. In Hytten F, Chamberlain G (eds): *Clinical Physiology in Obstetrics*. Oxford, Blackwell Scientific Publications, 1980, pp 3–42.
2. Horvath SM: Review of energetics and blood flow in exercise. *Diabetes* 28 (suppl):33–38, 1979.
3. Widlund G: Cardio-pulmonal function during pregnancy. *Acta Obstet Gynecol Scand* 25 (suppl 1), 1945.
4. Seitchik J: Body composition and energy expenditure during rest and work in pregnancy. *Am J Obstet Gynecol* 97:701–713, 1967.
5. Pernoll M, Metcalfe J, Schlenker T, et al: Oxygen consumption at rest and during exercise in pregnancy. *Respir Physiol* 25:285–293, 1975.
6. Pernoll M, Metcalfe J, Kovach P, et al: Ventilation during rest and exercise in pregnancy and postpartum. *Respir Physiol* 25:295–310, 1975.
7. Bader R, Bader M, Rose D, Braunwald E: Hemodynamics at rest and during exercise in normal pregnancy as studied by cardiac catheterization. *J Clin Invest* 34:1524–1536, 1955.
8. Rose D, Bader M, Bader R, et al: Catheterization studies of cardiac hemodynamics in normal pregnant women with reference to left ventricular work. *Am J Obstet Gynecol* 72:233–246, 1956.
9. Wiswell RA, Artal R, Romen Y, Kammula R: Hormonal and metabolic response to maximal exercise in pregnancy. *Med Sci Sports Exerc* 17:206, 1985.
10. Ueland K, Novy M, Peterson E, et al: Maternal cardiovascular dynamics; VI. The influence of gestational age on maternal cardiovascular response to posture and exercise. *Am J Obstet Gynecol* 104:856–864, 1969.
11. Guzman C, Caplan R: Cardiorespiratory response to exercise during pregnancy. *Am J Obstet Gynecol* 108:600–605, 1970.
12. Pomerance J, Gluck L, Lynch V: Physical fitness in pregnancy: its effect on pregnancy outcome. *Am J Obstet Gynecol* 119:867–876, 1974.
13. Erkkola R: The physical work capacity of the expectant mother and its effect on pregnancy, labor and the newborn. *Int J Gynaecol Obstet* 14:153–159, 1976.
14. Dressendorfer R: Physical training during pregnancy and lactation. *Physician Sports Med* 6:2, 1978.
15. Erkkola R, Rauramo L: Correlation of maternal physical fitness during pregnancy with maternal

and fetal pH and lactic acid at delivery. *Acta Obstet Gynecol Scand* 55:441–446, 1976.
16. Ihrman K: A clinical and physiological study of pregnancy in a material form northern Sweden; VIII. The effects of physical training during pregnancy on the circulatory adjustment. *Acta Soc Med Upsal* 65:335–347, 1960.
17. Erkkola R: Physical work capacity and pregnancy. Annales Universitatis Turkuensis, University of Turku, Finland, 1976.
18. Erkkola R, Makela M: Heart volumes and physical fitness of parturients. *Ann Clin Res* 8:15–21, 1976.
19. Blackburn M, Calloway D: Basal metabolic rate and work energy expenditure of mature pregnant women. *J Am Diet Assoc* 69:no 1:24–28, 1973.
20. Morris N: Frequency of sexual intercourse during pregnancy. *Arch Sex Behav* 4:501–507, 1975.
21. Falicov C: Sexual adjustments during first pregnancy and postpartum. *Am J Obstet Gynecol* 117:991–1000, 1973.
22. Sanström B: Adjustments of the circulation to orthostatic reaction and physical exercise during the first trimester of primipregnancy. *Acta Obstet Gynecol Scand* 53:1–5, 1974.
23. Davis J, Covertino V: A comparison of heart rate methods for predicting endurance training intensity. *Med Sci Sports* 7:295–298, 1975.
24. Genzell D, Robbe H, Stron G: Total amount of hemoglobin and physical working capacity in normal pregnancy and puerperium (with iron medication). *Acta Obstet Gynecol Scand* 36:93–136, 1957.
25. Dahlstrom H, Irhman K: Clinical and physiological study of pregnancy in material from northern Sweden; V. The results of work tests during and after pregnancy. *Acta Soc Med Upsal* 65:305–314, 1960.
26. Ueland K, Novy M, Metcalfe J: Cardiorespiratory responses to pregnancy and exercise in normal women and patients with heart disease. *Am J Obstet Gynecol* 115:4–10, 1973.
27. Knuttgen HG, Emerson Jr K: Physiological response to pregnancy at rest and during exercise. *J Appl Physiol* 36:549–553, 1974.
28. Browne J, Veall N: The maternal placental blood flow in normotensive and hypertensive women. *J Obstet Gynaecol Br Emp* 60:141–147, 1953.
29. Sovia K, Salmi A, Gronroos M, et al: Physical working capacity during pregnancy and effect of physical work test on fetal heart rate. *Ann Chir Gynaecol* 53:187–196, 1964.
30. Read C: Observation of a series of labours with special reference to physiological delivery. *Lancet* 1:721–726, 1949.
31. Thoms H, Wyatt R: One thousand consecutive deliveries under training for childbirth program. *Am J Obstet Gynecol* 61:205–209, 1951.
32. Rodway H: A statistical study of the effects of exercise on childbirth. *J Obstet Gynecol Br Commonw* 54:77–85, 1947.
33. Burnett C: The value of antenatal exercises. *J Obstet Gynecol* 63:40–57, 1955.
34. Curet L, Orr A, Rankin J, et al: Effect of exercise on cardiac output and distribution of uterine blood flow in pregnant ewes. *JAP*, 40:725–728, 1976.
35. Kasch F: San Diego State University, San Diego, Calif. (unpublished data), 1976.
36. Morris N, Osborn S, Wright H, et al: Effective uterine blood flow during exercise in normal and pre-eclamptic pregnancies. *Lancet* 2:481–484, 1956.
37. Hon E, Wohlgemuth R: Electronic evaluation of fetal heart rate; IV. The effect of maternal exercise. *Am J Obstet Gynecol* 81:361–371, 1961
38. Emmanouilides G, Hobel C, Yashiro K, et al: Fetal responses to maternal exercise in sheep. *Am J Obstet Gynecol* 112:130–137, 1972.
39. Orr J, Ungerer T, Will J, et al: Effects of exercise stress on carotid, uterine and iliac blood flow in pregnant and non-pregnant ewes. *Am J Obstet Gynecol* 114:213–217, 1972.
40. Blackburn M, Calloway D: Energy expenditure and consumption of mature pregnant and lactating women. *J Am Diet Assoc* 69:29–37, 1973.
41. Pomerance J, Gluck L, Lynch V: Maternal exercise as a screening test for uteroplacental insufficiency. *Obstet Gynecol* 44:383–387, 1974.

10
Hormonal Responses to Exercise in Pregnancy

Very few studies are available on the hormonal adaptation to exercise in pregnancy. Ample literature is available on the endocrine changes in pregnancy and the related pertinent literature has been reviewed in Chapter 5.

To properly assess the effects of physical activity on the endocrine system, a distinction has to be made between responses to acute exercise and physical training. The endocrine responses to exercise in pregnancy have to be examined against a background of various endocrine adaptations to pregnancy superimposed by acute oxygen and fuel requirements of exertion.

One of the major physiological requirements of pregnancy is the constant need for adequate supply of nutrients to the fetus. Pregnancy is characterized by a state of hyperinsulinemia that leads to an increase in peripheral glucose utilization, a decrease in plasma glucose levels, increased tissue storage of glycogen, and decreased hepatic glucose production. Late in pregnancy there is a sparing of maternal glucose utilization resulting in decreased maternal levels of glucose and amino acids, increased production of fatty acids and ketones, pancreatic islet hypertrophy, and increased insulin response to glucose. As such pregnancy has been described as a diabetogenic state during which various degrees of carbohydrate intolerance are observed (1–3) for additional details see Chapter 6.

To maintain even the lightest type of exercise there is a continuous uptake of glucose from the blood (4). To maintain such a steady glucose production there is a delicate interplay between an increased sympathoadrenal activity, elevation in plasma glucagon levels and a decrease in plasma insulin levels. In one study we have examined these complex responses to exercise in pregnancy. Figure 10.1 illustrates glucose, glucagon, and insulin levels prior to and after mild exercise, while Figure 10.2 illustrates the sympathoadrenal responses (norepinephrine, epinephrine, cortisol) to the same type of exercise (10).

With mild exercise, the mobilized energy stores come predominantly from fat. As the level of exercise increases, there is a greater contribution from carbohydrates. These events could be reflected in R (respiratory exchange ratio), a method of estimating food stuff utilization (Fig. 10.3) (5). Our studies confirm that with light exercise, plasma glucose concentrations are maintained at a remarkably constant level in pregnancy: this is facilitated by a fall in insulin and a rise in glucagon concentrations (6, 7). The decrease in plasma insulin level is proportionate to the duration and intensity of exercise. With mild exercise we have not observed a change in insulin concentrations, but we did observe a very small rise in glucagon. The interactions between glucose, glucagon, free fatty acids, (FFA), epinephrine, and norepinephrine are illustrated in Figure 10.4 (8).

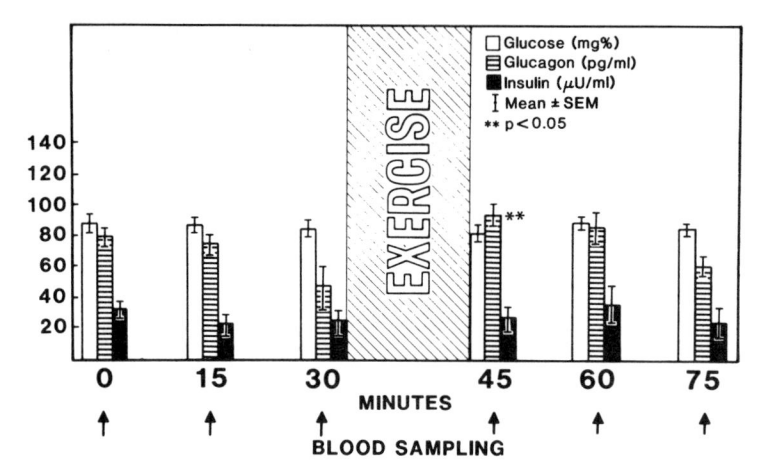

Figure 10.1. Effect of exercise on maternal glucose, glucagon, and insulin concentrations. The *asterisks* indicate a significant difference for that value when compared to the preexercise value. (From R. Artal et al.: *American Journal of Obstetrics & Gynecology*, 140:123, 1981 (10).)

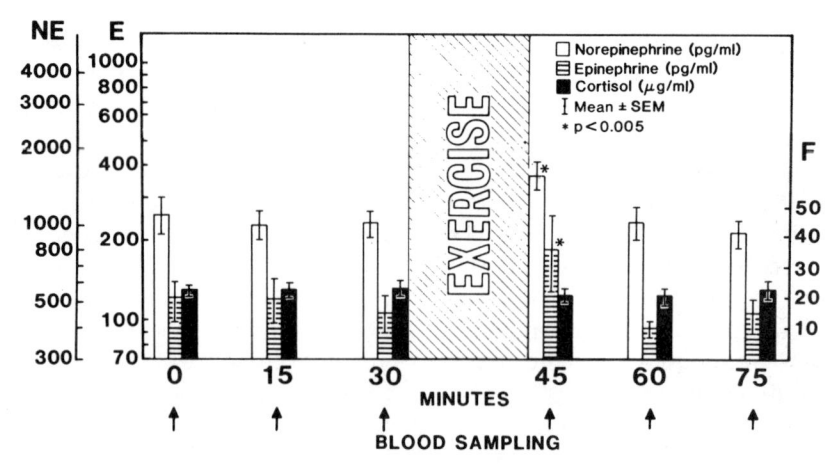

Figure 10.2. Comparison of preexercise and postexercise concentrations of norepinephrine, epinephrine, and cortisol. The data for norepinephrine (*NE*) and epinephrine (*E*) are illustrated on a logarithmic scale to the *left* of the figure and those for cortisol (*F*) are on a separate scale to the *right* of the figure. The *asterisks* indicate a significant statistical difference for that value when compared to the preexercise value. (From R. Artal et al.: *American Journal of Obstetrics & Gynecology*, 140:123, 1981 (10).)

With more intense exercise glucagon levels increase significantly. Glucagon increases glycogenolysis and gluconeogenesis in the liver and has an important role in the physiological adaptation to exercise. During recovery from exercise glucagon concentrations remain elevated for as long as 30 min, a reflection of the increased hepatic uptake of gluconeogenic precursors.

Acute changes in hormones are very sensitive to the type, intensity and duration of exercise. The physical fitness and the basic condition, i.e., fasting or postprandial, are crucial in determining hormonal responses. Figure 10.5 illustrates the percentage change in plasma glucose level to the peak of mild, moderate, and strenuous exercise. It appears that glucose levels are maintained at more stable levels during exercise in pregnancy (9). In addition, Figure 10.4 illustrates a comparison between the responses of healthy pregnant and pregnant type II diabetics to a 15-min walk on a motorized treadmill at a speed of 2 mph.

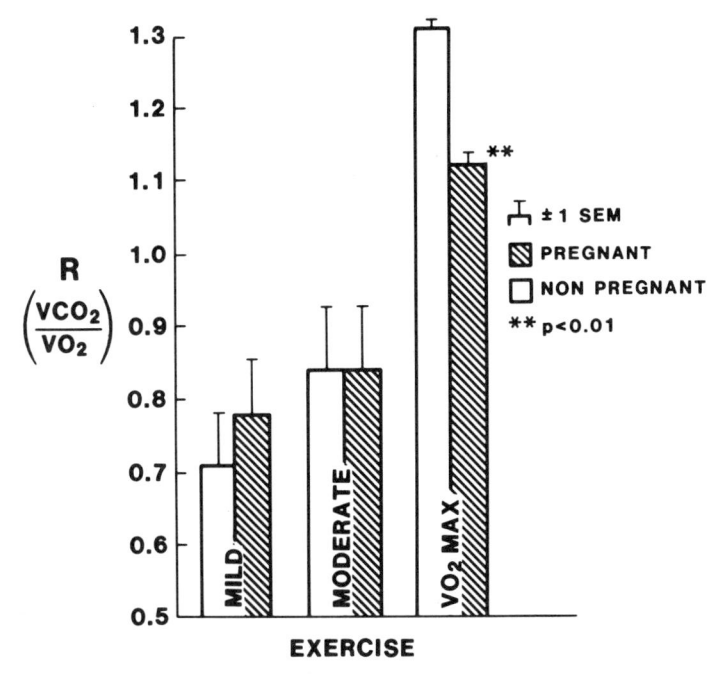

Figure 10.3. Comparison of R in pregnant and nonpregnant subjects during mild, moderate, and strenuous exercise.

Exercise has been often prescribed to achieve normoglycemia in the nonpregnant. Presently research is being conducted to establish exercise programs for the well controlled pregnant diabetics. It appears that under strict medical supervision pregnant diabetics can benefit from prescription exercise. Our own studies indicate that in such patients the response to mild exercise is similar to the one observed in the healthy pregnant subject. As illustrated in Figure 10.4, plasma glucose fell similarly with exercise in both groups and the changes are only minimal for glucagon and FFA.

The significant increase in glucose utilization during exercise is accompanied by simultaneous increases in glucose production, but hypoglycemia remains the major clinical problem in diabetics during and after exercise. Such occurrences are highly undesirable in pregnancy because of their adverse effect on the outcome. At this time, it is not known if pregnancy could be a contributing factor to exercise-related hypoglycemia, but it appears that prolonged strenuous exercise may induce hypoglycemia more rapidly in pregnancy.

We believe that the mild exercise level utilized in our study is of sufficient intensity to induce a training effect, sensitize insulin receptors, and increase glucose utilization (8). We consider this level of activity if repeated 3–4 times weekly to be of benefit to pregnant type II diabetics.

The catecholamines are known to promote both liver glycogenolysis and adipose tissue lipolysis. Epinephrine modulates both the release of glucagon and FFA. FFA provide an important energy substrate during prolonged exercise. In our laboratory studies of acute exercise we found very little change in FFA.

The level of the sympathoadrenal activity is determined by the severity of the work performed (11). Increases in circulating norepinephrine appear even at mild work loads as illustrated in Figure 10.2 and 10.6. The increments appear to be higher in pregnant women as compared to nonpregnant.

As stated many times in this text, the major hemodynamic response to exercise is the selective redistribution of blood flow to the working muscles, with a reduction in blood flow to the splanchnic organs and

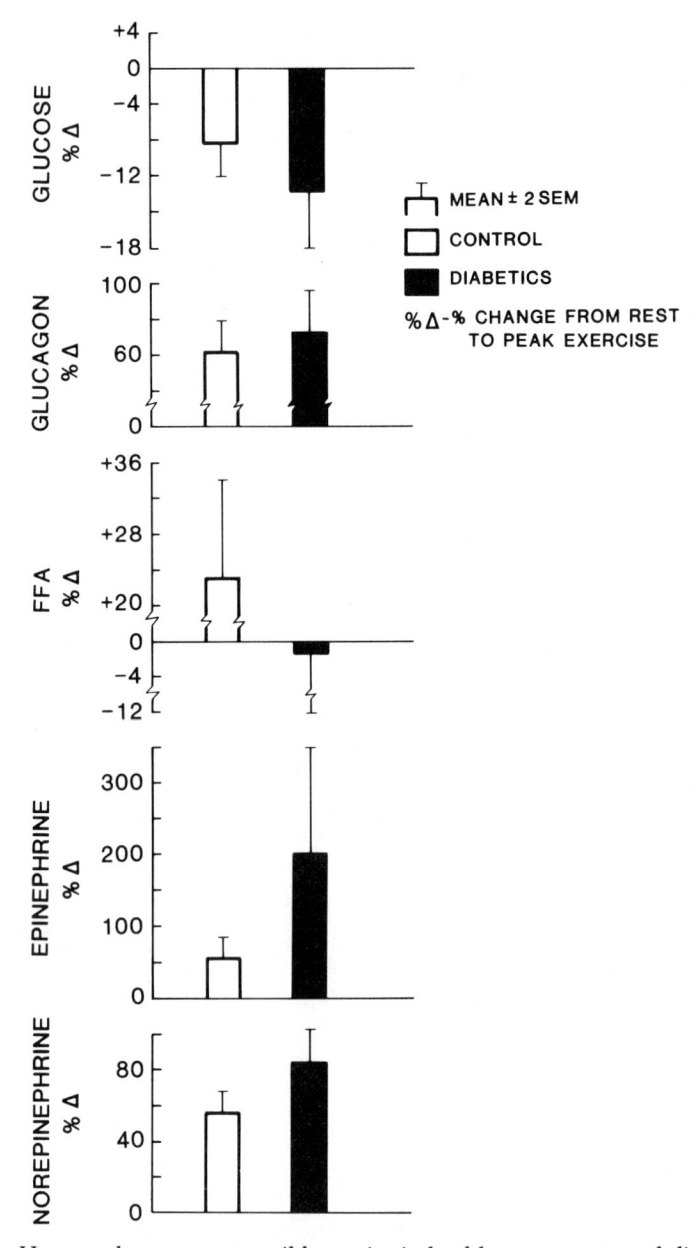

Figure 10.4. Hormonal responses to mild exercise in healthy, pregnant, and diabetic patients.

potentially to the pregnant uterus as well as to the fetus. The mechanism for blood flow redistribution is catecholamine mediated.

In all our studies we have observed a predominant rise in norepinephrine in comparision to epinephrine, confirming that exercise activates sympathetic nerves to a greater extent than the adrenal medulla, in both the pregnant and nonpregnant subjects alike. In addition it is of utmost importance to recognize that norepinephrine can act as a stimulant to the uterus and induce uterine activity (12).

During mild and moderate exercise the changes in circulating epinephrine are minimal. Under heavy strenuous exercise epinephrine increases significantly in the nonpregnant subject (11), but we have observed a significantly smaller increment in pregnancy (8) Figure 10.7. The smaller incre-

Hormonal Responses 143

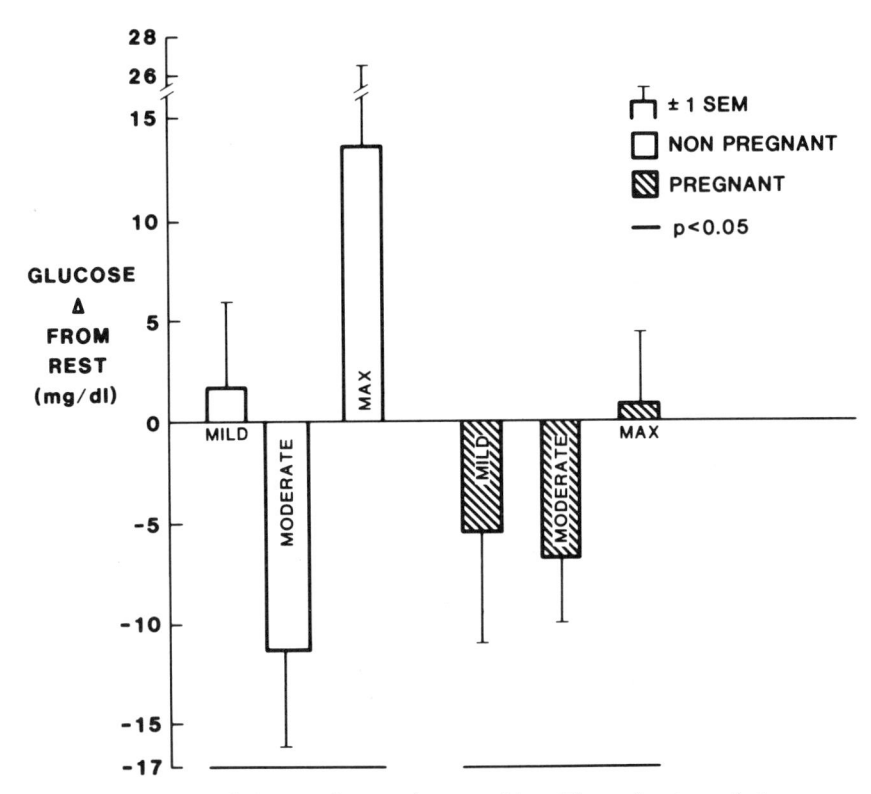

Figure 10.5. Comparison of plasma glucose change with mild, moderate, and strenuous exercise in pregnant and nonpregnant healthy subjects.

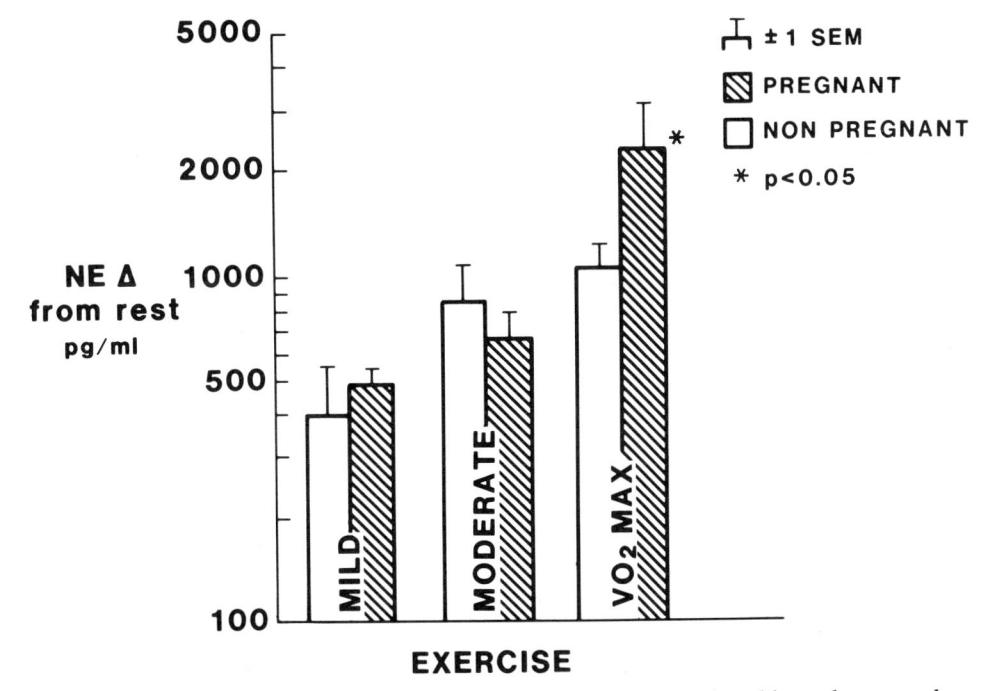

Figure 10.6. Comparison of plasma norepinephrine (NE) change with mild, moderate, and strenuous exercise in pregnant and nonpregnant healthy subjects.

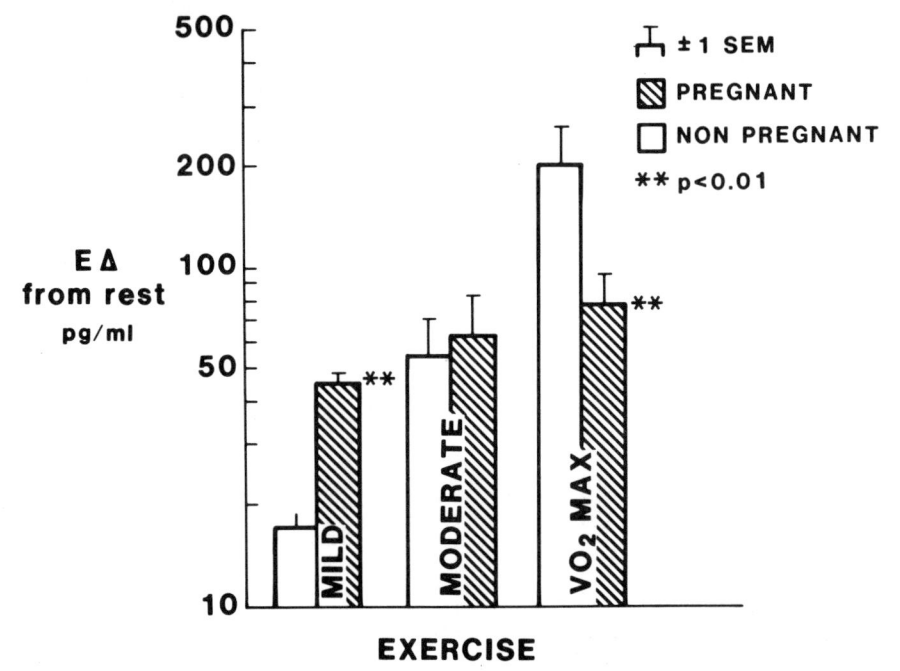

Figure 10.7. Comparison of plasma epinephrine (*E*) change with mild, moderate, and strenuous exercise in pregnant and nonpregnant healthy subjects.

ment in epinephrine would facilitate glucose uptake and maintain stable glucose levels. This steady state is desirable in pregnancy and essential to the well-being of the fetus. A further surge in epinephrine would inhibit glucose uptake and create a glut of circulating glucose. The hormonal changes observed during mild and moderate exercise are transient and return to control values within 15 min, with strenuous exercise the changes could last as long as 30 min and beyond (9).

The changes associated with exercise can be significantly diminished with training. Typical is a diminished catecholamine response in individuals after training (13). As a result, such training also blunts both the glucagon increase and the insulin decrease (14).

The role of glucocorticoids in exercise physiology has yet to be determined. Under normal conditions, glucocorticoids are known to increase, enhance liver gluconeogenesis, and induce lypolysis. In addition, anti-inflammatory properties have been attributed to them as well. It appears that short-term administration of glucocorticoids can improve exercise performance and this has been demonstrated under laboratory conditions (15). The mechanism behind the enhanced performance seems to be related to the increased ability to induce gluconeogenesis and provide further supply of glucose during exercise.

The ability of releasing glucocorticoids during exercise appears to be related to the work load itself, and to increase significantly during strenuous exercise (16). As with catecholamines, plasma glucocorticoids tend to increase less with exercise in trained subjects.

Plasma concentrations of cortisol increase with the advancement of gestation and primarily through an increase in the specific cortisol-binding protein, transcortin (17). Theoretically, along with increased levels of cortisol in pregnancy we should observe enhanced exercise performance and endurance; but there is no evidence for such effects. Mild exercise produces only a limited adrenal response, along with minimal changes in epinephrine levels, there are limited changes in circulating cortisol (Fig. 10.2) (10). Insignificant changes in circulating cor-

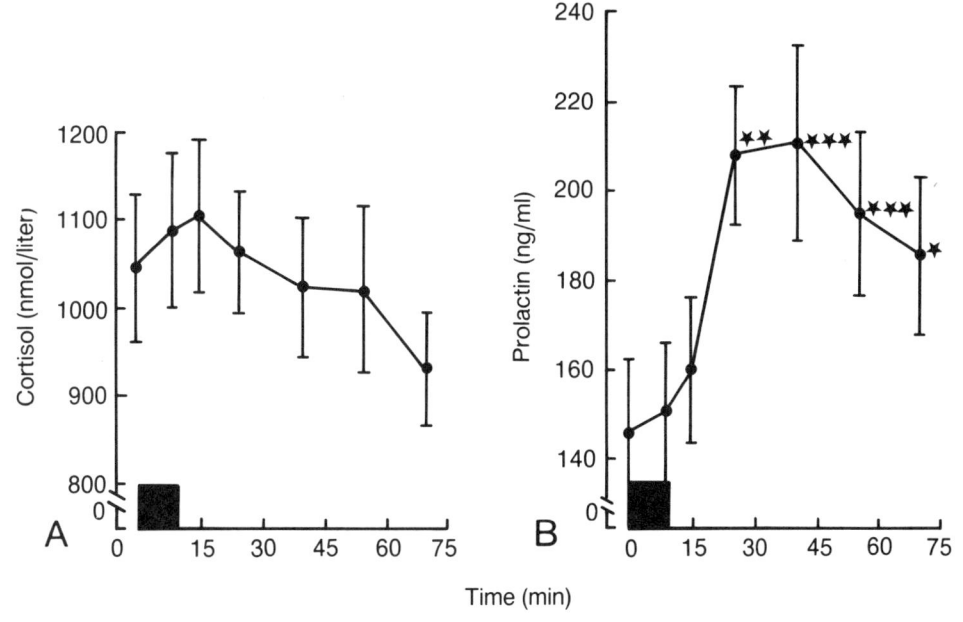

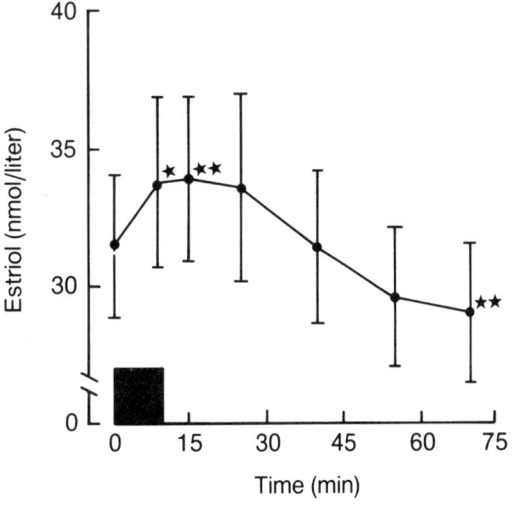

Figure 10.8. Serum cortisol (*A*) and prolactin (*B*) concentrations (means ± SEM). ■ = Submaximal exercise. Significance of differences: *P < 0.02; **P < 0.01; ***P < 0.005. (From I. Rauramo et al.: *British Journal of Obstetrics & Gynaecology*, 89:921, 1982 (18).)

tisol are also observed following submaximal exercise (Fig. 10.3) (18). Thus it appears that cortisol plays only a limited role in the physiology of exercise, both in pregnancy or not.

Prolactin is a peptide hormone with similarities to growth hormone. Prolactin has been reported to have a multitude of actions and because of its role in water electrolyte balance it has certain physiological significance in response to exercise (19). Submaximal exercise in pregnancy significantly elevates serum prolactin concentrations for at least 1 hour (Fig. 10.8) (18).

Ovarian hormones, estradiol and progesterone increase during exercise, with a most prominent response during strenuous exercise (20). It is unclear if the circulating hormones or their administration cause improved exercise performance. During normal human pregnancy there is a hyperestrogenic state, with a disproportionate increase in estriol. The close involvement of the fetus in the biosynthesis of estriol has been utilized in the past to monitor fetal status. Low values of estriol have been interpreted to reflect fetal distress. During submaximal ex-

Figure 10.9. Serum estriol concentration (means ± SEM). ■ = Submaximal exercise. Significance of differences: *P < 0.05; **P < 0.02. (From I. Rauramo et al.: *British Journal of Obstetrics & Gynaecology*, 89:921, 1982 (18).)

ercise in pregnancy a significant transient rise in serum estriol concentrations has been observed, as illustrated in Figure 10.9 (18). This temporary rise may be interpreted in different ways, it could reflect fetal well being and be considered a normal response to a state of increased sympathetic activity, or it could be explained by an increased flow of estriol-rich uteroplacental blood into the maternal circulation immediately after the exercise.

The endocrine responses to exercise in pregnancy are presently being investigated. The limited information that is available indicates that, in the healthy pregnant woman, the changes are transitory and reversible with no deleterious lasting effects. The complete complex interactions between mother and fetus, during maternal activity, have yet to be described.

REFERENCES

1. Kalkhoff RK, Schalch DS, Walker JL, et al: Diabetogenic factors associated with pregnancy. *Trans Assoc Am Physicians* 77:270, 1964.
2. Spellacy WN, Goetz FC: Plasma insulin in normal late pregnancy. *N Engl J Med* 268:988, 1963.
3. Kuhl C: Serum preinsulin in normal and gestational diabetic pregnancy. *Diabetologia* 12:295, 1976.
4. Wahren J, Ahlborg G, Felig P, Jorfeldt L: Glucose metabolism during exercise in man. In Pernow B, Saltin B (eds): *Muscle Metabolism during exercise*. New York, Plenum, 1971, p 189.
5. Artal R, Wiswell R, Romem Y: Pulmonary responses to exercise in pregnancy. *Am J Obstet Gynecol* (in press).
6. Pruett EDR: Plasma insulin concentrations during prolonged work at near maximal oxygen uptake. *J Appl Physiol* 29:155, 1970.
7. Bottiger I, Schlein FM, Faloona GR, et al: The effect of exercise on glucagon secretion. *J Clin Endocrinol Metab* 35:117, 1972.
8. Artal R, Wiswell R, Romen Y: Hormonal responses to exercise in diabetic and nondiabetic pregnant patients. *Diabetes* (in press).
9. Artal R, Wiswell R, Romen Y, Kammula R: Hormonal changes during exercise in pregnancy (submitted for publication).
10. Artal R, Platt LD, Sperling M, Kammula KR, Jilek J, Nakamura P: Exercise in pregnancy. Maternal cardiovascular and metabolic responses in normal pregnancy. *Am J Obstet Gynecol* 140:123, 1981.
11. Hartley LH, Mason JW, Hogan RP, Jones LG, Kotchen TA, Mongey EH, Wherry FE, Pennington LL, Rickets PT: Multiple hormonal responses to graded exercise in relation to physical training. *J Appl Physiol* 33:602, 1972.
12. Zuspan FP, Cibils LA, Pose SY: Myometrial and cardiovascular responses to alterations in plasmus epinephrine and norepinephrine. *Am J Obstet Gynecol* 84:841, 1962.
13. Scheuer J, Tipton CM: Cardiovascular adaptations to physical training. *Annu Rev Physiol* 39:221, 1977.
14. Gyntelberg F, Rennie MJ, Hickson RC, Holloszy JO: Effect of training on the response of plasma glucagon to exercise. *J Appl Physiol* 43:302, 1977.
15. Isekutz B, Allen M: Effect of methylprednisolone on carbohydrate metabolism of exercising dogs. *J Appl Physiol* 31:813, 1977.
16. Dessypris A, Kuoppasalmi K, Adlercrentz H: Plasma cortisol, testosterone, androstenedione and luteinizing hormone in a noncompetitive marathon run. *J Steroid Biochem* 7:33, 1976.
17. Rosenthal HE, Slaunwhite WR Jr, Sandberg AA: Transcortin: a corticosteroid-binding protein of plasma. Cortisol and progesterone interplay and unbound levels of these steroids in pregnancy. *J Clin Endocrinol Metab* 29:352, 1969.
18. Rauramo I, Andersson B, Laatikainen T: Stress hormones and placental steroids in physical exercise during pregnancy. *Br J Obstet Gynaecol* 89:921, 1982.
19. Yen SSC: Physiology of human prolactin. In Yen SSC, Jaffe RB (eds): *Reproductive Endocrinology*. Philadelphia, W. B. Saunders, 1978, pp 150.
20. Jurkowski JE, Jones NL, Walker WC, Younglai EV, Sutton JR: Ovarian hormonal responses to exercise. *J Appl Physiol* 44:109, 1978.

11
Pulmonary Responses to Exercise in Pregnancy

The physiological requirements and normal changes of pregnancy include close interactions between cardiovascular and respiratory functions. The mechanism by which O_2 and CO_2 are transported between the atmosphere and the cells, mother, and fetus is quite complex and is described in detail in Chapter 12.

As pregnancy progresses, individuals who exercise may experience increasing intolerance to exercise which is caused by the inability to transfer gas (O_2 and CO_2) between the atmosphere to cells. Such deficiencies are usually compensated in nonpregnant individuals by increased pulmonary diffusing capacity and increased alveolar ventilation. In addition, in pregnancy, hemoglobin, oxygen-carrying capacity and cardiac output increase significantly and in excess of demands, leading to decreased arteriovenous oxygen difference.

The purpose of this chapter is to review the adaptive changes in the respiratory system during exercise in pregnancy.

As described in Chapter 5, pregnancy is characterized by various anatomical changes and the most significant are summarized below. The upper respiratory tract is often affected by changes in the mucosa of the nasopharynx such as hyperemia, edema, and excessive secretion, all causing obstructive symptoms. The rib cage undergoes changes in pregnancy which result in an expansion of the chest circumference due to the elevation of the diaphragm by the growing uterus (1–4). These changes are more prominent during the second half of pregnancy, and lead to an increase in inspiratory capacity of 300 ml (tidal volume + inspiratory volume) and a reduction in functional residual capacity (5–6) to maintain intact total lung and vital capacity. Significantly, pregnancy is characterized by a 10–20% increase in oxygen consumption. The combination of reduced functional residual capacity and increased oxygen consumption results in lower oxygen reserve. If not properly compensated, the oxygen reserve could be further lowered during heavy exercise and potentially lead to hypoxia. The resting minute ventilation is increased by 40–50%, leading to a decrease of arterial P_{CO_2} to 30 mm Hg and an arterial P_{O_2} of approximately 105 mm Hg. The respiratory alkalosis is due to the effect of estrogen and progesterone on the respiratory center of the brain. Acid base status is maintained by a compensatory metabolic acidosis. This results in a decrease in serum bicarbonate of approximately 20 meq/liter. The arterial pH is approximately 7.44.

Arterial P_{O_2} can be significantly reduced in pregnancy in the supine position. Either supine position, hypoventilation of a lesser degree or hyperventilation leading to systemic maternal alkalosis in pregnancy can significantly increase the risk of hypoxia in the fetus.

Functionally, the pregnant woman compensates for all of the above changes by breathing more deeply. In pregnancy, even individuals with moderate to severe lung disease do well, in contrast to women with cardiac disease (9). In the nonpregnant state, subjects with lung disease, e.g., chronic obstructive lung disease, can exercise to a maximum breathing capacity of 80–100% while individuals with heart disease only to about 55% of their predicted maximum heart rate (7).

PULMONARY RESPONSES TO EXERCISE DURING PREGNANCY

As stated above, pulmonary functions change in pregnancy. Several studies have reviewed this topic and the findings are summarized in Table 11.1 (adapted from Alaily and Carrol (10)). Most of the measurements presented in this table were collected at rest at different stages in pregnancy and compared to postpartum states.

Few of the above studies have conducted the measurements in the same individuals in the pregnant and nonpregnant state. Furthermore, fewer have studied the same functions in humans during exercise. Several related studies have been completed in experimental animals and are described in detail in Chapter 3.

Exercise studies conducted or performed on pregnant women, by and large, lacked controls and standardization, ignored state of fitness or extrapolated it from estimated $\dot{V}_{O_2max}$ data. Only a few studies carried their subjects to $\dot{V}_{O_2max}$. Very little attention has been paid to distinguishing between weight- and non-weight-bearing exercise. The limitations and advantages of utilizing each such testing are detailed in Chapter 2.

Weight-bearing exercises are performed less efficiently and are more energy-costly in pregnancy, since they contain a component of body weight. Few studies have been published on pulmonary responses to exercise in pregnancy and postpartum (6, 8, 15–20). Since the methods, intensity of exercise, and level of fitness in the different studies cannot be compared in absolute values, we have summarized the data published by their relative changes (Table 11.2).

From the above studies, it appears that respiratory frequency tends to increase with either weight- or non-weight-bearing exercises. Such an increase is quite similar to that occurring in nonpregnant controls. Most of the studies have found a significant increase in minute ventilation and tidal volume, not only at rest, but also during and following exercise. The changes were significantly higher for the degree of exercise than in nonpregnant controls. The disproportionate increase in minute ventilation as compared to oxygen consumption is reflected in a relatively high ventilatory equivalent for oxygen.

In our studies (15), we compared the pulmonary responses to mild, moderate and $\dot{V}_{O_2max}$ exercise (Fig. 11.1). During mild exercise (approximately 210 kpm), the respiratory frequency of pregnant women (43 subjects) was found to be significantly higher when compared to controls (15 subjects) (Fig. 11.2). During the same type of exercise, minute ventilation appeared to be

Table 11.1. Comparison of Pulmonary Function of Pregnancy and Postpartum[a]

Author	No. of Patients	VC	IC	EC	MV	TV	RF	FRC	RV	TLC
Prowse and Gaensler (11)	9	—		↓				↓	↓	—
Gee et al. (12)	10	↓		↓				↓	↓	↓
Gazioglu et al. (5)	8	↑	↑	↓	↑	↑	—	↓	↓	
Lehmann and Fabel (13)	23	—	↑	↓	↑	↑	—	↓	↓	↓
Knuttgen and Emerson (6)	13	↑	↑		↑	↑	—	↓		—
Pernoll et al. (14)	12				↑	↑	↓			
Alaily and Carrol (10)	38	—	↑	↓	↑	↑	↓	↓		↓

[a] VC = vital capacity; IC = inspiratory capacity; MV = minute volume; TV = tidal volume; RF = respiratory frequency; FRC = functional residual capacity; RV = residual volume; TLC = total lung capacity; ↑ = increase; — = no difference; ↓ = decrease.

Table 11.2. Comparison of Pulmonary Responses to Exercise in Pregnancy Versus Controls[a]

Author	No. of Patients	RF	$\dot{V}_e$	$\dot{V}_{O_2}$	VT	$\dot{V}_e/\dot{V}_{O_2}$	R	Exercise	Intensity[b]
Bader et al. (8)	46			↑				Ergometer	Steady rate
Guzman and Caplan (16)	8	↑—	↑		—	—		Ergometer	150 kpm
Ueland et al. (17)	22			↑				Ergometer	100 kpm
Knuttgen and Emerson (6)	13	—	↑	↑	↑	↑	↑	Treadmill	380 kpm
Knuttgen and Emerson (6)	13	—	↑	—	;ua	↑	—	Ergometer	367 kpm
Pernoll et al. (18)	12	↑—	↑	↑	↑		—	Ergometer	306 kpm
Collings et al. (19)	20			↑				Ergometer	Submax
Artal and Wiswell (15)	58	↑	—↑	—	—	↑	—↑	Treadmill	~210 kpm
	34	↓	↓	—	—	—↓	—	Treadmill 10% grade	~350 kpm
	35	↓	↓	↓	↓	↑	↓	Treadmill	$\dot{V}_{O_2}$max ~650 kpm

[a] RF = respiratory frequency; $\dot{V}_e$ = minute ventilation; $\dot{V}_{O_2}$ = oxygen uptake; VT = tidal volume; $\dot{V}_E/\dot{V}_{O_2}$ = ventilatory equivalent; R = respiratory exchange ratio; ↑ = increase; — = no difference; ↓ = decrease.
[b] 100 kpm = 16.35 watts.

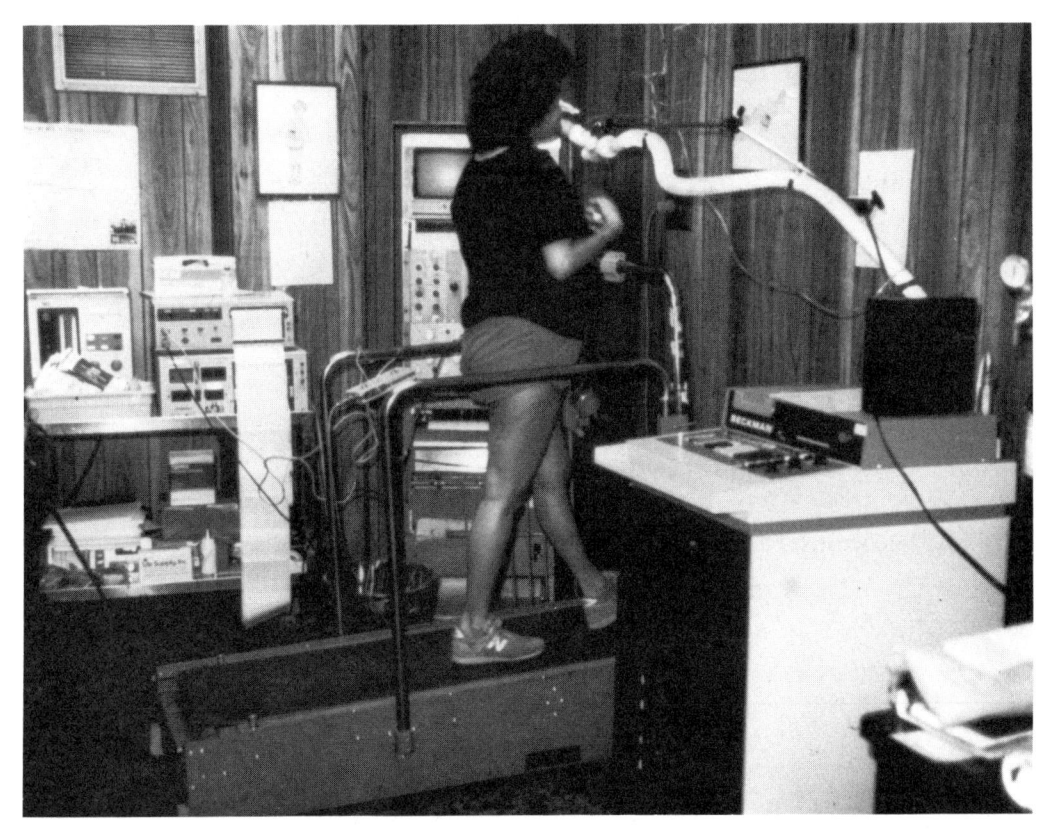

Figure 11.1. Pulmonary function testing in exercise laboratory.

slightly increased in pregnancy while $\dot{V}_{O_2}$ and tidal volume were found to be comparable for the same amount of work (Figs. 11.3 and 11.4). The relative increase in minute ventilation resulted in a higher ventilatory equivalent during this type of exercise in pregnancy when compared to controls (Fig. 11.5). During $\dot{V}_{O_2max}$ exercise (25 sub-

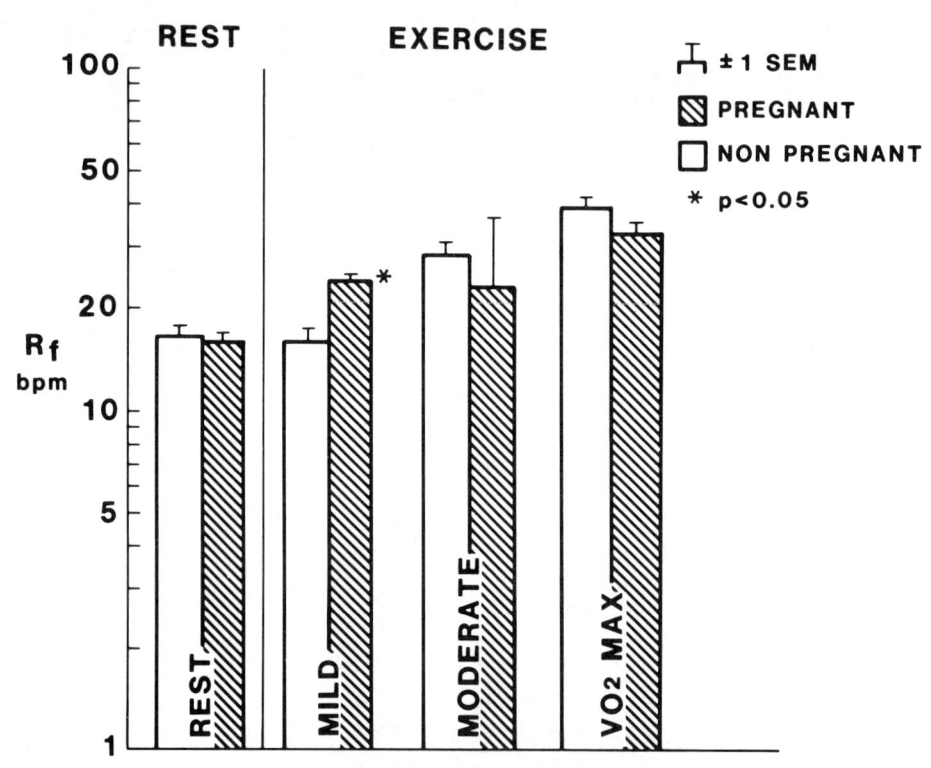

Figure 11.2. Respiratory frequency during mild, moderate, and $\dot{V}_{O_2max}$ exercise. (From R. Artal et al.: *American Journal of Obstetrics & Gynecology* (in press) (15).)

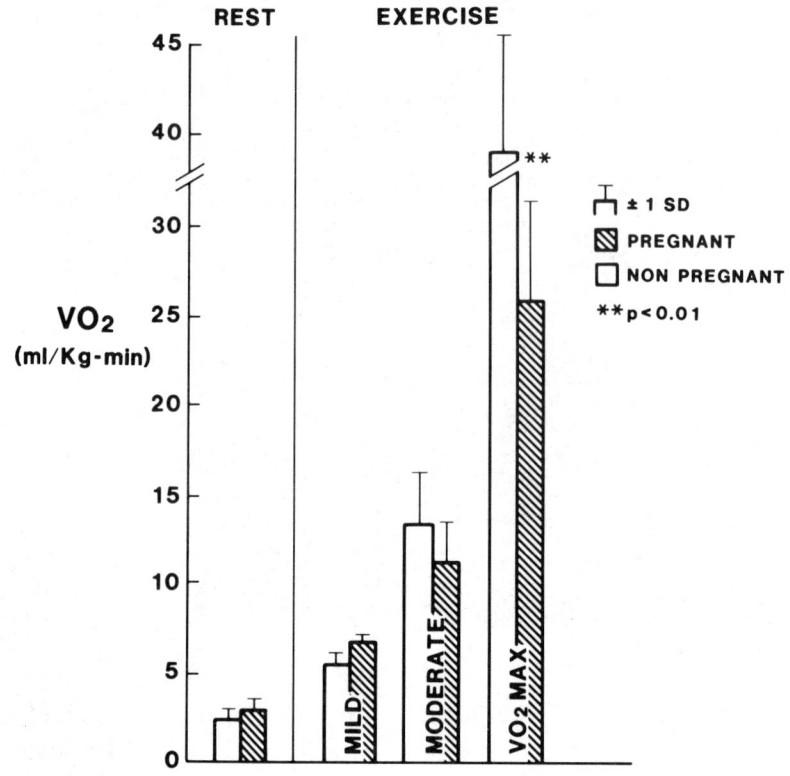

Figure 11.3. Oxygen consumption during mild, moderate and $\dot{V}_{O_2max}$ exercise. (From R. Artal et al.: *American Journal of Obstetrics & Gynecology* (in press) (15).)

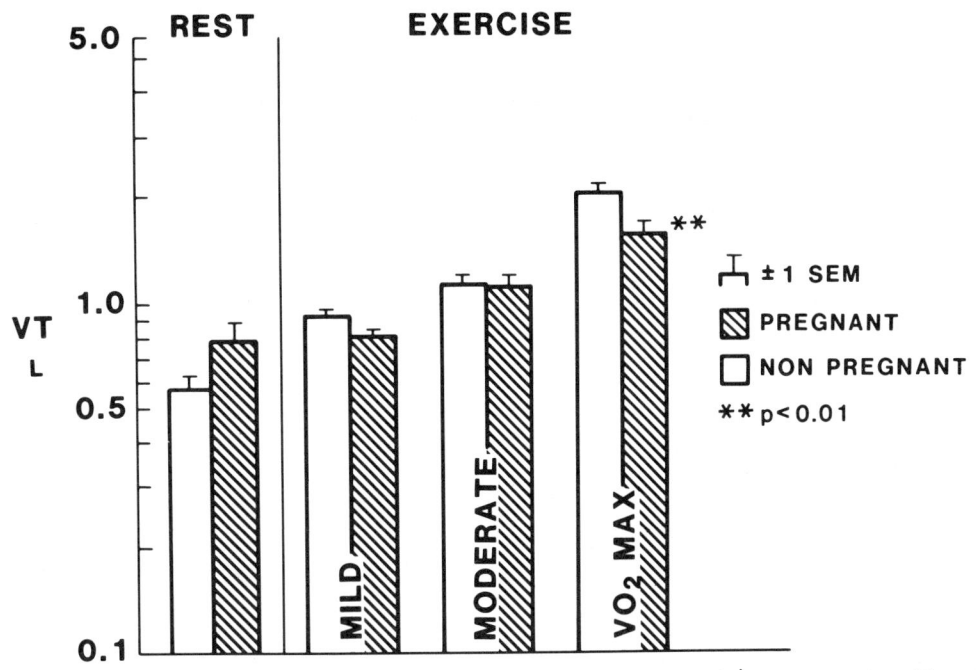

Figure 11.4. Comparison of tidal volumes during mild, moderate and $\dot{V}_{O_2}$max exercise. (From R. Artal et al.: *American Journal of Obstetrics & Gynecology* (in press) (15).)

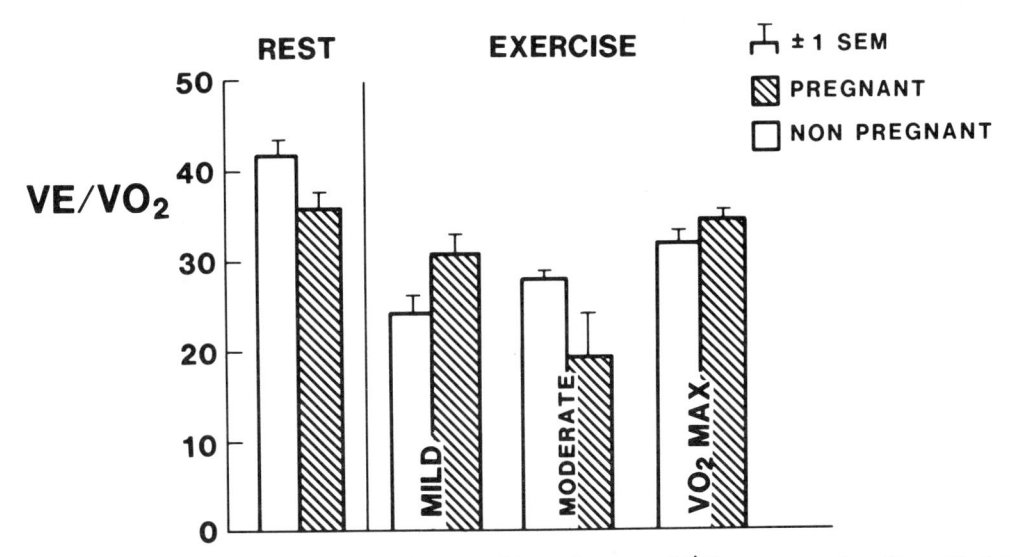

Figure 11.5. Ventilatory equivalents during mild, moderate and $\dot{V}O_2$ max exercise. (From R. Artal et al.: *American Journal of Obstetrics & Gynecology* (in press) (15).)

jects), the pregnant women were not capable of matching the responses of the nonpregnant controls (10 subjects).

By and large, the pregnant subjects responded to exercise with increased ventilation at mild and maximal exercise.

It appears that, contrary to our predictions, pregnant subjects demonstrate a more efficient ventilatory response to moderate exercise (3–4 METs) when compared to nonpregnant controls as demonstrated by a significantly lower ventilatory equivalent ($\dot{V}_E/\dot{V}_{O_2}$). It can be hypothesized that the improved response during moderate exercise is a result of the primary respiratory alkalosis of pregnancy. Tidal volumes were similar between the groups, but the pregnant subjects had significantly lower respiratory frequency. At $\dot{V}_{O_2max}$ exercise, the primary respiratory alkalosis is not sufficient to compensate for the developing metabolic lactic acidosis. Further support to the above findings is that CO_2 production during moderate exercise is slightly lower due to a favorable respiratory equivalent (Fig. 11.6).

This state of hyperventilation that occurs at rest in pregnancy persists and increases with exercise, resulting in lower CO_2 tension, lower bicarbonate concentrations, lower buffering capacity, a modest increase in pH, with negligible changes in O_2 tension.

It has been recognized for a long time that maternal hyperventilation, when producing respiratory alkalosis in the mother, may lead to fetal respiratory alkalosis (21). The fall in maternal and fetal P_{CO_2} is associated with a corresponding fall in fetal P_{O_2} (Fig. 11.7).

Our data indicate that, during intensive exercise, pregnant women utilize proportionately less carbohydrates as their fuel source and fat becomes the principal source of energy, as reflected in lower R during intensive exercise coupled by increased ventilation and respiratory acidosis. This may indicate an inability to exercise anaerobically, a protective mechanism from hypoxia, or reflect a protective mechanism to maintain steady levels of carbohydrates. In other words, the lower $\dot{V}_{O_2max}$ may be a result of decreased fuel or muscle mass, but also reflect the inability of the mother to allow a state of hypoxia or hypoglycemia (Fig. 11.8). However, caution must be exercised when trying to assess fuel substrate utilization pattern derived from R, in the presence of hyperventilation of pregnancy. We know of no studies that have evaluated substrate turnover during exercise in pregnancy and therefore we submit the above as a possible hypothesis.

PULMONARY HEMODYNAMICS

One unique study which is unlikely to be repeated was performed by Bader et al. (8)

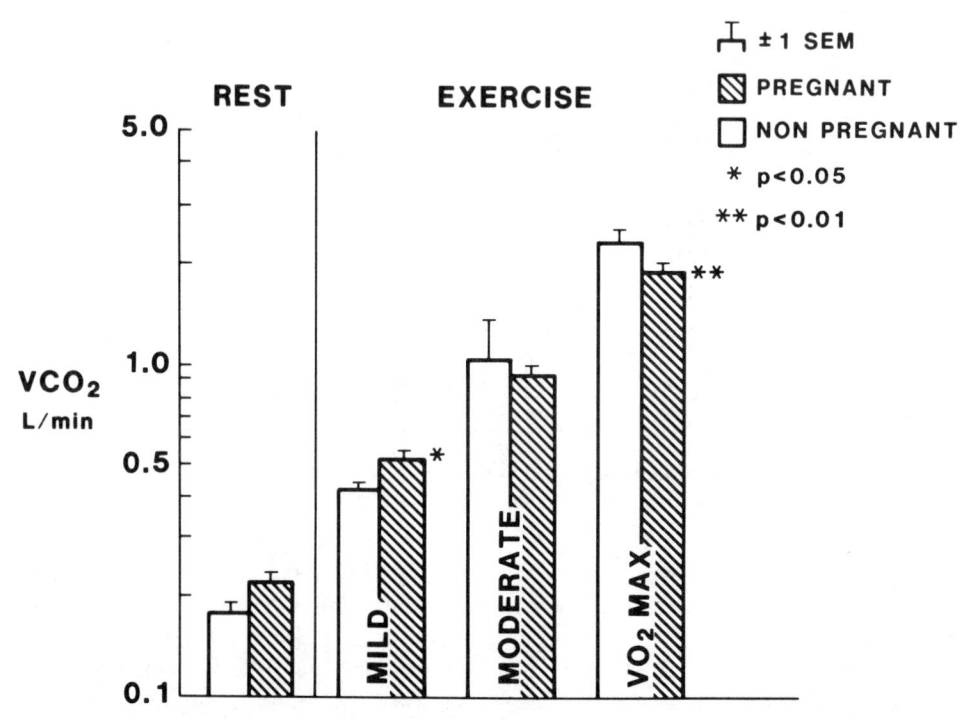

Figure 11.6. CO_2 production during mild, moderate, and $\dot{V}_{O_2}$max exercise. (From R. Artal et al.: *American Journal of Obstetrics & Gynecology* (in press) (15).)

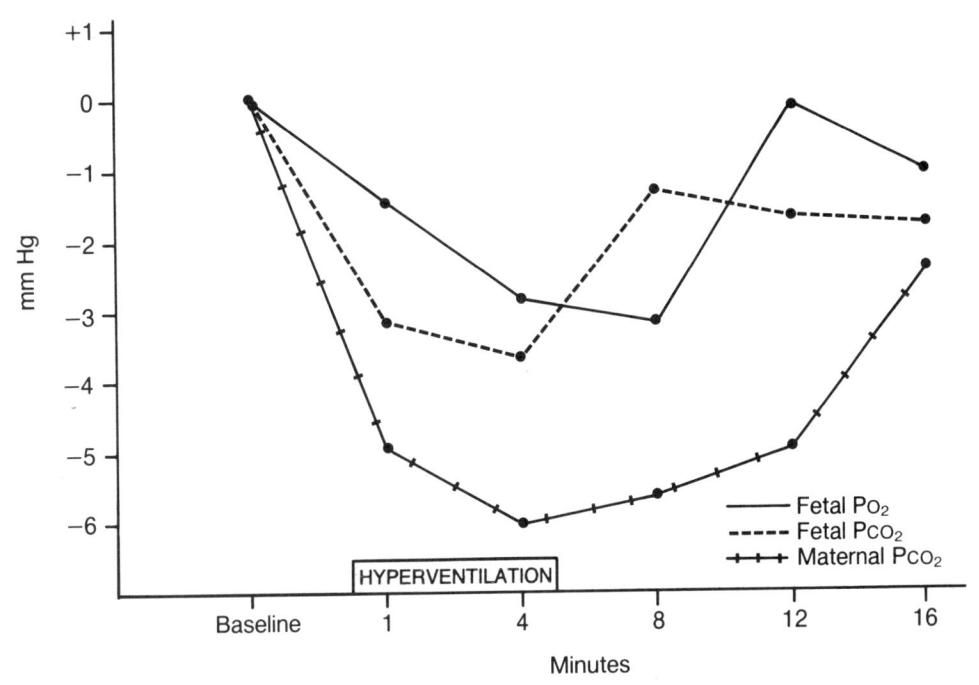

Figure 11.7. The relationship between maternal P_{CO_2}, fetal P_{CO_2}, and fetal P_{O_2} during maternal hyperventilation. (From F. C. Miller et al.: *American Journal of Obstetrics & Gynecology*, 120:489, 1974 (21).)

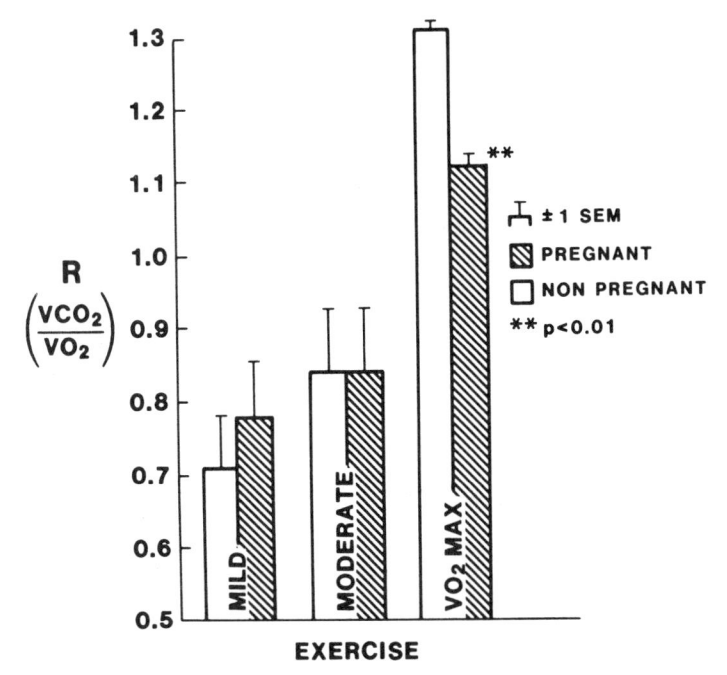

Figure 11.8. Comparison of respiratory exchange ratio (R) during mild, moderate, and $\dot{V}_{O_2 max}$ exercise. (From R. Artal et al.: *American Journal of Obstetrics & Gynecology* (in press) (15).)

in which 46 normal pregnant women had right heart and pulmonary artery catheterization at rest and during 10 min of exercise on a bicycle in a recumbent position. These authors found, at rest, increasing oxygen consumption levels as pregnancy progresses, and similar trends were maintained during exercise. Conversely, they found a decrease in cardiac output with exercise during pregnancy. In retrospect, such a decrease could be considered positional and attributed to impaired venous return to the heart.

The arteriovenous O_2 difference was significantly lower early in pregnancy when compared to late pregnancy. Pulmonary artery diastolic pressure was normal at rest, increased slightly with exercise, and exceeded 12 mm Hg in 5 subjects. Mean pulmonary artery pressure was normal through pregnancy, rose with exercise by 15 mm Hg in 6 subjects and, in 2 subjects the increment was 20 mm Hg. Pulmonary capillary pressure did not change either at rest or with exercise as pregnancy progressed.

An elevation in right ventricular and diastolic pressure at rest was noted in some patients, a finding consistent with a congested circulatory state. It also appears from this study that pregnant women respond to exercise with an increase in pulmonary diffusing capacity identical to nonpregnant subjects. Conversely, the pulmonary alterations associated with pregnancy and exacerbated by exercise (e.g., hyperventilation) are an important factor in regulating utilization of fuel and buffering the effect of lactate production that could limit exercise tolerance.

REFERENCES

1. Schofman MA: The nose and pregnancy. *J Fla Med Assoc* 48:160, 1961.
2. Thomson KJ, Cohen ME: Studies of the circulation in pregnancy: vital capacity observations in normal pregnant women. *Surg Gynecol Obstet* 66:591, 1938.
3. Marx GF, Orxin LR: Physiological changes during pregnancy: a review. *Anesthesiology* 19:258, 1958.
4. Leoutic EA: Respiratory disease in pregnancy. *Med Clin North Am* 61:111, 1977.
5. Gazioglu K, Kaltreider NL, Rosen M, Yu PN: Pulmonary function during pregnancy in normal women and in patients with cardiopulmonary disease. *Thorax* 25:445, 1970.
6. Knuttgen HG, Emerson K: Physiological response to pregnancy at rest and during exercise. *J Appl Physiol* 36:549, 1974.
7. Kanarek DJ, Hand RW: The response of cardiac and pulmonary disease to exercise testing. *Clin Chest Med* 5:181, 1984.
8. Bader RA, Bader ME, Rose DJ, Braunwald E: Hemodynamics at rest and during exercise in normal pregnancy as studied by cardiac catheterization. *J Clin Invest* 34:1524, 1955.
9. Bedell GN, Adams RW: Pulmonary diffusing capacity during rest and exercise. A study of normal persons and persons with atrial septal defect, pregnancy and pulmonary disease. *J Clin Invest* 41:1908, 1962.
10. Alaily AB, Carrol KB: Pulmonary ventilation in pregnancy. *Br J Obstet Gynaecol* 85:518, 1978.
11. Prowse CM, Gaensler EA: Respiratory and acid-base changes during pregnancy. *Anesthesiology* 26:381, 1965.
12. Gee BL, Packer BS, Millen EJ, Robin ED: Pulmonary mechanics during pregnancy. *J Clin Invest* 46:945, 1967.
13. Lehmann V, Fabel H: Lung enfunktion untersuchungen an schwangeren; Tell I: Lungenvolumina. *Z Geburtshilfe Perinatol* 177:387, 1973.
14. Pernoll ML, Metcalfe J, Schlenker TL, Welch JE, Matsumoto JA: Oxygen consumption at rest and during exercise in pregnancy. *Respir Physiol* 25:285, 1975.
15. Artal R et al.: Pulmonary responses to exercise in pregnancy. *Am J Obstet Gynecol* (in press).
16. Guzman CA, Caplan R: Cardiorespiratory response to exercise during pregnancy. *Am J Obstet Gynecol* 108:600, 1970.
17. Ueland K, Navy JM, Metcalfe J: Cardiorespiratory responses to pregnancy and exercise in normal women and patients with heart disease. *Am J Obstet Gynecol* 115:4, 1973.
18. Pernoll ML, Metcalf J, Kovach PA, Wachtel R, Dunham MJ: Ventilation during rest and exercise in pregnancy and postpartum. *Respir Physiol* 25:295, 1975.
19. Collings CA, Curet LB, Mullin JP: Maternal and fetal responses to a maternal aerobic exercise program. *Am J Obstet Gynecol* 145:702, 1983.
20. Edwards MJ, Metcalfe J, Dunham MY, Paul MS: Accelerated respiratory response to moderate exercise in late pregnancy. *Respir Physiol* 45:229, 1981.
21. Miller FC, Petrie RH, Arce JJ, Paul RH, Hon EH: Hyperventilation during labor. *Am J Obstet Gynecol* 120:489, 1974.

12

Placental Oxygen Transfer with Considerations for Maternal Exercise

The fetus requires virtually a continuous supply of oxygen to maintain normal metabolism, growth, and development. Averaging 8 ml·min^{-1}·kg^{-1}, this oxygen requirement is derived from the maternal circulation by diffusion across the placenta. Questions arise as to what controls placental oxygen transfer under normal conditions, and how it might be affected by maternal exercise.

A number of factors contribute to oxygen transfer across the placenta and are summarized in Table 12.1. Some of these include: maternal and fetal arterial O$_2$ partial pressures, maternal and fetal hemoglobin affinities for O$_2$, maternal and fetal placental hemoglobin flow rates, the diffusing capacity of the placenta, the vascular relations of maternal to fetal vessels, and the quantity of carbon dioxide exchanged (93). This chapter will explore the role of each of these variables on oxygen transfer and identify the factors which normally limit oxygen exchange across the placenta. The possible effects of maternal exercise on these transfer mechanisms will also be discussed.

MATERNAL BLOOD

Hemoglobin

After birth, tissue oxygenation depends upon a virtually continuous diffusion of oxygen from the alveolar spaces to blood. Similarly, oxygenation of fetal tissues depends upon oxygen in maternal blood diffusing across the placenta into fetal blood. Hemoglobin in maternal blood contributes considerably to the transfer of oxygen across the placenta.

Oxygen Affinity

Reduced hemoglobin binds with oxygen to form oxyhemoglobin. Since this binding is reversible, hemoglobin is able to unload oxygen as the O$_2$ partial pressure decreases. The ability of hemoglobin to bind oxygen depends not only upon the oxygen partial pressure but also upon the affinity of hemoglobin for O$_2$, as indicated by the sigmoid-shaped oxyhemoglobin saturation curve (30).

The P$_{50}$ describes the partial pressure of oxygen required to half saturate hemoglobin. Under standard conditions (pH 7.4, PCO_2 = 40 torr, 37°C) the P$_{50}$ for normal adult human blood is 26.5 torr (Fig. 12.1). However, under other conditions the position of the oxygen dissociation curve (and P$_{50}$) may be changed. For example, the curve shifts to the right in association with increased concentrations of CO$_2$, hydrogen ion (H$^+$), 2,3-diphosphoglycerate (2,3-DPG), adenosine triphosphate, or chloride ion.

A number of physiologic changes occur during pregnancy which might be expected to alter the maternal oxyhemoglobin dissociation curve. The hyperventilation which normally develops early in pregnancy decreases the mean arterial PCO_2 from nonpregnant values of about 40 torr to a mean

Table 12.1. Major Factors Affecting Placental Oxygen Transfer

Mother	Placenta	Fetus
Arterial Po₂	*Diffusing capacity*	*Arterial Po₂*
Inspired Po₂	Area	Umbilical venous Po₂
Alveolar ventilation	O₂ diffusivity	Fetal O₂ consumption
Mixed venous Po₂	Hb reaction rates	Peripheral blood flow
Pulmonary blood flow and diffusing capacity	Thickness	Maternal arterial Po₂
	O₂ solubility	Maternal placental Hg flow
		Placental diffusing capacity
Hb O₂ affinity	*Spatial relation of maternal to fetal flow*	*Hb O₂ affinity*
pH		pH
Temperature		temperature
Pco₂		Pco₂
2,3-DPG concentration		2,3-DPG concentration
CO concentration		CO concentration
Placental Hb flow rate	*Amount of CO₂ exchange*	*Placental Hb flow rate*
Arterial pressure		Umbilical arterial pressure
Placental vascular resistance		Umbilical venous pressure
Venous pressure		Placental vascular resistance
Blood O₂ capacity		Blood O₂ capacity

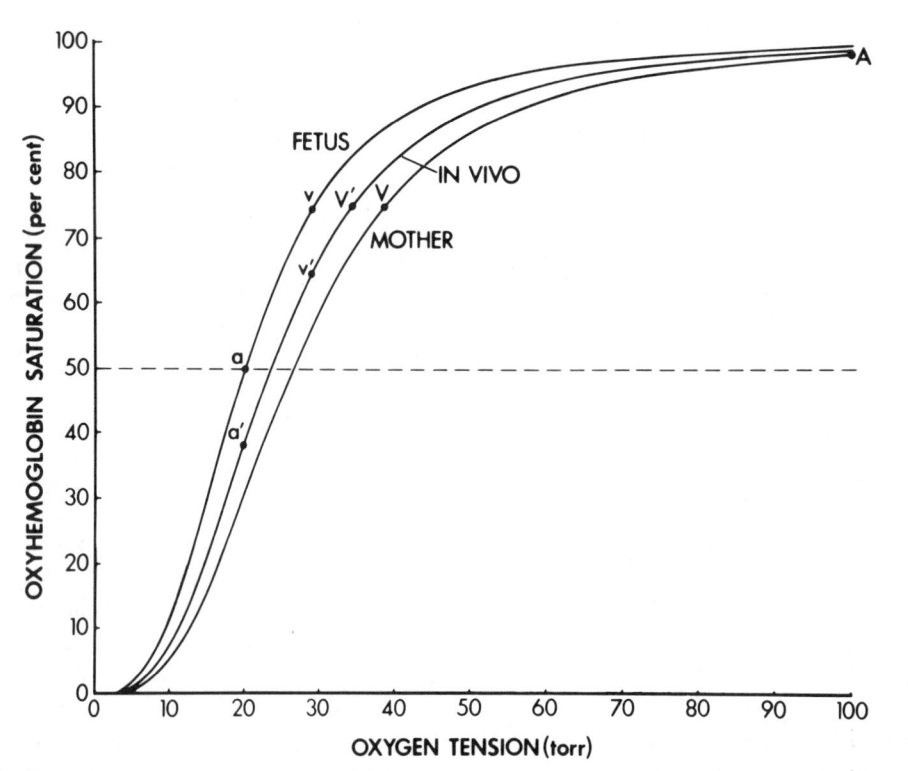

Figure 12.1. Oxyhemoglobin saturation curve under standard conditions for human maternal and fetal blood. Maternal arterial and venous values are indicated by *A* and *V*, respectively, while umbilical arterial and venous figures are represented by *a* and *v*. Maternal venous, and umbilical arterial and venous values which probably occur in vivo are indicated by *V'*, *a'*, and *v'*, respectively.

of about 32. As a result of increased renal excretion of bicarbonate, plasma bicarbonate concentrations decrease to about 23 meq·liter^{-1} from a nonpregnant concentration of 26. This small base deficit would shift the oxygen saturation curve to the left by about 0.5 torr.

Some investigators have reported that the 2,3-DPG concentration in erythrocytes increases during pregnancy (23). This would tend to shift the dissociation curve to the right. However, despite these observations, the P$_{50}$ of maternal blood either remains unchanged or is increased slightly when compared to nonpregnant values (20, 45, 65, 98, 124, 141).

The oxygen dissociation curve under physiologic conditions differs from the observations made under standard conditions. Maternal blood is normally slightly alkalotic (pH 7.42) and hypocarbic (Pco$_2$ = 32 torr). This tends to shift the maternal oxyhemoglobin dissociation curve slightly to the left as shown in Figure 12.1.

Oxygen Capacity

The capacity of blood for oxygen is the maximum amount of oxygen which can reversibly bind with hemoglobin. A lesser amount of O$_2$ (about 2% of the total) is carried as physically dissolved in the blood. Because one hemoglobin molecule can combine with four molecules of oxygen, 1 g of hemoglobin can theoretically bind 1.39 ml of oxygen. However, experimental values have been slightly less, from 1.34 ml (72) to 1.368 ml (132). Small amounts of methemoglobin and carboxyhemoglobin likely account for these differences in theoretical and experimental values.

The nonpregnant woman has a hemoglobin concentration of about 14 g·dl^{-1} and an oxygen capacity of 19.1 ml·dl^{-1}. During pregnancy the red cell mass increases about 25% while plasma volume increases even more at 54% (91). As a result of this hemodilution, the hemoglobin concentration decreases to about 12 g·dl^{-1} with an oxygen capacity of 16.4 ml·dl^{-1} (122).

FETAL BLOOD
Hemoglobin

The human embryo produces a distinct hemoglobin (50, 59–61) which actually consists of three separate hemoglobins (38, 39, 71, 78). These embryonic hemoglobins are produced sequentially as Hb Gower I ($\beta_2\epsilon_2$), Hb Gower II ($\alpha_2\epsilon_2$), and Hb Portland ($\beta_2\gamma_2$).

During fetal life another hemoglobin (HbF) predominates. This was perhaps first suggested in 1866 when von Korber (81) observed that human newborn blood had greater resistance to alkaline denaturation than adult blood. Later, Huggett (73) showed that fetal blood oxygen affinity differed from that of the adult, and Brinkman and Jonxis (33) conclusively demonstrated the existence of human fetal hemoglobin. Amino acid sequencing has shown that fetal hemoglobin consists of two alpha and two gamma chains. While having the same number of amino acids, gamma and beta chains differ in the types of amino acids present in 39 of the 146 positions (135). More recently three types of gamma chains have been identified in fetal blood which differ only slightly in the amino acid sequence (134). During the last few months of pregnancy, an increasing number of beta chains are produced, so that at birth the newborn blood contains about 80% fetal and about 20% adult hemoglobin (34, 79).

Although a specific fetal hemoglobin exists for humans, this is not the case for all species. For example, no separate fetal hemoglobin has been identified in the horse (58, 138), camel (128), hamster (58), dog (87, 108) cat (110), or pig (140).

Oxygen Affinity

In humans (51) and several other species (8, 62, 63, 99) the fetal hemoglobin dissociation curve is shifted to the left compared to that of maternal blood under standard conditions. Figure 12.1 shows that the P$_{50}$ for human fetal blood equals about 20 torr (65). The actual P$_{50}$ depends on gestational age. The P$_{50}$ of about 15 torr for human fetal blood at 20 weeks of gestation is about 5 torr less than the value near term (43). This increase in P_{50} with gestational age results from the increase in hemoglobin A relative to that of hemoglobin F.

The different oxygen affinities of HbA and HbF exist in erythrocytes, but not in hemoglobin solutions free of 2,3-DPG (4, 18, 136). 2,3-DPG decreases the O_2 affinity of hemoglobin by binding to four positively charged amino acids on the beta chain (22, 40). While equal 2,3-DPG concentrations exist in fetal and maternal erythrocytes, the 2,3-DPG in fetal red cells is less effective since fetal hemoglobin has one less binding site for this phosphate (18, 49, 144).

Although reduced interaction of 2,3-DPG and fetal hemoglobin explains the increased oxygen affinity of fetal blood in humans and, to a certain extent, in rhesus monkeys (105, 139), this is not true for some other species. For example, in goats and sheep fetal hemoglobin itself has a greater oxygen affinity as well as having a reduced interaction with intracellular phosphates (105). In fetuses which produce only adult hemoglobin, such as the dog, horse, and pig, the increased oxygen affinity apparently results from a reduced 2,3-DPG concentration in erythrocytes (19, 42, 108, 142, 143).

Not all fetuses have blood with increased oxygen affinity. The fetal cat, which only synthesizes adult hemoglobin, has a P_{50} similar to that of the mother (110).

Under physiologic conditions in vivo the fetal oxyhemoglobin curve is shifted to the right as it is slightly acidotic (pH 7.34) and hypercarbic (P_{CO_2} = 45 torr) as compared to standard conditions (Fig. 12.1).

Oxygen Capacity

In humans the fetal hemoglobin concentration increases from about 8.5 g·dl^{-1} at 10 weeks of gestation (111, 145) to a mean value of about 16.5 g·dl^{-1} at term. During this time the maternal hemoglobin concentration decreases from about 13 to 11.5 g·dl^{-1}. As a result the oxygen capacity of fetal blood exceeds that of maternal blood during the last trimester. However, this phenomenon has not be observed in all species. For example, similar oxygen capacities for maternal and fetal blood exist for the guinea pig and sheep; and a decreased oxygen capacity for fetal blood relative to that of the mothers occurs in the rabbit and cow (105).

INTERRELATIONS OF MATERNAL AND FETAL O_2 DISSOCIATION CURVES

Oxygen Affinity

Figure 12.1 shows the oxyhemoglobin dissociation curves for human maternal and near-term fetal blood. Notice that under physiologic conditions in vivo the fetal curve shifts to the right while the maternal curve shifts to the left. As a result the maternal and fetal dissociation curves are probably superimposed. As previously indicated, these departures from the standard dissociation curves largely result from the slightly alkalotic and hypercarbic maternal blood and the slightly acidotic and hypercarbic fetal blood. The greater temperature of the fetus (0.5°C) relative to the mother also contributes to similar oxyhemoglobin dissociation curves in vivo.

O_2 Saturation

Figure 12.2 depicts the O_2 content for human maternal and fetal blood as a function of the oxygen partial pressure. This shows that normal fetal umbilical venous P_{O_2} of only about 28 torr is associated with an O_2 content of 16.5 ml·dl^{-1}, a value which actually exceeds the maternal content of 15.4 ml·dl^{-1}. This occurs despite the fetal hemoglobin being only 75% saturated compared to 98% in the adult because of the higher O_2 capacity (greater hemoglobin concentration) of fetal blood. In some species, the O_2 capacity of the mother and fetus are about equal (rat, guinea pig, sheep), while in others (cow, goat, pig, rabbit) the fetal O_2 capacity is actually less than that of the mother.

The oxyhemoglobin saturation of maternal and fetal blood has important implications for placental oxygen transfer. An in-

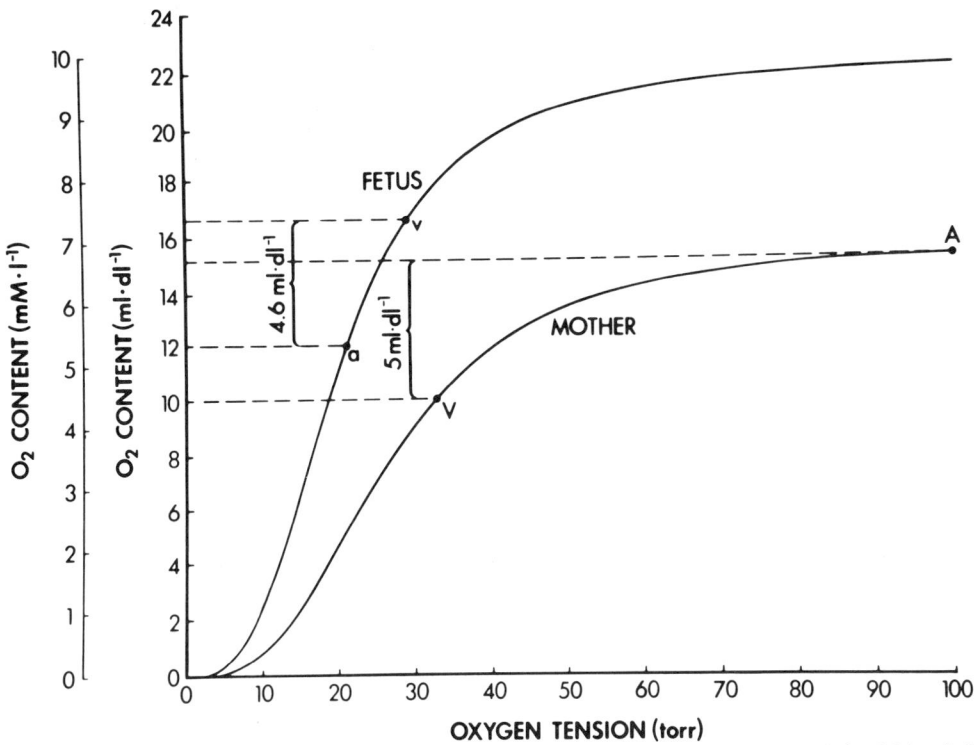

Figure 12.2. Oxygen content as a function of oxygen tension for maternal and fetal blood. The letters A and V represent values for maternal arterial and venous blood, while a and v represent those for umbilical arterial and venous blood, respectively.

crease of either maternal or fetal O_2 capacity will promote placental O_2 exchange (14, 93). All other factors remaining constant, the larger the sum of maternal and fetal blood O_2 capacities, the more oxygen will be exchanged before equilibrium is reached.

Effects of Respiratory Gas Exchange

BOHR EFFECT

As fetal blood courses through the placental exchange vessels, hydrogen ions and CO_2 diffuses across the placenta resulting in a fall in P_{CO_2} and a rise in pH. This results in maternal blood becoming more acidotic and hypercarbic as it passes through the exchange areas. This increase in hydrogen ions in maternal blood shifts the oxyhemoglobin dissociation curve to the right, making more oxygen available for transfer, while in fetal blood, the decreased hydrogen ion concentration shifts the dissociation curve to the left, promoting O_2 uptake by fetal hemoglobin. Theoretical studies by Hill and associates (68) suggest that this mechanism accounts for about 8% of the oxygen transferred to the fetus.

HALDANE EFFECT

As a result of this exchange process the deoxyhemoglobin concentration in maternal blood increases while that in fetal blood decreases. Deoxyhemoglobin binds CO_2 to a greater extent than oxyhemoglobin; consequently, the increased concentrations of deoxyhemoglobin in maternal blood and decreased levels in fetal red cells promote CO_2 transfer from fetal to maternal blood. In fact, this "double Haldane effect" is calculated to account for 46% of placental exchange of carbon dioxide (67).

TRANSPLACENTAL DIFFUSION

Maternal and Fetal Oxygen Tensions

As shown in Table 12.1, placental oxygen exchange depends upon a number of factors. One important variable is the mean O_2

partial pressure difference between maternal and fetal exchange vessels.

In an attempt to understand the transfer process, early investigators measured the oxygen tensions in the uterine and umbilical arteries and veins. From these data the mean driving gradient between maternal and fetal blood vessels was calculated to equal 40–50 torr (5, 10–12, 73, 130, 131). Although in rabbits umbilical venous P_{O_2} has been reported to be higher than that in the uterine vein (13), umbilical venous oxygen tension usually has been found to be less than uterine venous values. For example, the partial pressure of O_2 in human umbilical venous blood has been observed to be about 2 torr less than that of uterine venous blood (148), although this difference probably does not reflect steady state values since the blood samples were collected at the time of cesarean section (46). However, the umbilical to uterine venous difference has been determined under stable conditions in chronically catheterized fetal lambs and has been reported to range between 10 and 20 torr (125, 146), suggesting that the P_{O_2} in placental exchange vessels might not equilibrate (Fig. 12.3), and that the placenta might not equilibrate (Fig. 12.3), and that the placenta might represent a significant barrier to gas exchange. A number of factors, however, could theoretically affect placental oxygen transfer and might invalidate conclusions from the P_{O_2} gradient between umbilical and uterine venous blood.

GEOMETRY OF VESSELS

Placental oxygen transfer depends to a certain extent upon the geometric interrelations of maternal and fetal placental vessels, as shown in Figure 12.4 (15, 16, 52). For instance, if the vessels are arranged so that fetal and maternal blood flows are concurrent (Fig. 12.4A), fetal and maternal end-

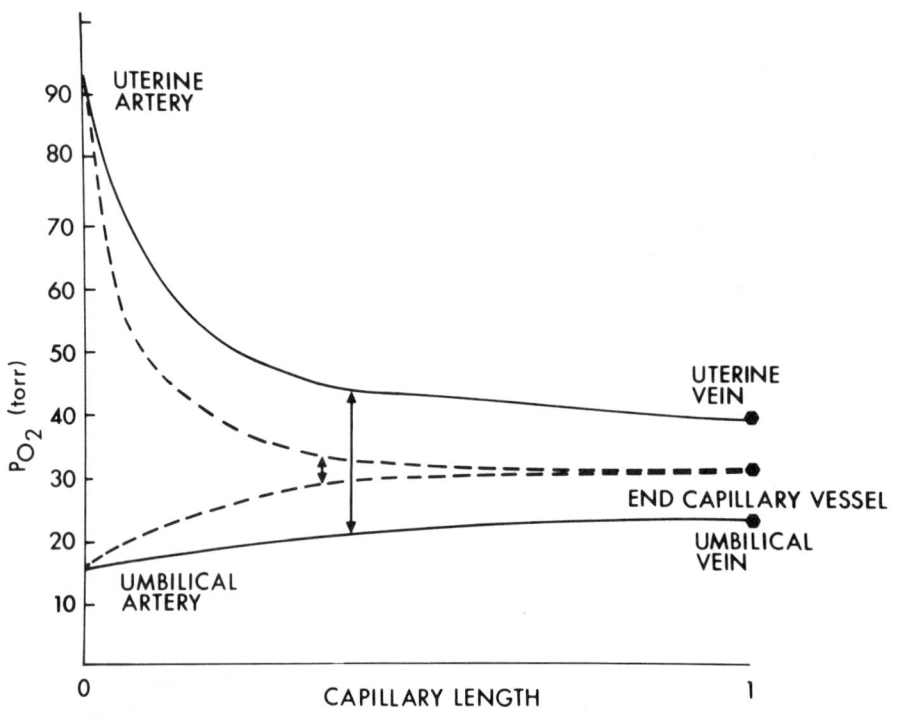

Figure 12.3. Predicted oxygen tensions in maternal and fetal placental exchange vessels. The *solid lines* represent values assuming that uterine and umbilical venous tensions are the same as those of maternal and fetal end-capillaries. The *broken lines* show the oxygen tensions assuming end-capillary equilibration, and are calculated from measurements of placental CO diffusing capacity. The *arrows* show the mean maternal to fetal O_2 differences under these two circumstances.

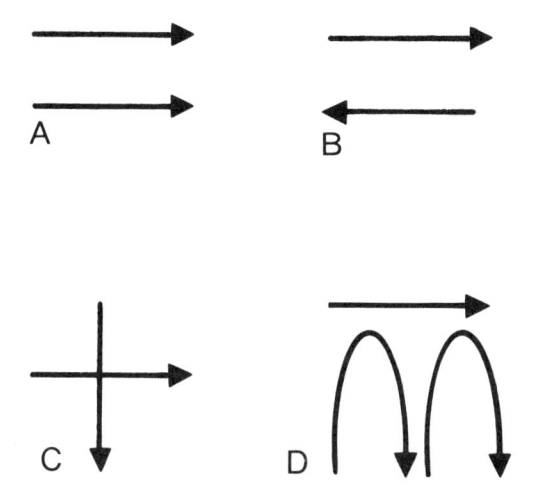

Figure 12.4. Possible relationships of maternal and fetal blood flow within placental exchange vessels. (*A*) Concurrent, (*B*) countercurrent, (*C*) crosscurrent, and (*D*) pool flow.

capillary P_{O_2} values would equilibrate, assuming there is no diffusional limitation. Such a relationship is thought to exist for the goat and sheep placenta (125, 146). If fetal and maternal blood flow in a countercurrent manner (Fig. 12.4*B*), then fetal end-capillary P_{O_2} would equilibrate at a higher value than that in the maternal vessels. Experimental evidence suggests that the placentas of guinea pigs (133) and rabbits (53) probably function as countercurrent exchangers. A crosscurrent relationship is also possible in which fetal and maternal blood flow at right angles to each other (Fig. 12.4*C*). Another possibility is pool flow in which capillaries on one side of the placenta are bathed in a reservoir of blood filled by arteries and drained by veins (Fig. 12.4*D*). Such a relationship functions similarly to that of a concurrent exchanger (15) and may be the most representative of the human placenta. In actual fact, however, rather than a specific pattern of blood flow, the placenta probably contains areas of exchange with each of these patterns. In addition, a clear demonstration of the type of transfer relationship in the hemochorial placenta is difficult because of other factors such as uneven distribution of maternal and fetal blood flows (52, 116).

PLACENTAL OXYGEN CONSUMPTION

A metabolically active organ, the sheep placenta consumes O_2 at a rate of 10 (36) or as much as 25 ml·min^{-1}·kg placenta^{-1} (103). Theoretically this oxygen consumption near or within the exchange area could contribute to the uterine to umbilical venous P_{O_2} difference and to the calculated mean maternal-fetal oxygen tension gradient. The oxygen which is metabolized could be supplied to placental tissue from either maternal or fetal blood. The placenta could also receive oxygen from maternal or fetal blood after the blood had left the exchange area.

The relative contribution of placental oxygen consumption to the magnitude of the oxygen tension gradient in umbilical and uterine venous blood has been explored by Hill and associates (66). Assuming that the placenta receives O_2 from the maternal and fetal circulations, these investigators showed that placental oxygen requirements could be met without significantly contributing to the umbilical-uterine venous oxygen tension difference (66).

On the other hand, it is possible that the placenta receives most of its oxygen supply from fetal blood. Under these conditions, placental metabolism might account for part of the O_2 tension difference between umbilical and uterine venous blood.

PLACENTAL SHUNTS

The O_2 tension of uterine venous blood could be increased and that of umbilical venous blood could be lowered if some arterial blood (uterine or umbilical, respectively) entered the venous circulation without passing through placental exchange areas. This then could account for the uterine to umbilical venous oxygen tension difference. Using an in vivo perfusion method, Metcalfe (106) has reported an effective shunt of 19% on the fetal side of the sheep placenta. Rankin and Peterson (127) have demonstrated a 23% shunt on the fetal side and a 36% shunt on the maternal side of the sheep placenta. These estimations, however, may be on the high side due to experimental conditions. But more important, morphologic studies have not shown that arterial-venous anastomoses exist in the sheep or human (29, 44) placenta to the extent necessary to account for this degree of shunting. Nevertheless, vascular shunts in the placenta might explain part of the uterine to umbilical venous O_2 tension difference.

PERFUSION-PERFUSION INEQUALITIES

In the lung, maximum oxygen transfer depends upon optimal matching of areas of oxygen supply (alveoli) with areas of oxygen uptake (blood flow). Similarly, in the placenta optimal oxygen diffusion occurs when uterine blood flow in an exchange area matches umbilical flow. For example, less oxygen would diffuse across the placenta under conditions in which a relatively high maternal blood flow occurred in an area supplied by a low fetal blood flow. Reduced oxygen transfer would also occur in the reverse circumstances, that is increased fetal and reduced maternal blood flow.

Using radiolabeled albumin aggregates, Power and associates (121) first demonstrated that perfusion-perfusion inequalities exist in 1-g samples of sheep placenta. Others subsequently observed a more homogeneous relation of maternal to fetal blood flow in the sheep placenta in similarly large tissue samples (1–4 g) using microsphere techniques (126). However, the size of the placental samples in these studies was very large compared to the size of individual exchange vessels and the distance over which gas diffusion takes place (116). The larger the sample size, the more the tendency to average flows and, therefore, to obscure variations occurring at the capillary level. In an effort to address this question, Power et al. (116) repeated their studies by measuring blood flow with microspheres in very small tissue samples of about 30 mg in which the XYZ coordinates were recorded. These polar coordinates were used to calculate the maternal to fetal flow ratios as a function of sample size. Figure 12.5 shows that in the average cotyledon the maternal-fetal blood flow ratio differs significantly from unity. This perfusion-perfusion inequality may represent variations in capillary volume and/or variations in blood flow velocity (115). Based on experimental data, Power and associates (116) calculated that this uneven distribution of blood flow in the placenta could account for about 6 torr O_2 tension difference in the umbilical and uterine venous blood, or roughly 50% of the value normally observed. Theoretically it might even explain a greater proportion of the O_2 tension difference since 30-mg tissue samples are still very large compared to the size of the individual exchange vessels (115).

CONCLUSION

Clearly uterine and umbilical venous blood do not reflect those gas tensions at the end of a capillary transit. Ideally one would like to sample inflowing and end-capillary blood within a single exchange unit. However, this is virtually impossible to do from a technical standpoint. As a result the question of whether the placenta actually represents a barrier to oxygen diffusion must be answered using indirect methods.

Placental Diffusing Capacity

CARBON MONOXIDE

Unlike oxygen and carbon dioxide, carbon monoxide (CO) transfer across the lung and other membranes is limited by diffusion rather than blood flow. Krogh (83) took advantage of this diffusion limitation to determine the carbon monoxide diffusing capacity in the lung as an index of the efficiency of pulmonary gas exchange. Longo et al. (95) applied this method to quantify gas exchange across the placenta.

Placental diffusing capacity depends upon the membrane diffusion characteristics of the placenta, such as the area, permeability, diffusivity, and thickness of the placenta. These properties can be expressed collectively in the equation:

$$D_p = dQ \cdot dt^{-1} \cdot (P_1 - P_2)^{-1}$$

where D_p is the placental diffusing capacity

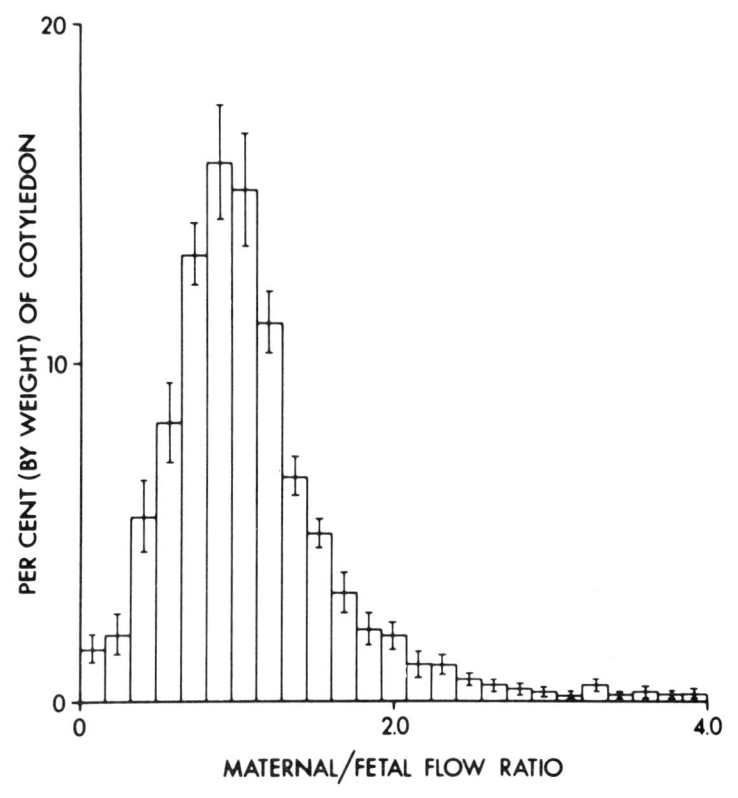

Figure 12.5. Maternal to fetal blood flow ratios within an average cotyledon. (From G. G. Power et al.: American Journal of Physiology, 241:H486–H496, 1981 (116).)

in ml·min^{-1}·torr^{-1}, $dQ·dt^{-1}$ is the volume of carbon monoxide transferred per minute, and (P_1-P_2) represents the carbon monoxide partial pressure difference.

In 1967 Longo and associates determined maternal-fetal carbon monoxide exchange in sheep and dogs. Since then the CO diffusing capacity for several other species has been determined as shown in Table 12.2. Expressed per gram of fetal weight, the placental diffusing capacity of the sheep of about 0.55 ml·min^{-1}·torr^{-1} (89, 95) is similar to that of the monkey (26) but significantly less than that of rodents such as the rat (B. J. Koos, R. D. Gilbert and L. D. Longo, unpublished data), rabbit (129), and guinea pig (27, 57). The differences in cellular layers and vascular morphology probably contribute to the observed differences in the capacity for respiratory gas transport (26). In sheep the diffusing capacity expressed as per gram fetal weight remains remarkably constant over the last third of gestation (89).

Table 12.2. Placental Diffusing Capacities for Carbon Monoxide[a]

Species	Diffusing Capacity (ml·min^{-1}·torr^{-1}· g fetal wt^{-1})	Reference
Rat	1.73 ± 0.33	—[b]
Guinea pig	3.27 ± 0.10	57
	2.28 ± 0.13	27
Rabbit	2.33 ± 0.21	129
Sheep	0.55 ± 0.02	89
Monkey	0.65 ± 0.06	26

[a] Means ± SEM for at least seven determinations.
[b] Unpublished observations of B. J. Koos, L. D. Longo and R. D. Gilbert.

OXYGEN

From theoretical calculations based on the difference between CO and O_2 in diffusivity and hemoglobin reaction rates, Longo and associates (95) calculated that the placental diffusing capacity for oxygen equalled about 0.5 ml·min^{-1}torr^{-1}·kg fetal weight^{-1}, a value 3–6 times greater than previous estimates (9, 11, 13, 86). They also calculated that mean maternal to fetal oxygen tension gradient in the exchange vessels to equal only 5–9 torr (95) rather than a value as high as 50 torr (9).

From these observations Hill et al. (66) determined that maternal and fetal O_2 tensions closely approach equilibrium during the course of a single capillary transit (Fig. 12.6). Thus, it became clear that under normal conditions uteroplacental blood flow limits the total quantity of oxygen exchanged each minute across the placenta, and not the diffusion rate through the membranes. Other investigators (54, 55, 90, 102) carried out different experiments which also suggested that placental O_2 transfer is flow limited.

SITE OF DIFFUSION RESISTANCE

While placental oxygen transfer is perfusion limited, a definite resistance to diffusion does exist. Theoretically this resistance includes the resistance of the maternal and

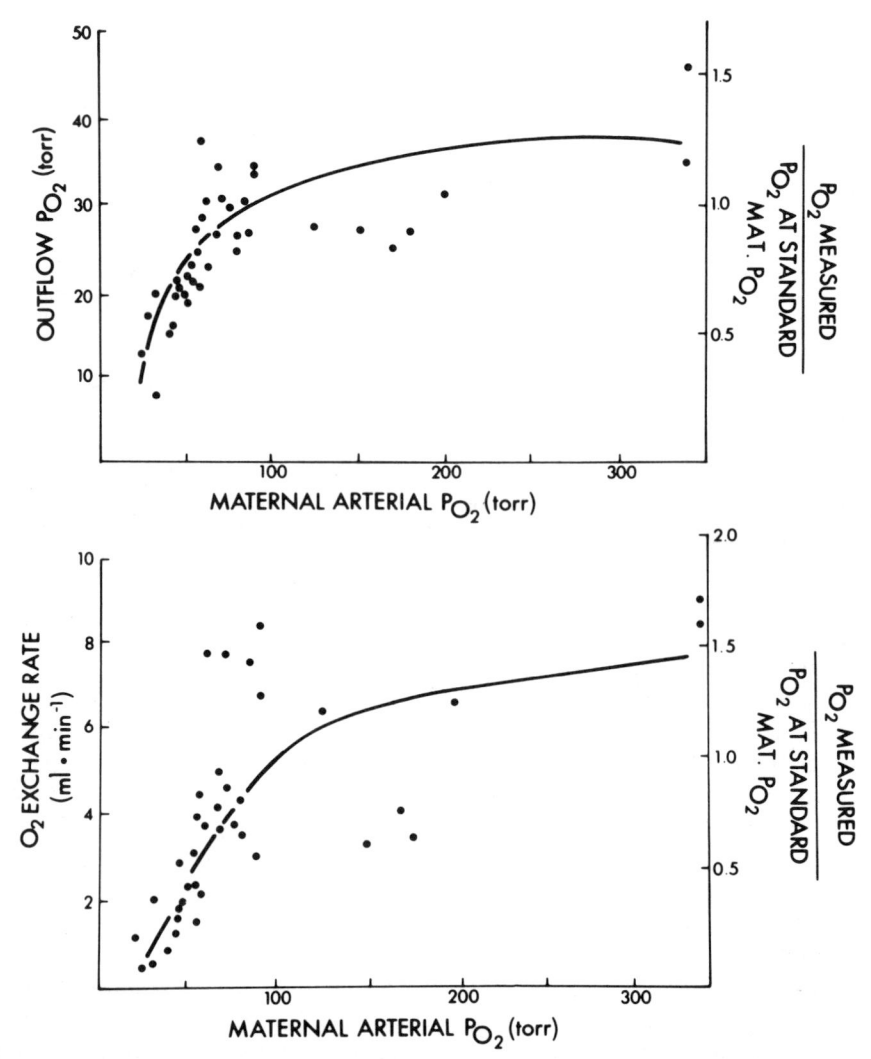

Figure 12.6. The effect of changes in maternal arterial Po_2 on umbilical venous O_2 tension and exchange rate across the placenta. Samples were collected from isolated cotyledons perfused at constant umbilical flow. (From G. G. Power and F. Jenkins: *American Journal of Physiology*, 229:1147–1153, 1975 (119).

fetal red cells (which depends on the rate of combination of oxygen with reduced hemoglobin) and the resistance of the placental membranes. These resistances may be expressed as:

$$1/D_p = 1/\phi_m V_m + 1/D_m + 1/\phi_f V_f$$

where ϕ_m and ϕ_f are the diffusing capacities of maternal and fetal blood, respectively, in ml·ml^{-1}·min^{-1}·torr^{-1}, V_m and V_f are the maternal and fetal blood volumes in the placental exchange vessels in ml, and D_m is the diffusing capacity of the placental membranes in ml·min^{-1}·torr^{-1}.

In 1969 Longo et al. (94) carried out experiments which determined the distribution of oxygen diffusion resistance between blood and the placenta. Under hyperbaric conditions they observed that D_p varied as a function of oxygen partial pressure. From this they determined that the reaction rates of O_2 with hemoglobin in maternal and fetal erythrocytes comprise 40% of the total resistance to diffusion, while the placental membranes contribute about 60%.

The diffusing capacity depends to a certain extent upon capillary volumes in maternal and fetal exchange vessels (95). From their studies of placental transfer of CO under varying partial pressures of oxygen, Longo et al. (94) estimated that placental exchange area in the sheep approximates 5 m^2 with a maternal and fetal capillary volume of about 10 ml each. These volumes may be underestimates, however, because recent findings for ϕ for whole blood in vivo suggest that capillary volumes are likely to be 2–3 times greater than previously thought (E. P. Hill and G. G. Power, personal communication). Such larger volumes would agree more closely with those determined experimentally using a multiple isotope indicator dilution method in which maternal and fetal sheep capillary volumes were calculated to be 45 ml each (24). Using stereologic methods, Laga et al. (85) estimated the villous capillary volume and the intervillous space in the human placenta to equal 30 and 45 ml, respectively.

EFFECT OF VARYING FACTORS AFFECTING OXYGEN TRANSFER

The above discussion relates oxygen transfer to the fetus under normal conditions. However, the question arises as to what extent varying individual factors important in respiratory gas exchange affect oxygen transfer. Such predictions can be made using mathematical equations describing placental O_2 transfer (93). An understanding of the relative importance of variables affecting placental O_2 exchange can also be determined experimentally. The observed changes in O_2 transfer would result from the experimentally altered variable as well as compensatory changes in other factors which might occur to limit the change in placental O_2 exchange.

Placental Diffusing Capacity

Under normal conditions placental diffusing capacity does not limit the rate of oxygen transfer across the placenta. However, theoretically oxygen transfer could be affected if the diffusing capacity was reduced below a critical value. The effect on fetal blood gases of reducing the placental diffusing capacity in sheep by embolizing the uteroplacental vascular bed with microspheres was examined by Boyle et al. (32). Fetal arterial O_2 tensions did not significantly decrease until the placental diffusing capacity was reduced by about 50%. This study suggests that the placental diffusing capacity becomes critical at values about one half that of normal. However, this effect may not be solely the result of reduced diffusing capacity since decreased placental blood flow and/or increased perfusion-perfusion inequalities might also have contributed.

Arterial Oxygen Tension

MATERNAL OXYGEN TENSION

The extent to which changes in maternal Po_2 affect fetal O_2 tensions depends upon the shape of the maternal and fetal oxyhemoglobin saturation curves (Fig. 12.1). For example, reducing the maternal arterial Po_2

from normal values (95–100 torr) to about 70 torr results in only about a 5% decrease in the oxyhemoglobin concentration of maternal blood. Such moderate reductions in maternal arterial O_2 tension would be expected to have only a small effect on placental oxygen transfer and fetal arterial Po_2. Further uncompensated decreases in maternal Po_2 are associated with much larger reductions in oxyhemoglobin concentrations and, consequently, a fall in fetal arterial oxygen tensions.

Increasing maternal arterial Po_2 above normal values would be expected to have a small effect on the partial pressure of O_2 in fetal blood. For example, elevating the ewe's arterial O_2 tension to 3,000 torr in a hyperbaric chamber only raised the fetal arterial Po_2 to about 750 torr (94). Under these conditions, the increase in O_2 carrying capacity of maternal blood occurred primarily as a result of increased physically dissolved oxygen (0.003 ml·100 ml^{-1}·torr^{-1}), since hemoglobin is virtually saturated with oxygen at 100 torr. As a result large increases in maternal arterial oxygen tension cause only small increases in fetal arterial Po_2.

The effect of uncompensated changes in maternal arterial O_2 tensions on placental oxygen transfer has been determined experimentally by Power and Jenkins (119). Using an isolated placental cotyledon preparation, these investigators showed that the minor effect on oxygen exchange of increases in maternal arterial oxygen tension for values greater than 70 torr, while a significant reduction in umbilical venous oxygen tensions occurred when maternal Po_2 fell below 70 torr (Fig. 12.6).

UMBILICAL ARTERIAL Po_2

Once fetal blood has left the placenta and supplied the fetal tissues it returns to the placenta in the umbilical arteries. Thus umbilical arterial oxygen tension is a function predominantly of placental oxygen transfer, umbilical venous O_2 tension, and fetal oxygen consumption. However, umbilical arterial Po_2 itself is also a major determinant of placental O_2 transfer. As umbilical arterial Po_2 decreases, the transplacental O_2 tension gradient increases, resulting in an increase in placental oxygen exchange rate and a fall in the end-capillary O_2 tension. Conversely, increasing umbilical arterial oxygen tension reduces the transplacental oxygen gradient and lowers the oxygen exchange rate. Theoretically, percent changes in umbilical arterial Po_2 affect placental oxygen transfer rate and end-capillary oxygen tension to a greater extent than similar changes in any other determinant of oxygen exchange (93). The importance of umbilical arterial oxygen tensions on transplacental oxygen transfer has also been shown experimentally by in situ perfusions of isolated cotyledons in sheep (119), as shown in Figure 12.7.

Placental Blood Flows

Oxygen transfer across the placenta depends to a great extent on the rate of placental blood flow. Both maternal and fetal blood flows contribute to this exchange, and their relative importance to placental oxygen transfer will now be considered.

MATERNAL FLOW

Uteroplacental blood flow increases during pregnancy from 50 ml·min^{-1} at 10 weeks (6) to about 500 ml·min^{-1} at term (7, 28, 107). Evidence from animal studies suggests that 80–90% of this flow supplies the placenta and thus is available for transfer of oxygen and nutrients to the fetus. The maternal placental vascular anatomy varies with species. For example, in ruminants maternal blood courses through its own vascular system lined by capillary endothelium. In other species, such as rodents and primates, blood flows from maternal vessels into a reservoir directly bathing trophoblastic tissue. In the human, blood from spiral arteries enters the intervillous space and is directed in spurts toward the chorionic plate. As the blood encounters villi it is slowed and flows laterally into venous sinuses.

Several investigators have experimentally determined the importance of uterine blood flow on oxygen uptake by the pregnant

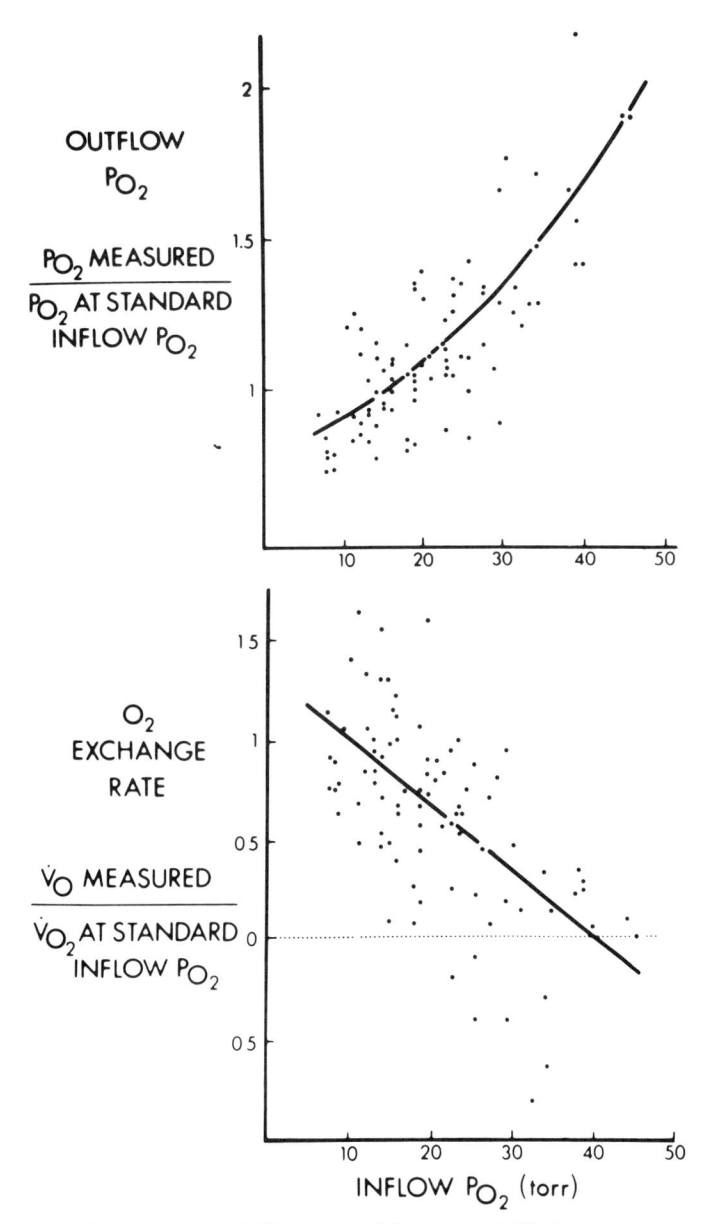

Figure 12.7. Effect of changes in umbilical arterial P_{O_2} on umbilical venous oxygen tension and O_2 exchange rate. Umbilical blood flow through the isolated cotyledon was kept constant. (From G. G. Power and F. Jenkins: *American Journal of Physiology*, 229:1147–1153, 1975 (119).)

uterus. Perfusing the uterine vessels of sheep in a controlled manner in vivo, Fuller et al. (56) showed that uterine oxygen uptake varied directly as a function of uterine blood flow for animals at 132–145 days of gestation. However, earlier in gestation (50–118 days) this relation did not hold for uterine blood flows in excess of about 250 ml·min^{-1}kg^{-1}. Oxygen transfer at this early gestational age was likely limited by a much smaller oxygen consumption of the uterus, placenta, and fetus. This agrees with acute studies in monkeys (113) and chronic investigations in fetal lambs (37) in which higher uterine blood flows were generally associated with a greater placental O_2 transfer as indicated by fetal oxygen consumption.

On the other hand, some studies in chronically catheterized fetal sheep indicate that changes in uteroplacental blood flow can occur without affecting fetal oxygen consumption. For example, Caton et al. (37) observed a high O_2 consumption in some fetuses despite low uterine blood flows. In these cases, placental O_2 transfer was maintained at the expense of a lower O_2 saturation in uterine venous blood. In addition, other studies in chronically catheterized sheep have shown that the oxygen supply to the fetus as judged by placental blood flow normally exceeds fetal oxygen requirements. For example, no significant change in oxygen uptake has been observed in fetal lambs in association with normal biologic variations in uterine blood flow (41). Furthermore, when oxygen delivery (blood flow × O_2 content) was reduced experimentally by partial occlusion of the maternal aorta, the fetal O_2 uptake did not fall until uterine blood flow (and O_2 delivery) fell by about 50% (146), as shown in Figure 12.8.

The importance of uterine blood flow on fetal oxygenation has many clinical implications. For example, placental blood flow could be reduced in women with vascular disease or pregnancy-induced hypertension. Uterine blood flow also decreases with contractions during labor, and experimental evidence in sheep indicates that the occasional mild contraction which normally occurs before labor can cause transient decreases in oxygen transfer to the fetus (64, 76).

FETAL FLOW

Dawes and Mott (47) studied the effects of variations of umbilical blood flow on femoral arterial O_2 tensions and fetal O_2 consumption. Using acute experimental methods in young fetal lambs (77–86 days of gestation), they observed a decrease in oxygen saturation in femoral arterial blood associated with partial occlusion of the umbilical vein. Under these conditions the umbilical venous O_2 tension remained largely unchanged although it increased if umbilical blood flow was reduced by hemorrhage. Fetal oxygen consumption fell when umbilical blood flow was less than 100 ml·min^{-1}·kg^{-1}. However, this finding was not consistently observed in mature lambs. Other studies (75) in chronically catheterized fetal lambs (120–130 days of gestation) have also shown that partial cord occlusion did not lower the oxygen content of umbilical venous blood, but did reduce the oxygen

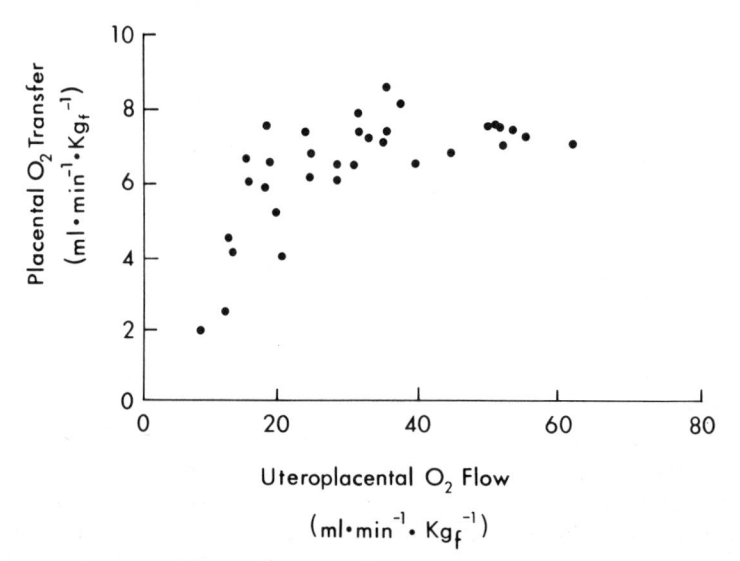

Figure 12.8. Dependence of placental O_2 transfer on uteroplacental O_2 flow. Uteroplacental O_2 delivery normally ranges between 36 and 63 ml·min^{-1}·kg^{-1}. (Redrawn from R. B. Wilkening and G. Meschia (146).)

content of blood in the descending aorta. Fetal oxygen delivery was found to be highly correlated with umbilical blood flow. In contrast, natural variations in umbilical blood flow (154–444 ml·min^{-1}·kg^{-1}) have been observed with changes in arteriovenous oxygen content but without changes in fetal oxygen uptake (41). These observations indicate the importance of umbilical blood flow on placental O_2 transfer; however, quantitative understanding of the importance of umbilical blood flow alone on oxygen transfer is difficult to achieve experimentally because of compensating changes in other factors affecting oxygen transfer to the fetus.

In an effort to minimize these problems, Power and Jenkins (119) perfused in situ an isolated cotyledon of the sheep placenta with blood of known oxygen tension and flow rate. Figure 12.9 shows the dependence of venous outflow oxygen tension and oxygen transfer on fetal cotyledonary blood flow. Outflow Po_2 varied inversely with cotyledonary blood flow, with higher values at lower rates of flow. In contrast, oxygen exchange rate increased with higher rates of flow.

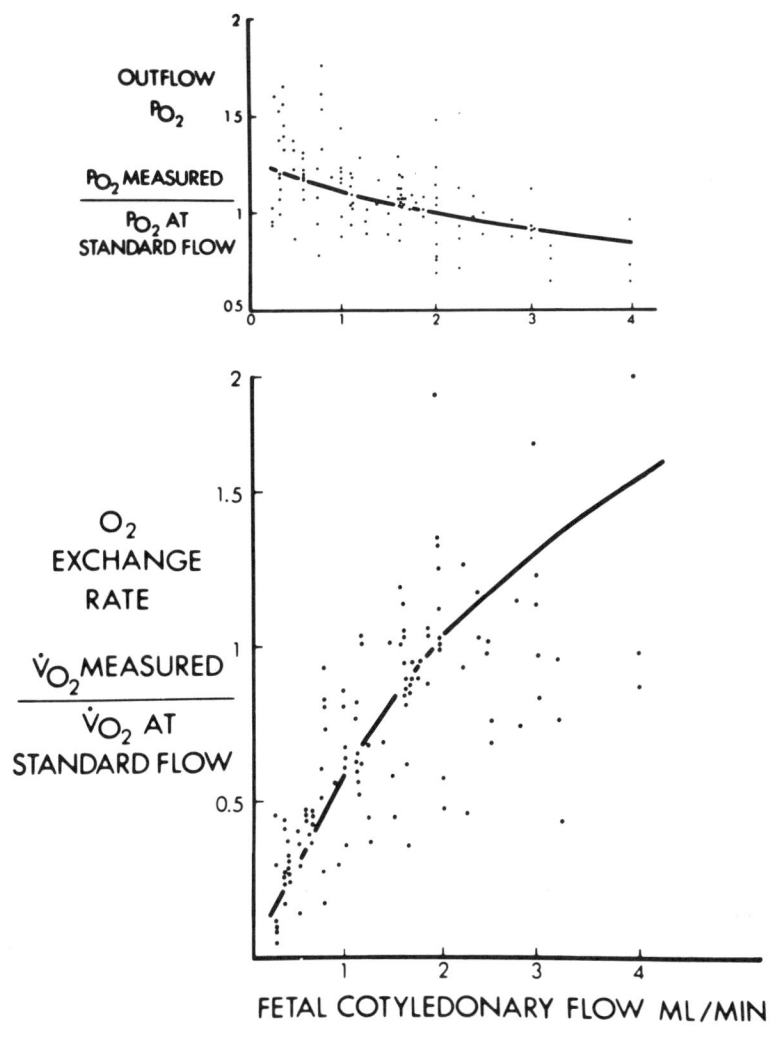

Figure 12.9. Dependence of fetal cotyledonary venous Po_2 and placental O_2 exchange rate on fetal cotyledonary blood flow. Umbilical arterial Po_2 was kept constant. (From G. G. Power and F. Jenkins: *American Journal of Physiology*, 229:1147–1153, 1975 (119).)

Fetal placental blood flow normally is thought to be proportional to the pressure difference between the umbilical arterial and umbilical venous vessels. However, because of the close association of maternal and fetal placental circulations, it is possible that changes in dimensions of one vascular bed might alter the size and thus the resistance of the other. For instance, an increase in the maternal placental blood volume might reduce the volume in fetal exchange vessels. Under these conditions, fetal placental blood flow would be proportional to the fetal inflow pressure minus that of the surrounding maternal blood. Such a "sluice" flow relation in which surrounding pressure affects vascular resistance has been described in the lung (114), and experimental evidence suggests that it also exists in the placenta. By perfusing an isolated sheep cotyledon, Power and Longo (120) showed that, at a constant perfusion rate, fetal inflow pressure increased when maternal placental pressure was elevated by clamping the inferior vena cava. Bissonnette and Farrell (25) subsequently confirmed the sluice flow phenomenon in sheep placenta. Other evidence exists for maternal-fetal vascular interaction. For instance, fetal placental vascular compliance in sheep increased with reductions in maternal vascular pressure (117).

As a result of the sluice mechanism, elevations in uterine venous pressure might reduce umbilical blood flow. However, increasing uterine venous pressure to values up to 70 torr had no significant effect on fetal limb umbilical blood flow as measured by an electromagnetic flowmeter (21). This suggests that either the sluice effect in sheep is small compared to the sensitivity of the method used to measure flow or that umbilical flow was maintained by a small rise in umbilical arterial pressure.

Although demonstrated in animals, sluice flow also likely occurs in humans. Fetal capillary tufts in the human placenta are surrounded by maternal blood. This arrangement should result in a greater sluice effect than observed in the sheep where stroma separates maternal and fetal capillaries. At the present time, the clinical significance of sluice flow in the placenta is not known. However, it is most likely to be of importance in postural changes of the mother which result in alterations in intervillous pressure. In the supine position, the pregnant uterus of some women compresses the inferior vena cava (100). This reduces venous return to the heart, resulting in decreased cardiac output and arterial pressure. With caval compression, uterine venous outflow would be impeded, and intervillous pressure should rise. Under these conditions fetal vessels within the placenta would be compressed, resulting in increased vascular resistance and, at least initially, a reduction in fetal placental blood flow. Of course, flow might be maintained in the long-term if fetal umbilical arterial blood pressure increased sufficiently.

Hemoglobin Concentration

Alterations in the hemoglobin concentration of maternal or fetal blood could affect oxygen transfer to the fetus in several ways. For example, decreased hemoglobin concentration reduces the buffer capacity and influences oxygen transfer by the Bohr effect. A reduced hemoglobin concentration also decreases slightly the placental diffusing capacity (94) and theoretically could change the distribution of flow within placental vessels as a result of altered blood viscosity. However, these effects are minor. The principal effect on oxygen exchange relates to the effect of changes in oxygen carrying capacity of blood. Since the hemoglobin concentration determines the oxygen-carrying capacity of blood, the amount of oxygen transferred across the placenta depends to a great extent on maternal and fetal hemoglobin concentrations.

MATERNAL HEMOGLOBIN

Oxygen delivery to the placenta equals the product of placental blood flow and the O_2 content of maternal blood. A 50% reduction in maternal hemoglobin concentration would theoretically decrease by the same amount of oxygen delivery to the placenta, assuming uteroplacental blood flow remained unchanged. Therefore, reducing the hemoglobin concentration of maternal blood would be expected to have a similar effect on placental O_2 transfer as decreasing placental blood flow (Fig. 12.8). However, normal placental oxygen delivery and transfer could be maintained if a compensatory increase occurred in uteroplacental blood flow.

FETAL HEMOGLOBIN

Since oxygen-carrying capacity and placental blood flow determine the "oxygen flow" to the placenta, changes in fetal hemoglobin concentrations also would be expected to have similar effects on placental oxygen exchange as do changes in umbilical blood flow (Fig. 12.9). The effects of reducing hemoglobin concentrations in fetal monkeys has been determined by Adamsons and associates (3). They observed that fetal hemoglobin concentrations could be lowered 50% before signs of fetal compromise developed. Human fetuses with hemolytic anemia (Hgb < $g \cdot dl^{-1}$) have also been shown to have normal blood gases and pH in scalp blood at the onset of labor (70).

Increased fetal hemoglobin concentrations occur during hypoxia (31) or asphyxia (2). This results from a shift of water from the vascular space to the interstitial fluid compartment which accompanies vasoconstriction of certain fetal vascular beds (48). An increased number of circulating erythrocytes may also contribute. Such an increase in fetal oxygen carrying capacity should favorably affect placental O_2 transfer under these conditions.

Variation in Hemoglobin Oxygen Affinity

As discussed earlier, hemoglobin oxygen affinity can be affected by a number of factors such as acid-base status, intraerythrocyte concentrations of 2,3-DPG, and temperature. Furthermore, the P_{50} of hemoglobin can differ from normal as the result of inherited abnormalities in hemoglobin production or as a consequence of blood transfusion.

MATERNAL BLOOD

Women with altered blood oxygen affinity due to a hemoglobinopathy apparently can give birth to normal infants. For instance, cases have been reported of women with hemoglobin Ranier (P_{50} = 12.8 torr) delivering infants with hemoglobin F and a normal oxygen affinity (1, 112). A normal fetus has also been reported in a mother with hemoglobin McKees Rocks, which has a P_{50} of 10 torr (147). On the other hand, a mother with hemoglobin Yakima (P_{50} = 12 torr) had four abortions and three stillbirths in eight pregnancies (77). However, the significance of this poor reproductive history is unknown.

FETAL BLOOD

Intrauterine transfusion of the human fetus with adult red cells has developed as part of the modern management of erythroblastosis fetalis (88). This has raised questions as to what extent varying fetal hemoglobin P_{50} affects placental oxygen transfer. In 1969 Battaglia et al. (17) first studied this question by exchange transfusing chronically catheterized fetal lambs with maternal sheep blood with a P_{50} of 37 torr, a value about twice that of fetal blood. This reduced fetal oxygen affinity while keeping blood oxygen capacity constant. With this unknown increase in fetal P_{50}, umbilical venous oxygen tension increased about 4 torr, and the oxyhemoglobin saturation fell 28%, from 79% to 51%. In a separate paper, Meschia et al. (104) reported that the increase in umbilical venous O_2 tension occurred without a change in umbilical blood flow or placental O_2 transfer, as determined by fetal oxygen consumption. These observations have been confirmed in anesthetized fetal sheep by Kirschbaum et al. (80).

In 1970 Mathers et al. (101) reported that adult hemoglobin (P_{50} = 27.5 torr) comprised about 75% of the total hemoglobin in newborn infants who had undergone intrauterine transfusion for hemolytic anemia within 2 weeks of delivery. Five of these six infants had a P_{50} which was within 0.5 torr of the maternal value. Novy et al. (109) also have examined the effects of intrauterine transfusion in 15 infants with severe erythroblastosis fetalis. The P_{50} of cord blood in these infants at delivery averaged 27.1 torr, a value about 6 torr greater than the mean of 20.8 in seven erythroblastotic infants who were not transfused. The transfused infants grew normally in utero and were not acidotic at birth. Thus, it is clear that decreased blood oxygen affinity is well tolerated by the human fetus.

The human fetus can also survive with blood of increased oxygen affinity. For example, hemoglobin variants compatible with intrauterine development include hemoglobin Ranier ($P_{50} = 12$ torr), hemoglobin Yakima ($P_{50} = 12$ torr), and hemoglobin McKees Rocks ($P_{50} = 10$ torr). However, the fetus does not tolerate blood with very high oxygen affinity such as hemoglobin Bart's ($P_{50} = 3$ torr). This hemoglobin consists of four gamma chains (74) and comprises almost all of hemoglobin in α-thalassemia major. This high oxygen affinity prevents oxygen unloading except at very low oxygen tensions and makes it of little use in oxygenating fetal tissues. Therefore, it is not surprising that fetuses with hemoglobin Bart's develop a fatal hydrops fetalis syndrome.

MATERNAL EXERCISE

As indicated above, placental oxygen exchange is a function of maternal and fetal blood flows, placental blood hemoglobin concentrations, and arterial O_2 tensions. Several other factors affect oxygen exchange as summarized in Table 12.1. The question arises as to which of these factors are altered during maternal exercise and how such changes affect oxygen delivery to the fetus.

Lotgering et al. (96, 97) have studied the effects of exercise on pregnant ewes and their fetuses under chronic experimental conditions. Figure 12.10 shows some of the maternal effects of 10 min of exercise at 70% maximal oxygen consumption. During exercise the mean maternal arterial P_{O_2} increased by about 8%, and the maternal hemoglobin concentration rose by about 25%. However, uterine blood flow as measured by an electromagnetic flowmeter decreased by about 21% by the end of exercise period. Despite this fall in uterine blood flow, uteroplacental oxygen delivery remained unchanged as a result of the increase in maternal hemoglobin concentration.

Other changes also accompanied exercise. For example, the control values of maternal (7.45) and fetal (7.33) arterial pH increased slightly to 7.48 and 7.36, respectively. These pH changes would be expected in association with exercise hyperventilation. No significant changes occurred in fetal arterial P_{O_2} or hemoglobin concentration. The temperature of the ewe increased progressively during exercise, reaching a value of about 0.9°C greater than the control mean of 39.2°C at the end of the exercise period. Following a recovery period of 20 min, the maternal temperature returned to virtually control values. As might be expected the temperature of the fetus followed the maternal trend during exercise, but with some time lag.

Obviously maternal exercise affects a number of variables which determine oxygen transfer across the placenta. The net effect of these changes on oxygen exchange can be predicted using a mathematical model which describes the relative importance of these factors (93). However, the mathematical analysis requires the numerical solution of many differential equations, which consumes considerable time. In an effort to simplify such calculations, G. G. Power and P. S. Dale (unpublished data) have reduced the complex mathematical model (66) to an algebraic representation which is more easily applied to determine effects on placental oxygen transfer. As a result, placental oxygen transfer can be predicted for changes in the following: maternal and fetal arterial P_{O_2}, maternal and fetal hemoglobin concentrations, maternal and fetal arterial pH, maternal and fetal blood flow, and placental diffusing capacity (Table 12.3). The fraction change, p, from the

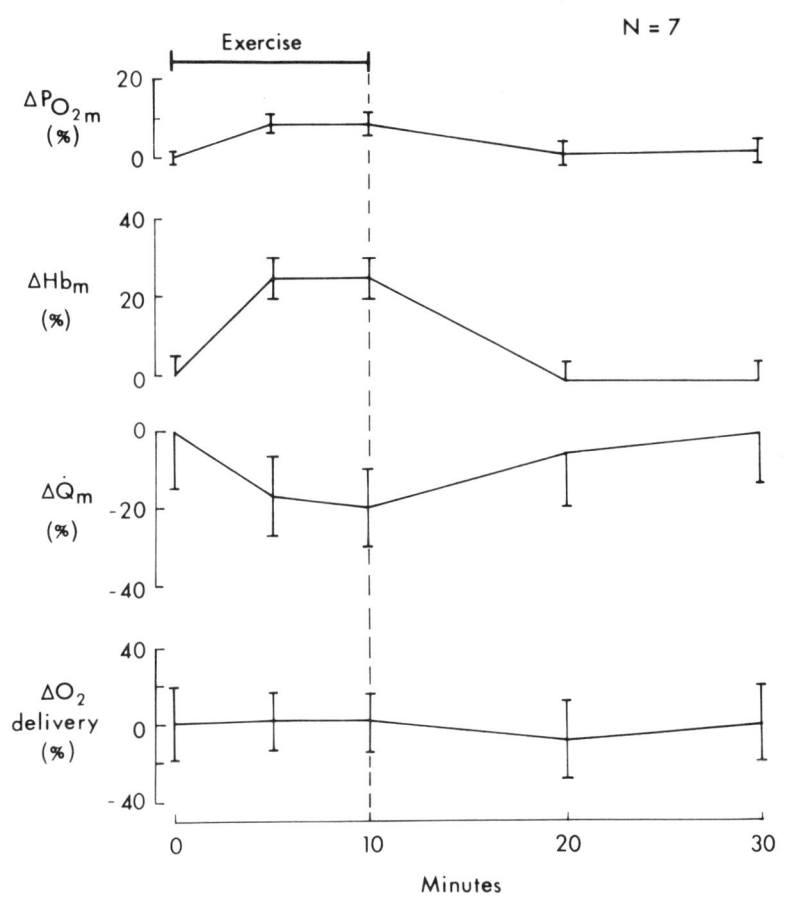

Figure 12.10. Effect of exercise in pregnant ewes on maternal arterial O₂ tension and hemoglobin (Hb) concentration, uteroplacental blood flow ($\dot{Q}_m$), and uteroplacental oxygen delivery. (From F. K. Lotgering et al.: *Journal of Applied Physiology*, 55:834–841, 1983 (96).)

Table 12.3. Values Relating to Equation 1 for Sheep

Variable	Standard Value	Range	A	k	Typical Error[a]	Maximum Error[a]
Maternal arterial Po₂ (torr)	95.0	±30.0	0.02031	0.04998	0.02	0.04
Umbilical arterial Po₂ (torr)	20.0	±10.0	−1.839	0.04007	0.75	1.67
Maternal hemoglobin (g·100 ml⁻¹)	11.0	±4.0	0.1079	0.1968	0.02	0.03
Fetal hemoglobin (g·100 ml⁻¹)	12.0	±4.0	1.053	0.05997	0.02	0.04
Maternal pH	7.40	±0.30	0.1862	−2.017	0.03	0.05
Fetal pH	7.35	±0.30	0.7039	−1.627	0.30	0.53
Maternal blood flow (ml·min⁻¹)	486.0	±300	0.1100	0.004555	0.08	0.18
Fetal blood flow (ml·min⁻¹)	486.0	±300	0.9967	0.001518	0.11	0.20
Membrane diffusing capacity (ml·min⁻¹·torr⁻¹)	2.73	±2.00	0.0005651	2.776	0.08	0.30

[a] Typical error is the standard deviation of the values calculated from Equation 1 about the actual values predicted by the model. Both typical and maximum error are in units of ml·min⁻¹ oxygen flux and are valid for the ranges specified.

standard rate of oxygen transfer may be calculated from the equation:

$$p = A(1 - e^{-k\Delta x}) \quad (1)$$

where Δx is the absolute change in a single variable, and A and k are constants, the values of which depend on the variable. Table 12.3 lists the values of these variables taken as standard for the sheep and the A and k values for each variable. Ranges for each factor along with typical and maximum errors in oxygen transfer rate when compared to the mathematical model (66) are also shown for changes in each single variable. An oxygen consumption of 24 ml·min^{-1} is taken as standard for a fetus weighing 3 kg.

When more than one factor changes, predictions can be made from the equation:

$$\dot{V}_{O_2} = 24 \; \pi_{i=1}^{n} (1 + p_i) \quad (2)$$

when n variables differ from their standard values. Placental oxygen flux ($\dot{V}_{O2}$) can be predicted by using Equation 1 to calculate p_i for i equaling one to n. One is added to each p_i, and the results are multiplied, giving the predicted fraction of the standard $\dot{V}_{O2}$.

We have simplified the method of determining placental oxygen transfer that was used to predict the effects of exercise on placental oxygen exchange. Values for each variable were taken for control, exercise and recovery periods for sheep exercising on a treadmill for 10 min at 70% maximum oxygen consumption (96, 97). Maternal and fetal temperature effects were included in the prediction. While decreased placental diffusing capacity has been reported in chronically exercised guinea pigs (57, 137), placental diffusing capacity was held constant since Lotgering et al. (97) observed no change in diffusing capacity during these experiments in sheep. Fetal placental blood flow was not measured and was assumed constant at 486 ml·min^{-1}. Umbilical arterial P_{O2} also was unknown and was taken to be the standard value of 20 torr.

Figure 12.11 shows the effects of each variable on the instantaneous oxygen transfer rate. Notice that placental oxygen exchange is favorably affected by several factors. After 10 min of exercise, increased maternal hemoglobin concentration accounts for about 60% of this effect, while the rise in maternal and fetal temperatures is responsible for about 15% and 20%, respectively. The increase in maternal P_{O2} also contributes, but to a lesser extent. During the recovery period, placental O_2 transfer is still favored, principally as the result of increased maternal and fetal temperatures and the slight decrease in fetal pH.

During exercise other factors tend to reduce oxygen exchange. Decreased uterine blood flow is predicted to contribute about 31% of the total negative effect at 10 min. However, this was surprisingly less than the 49% contributed by the small rise in fetal arterial pH. The increase in maternal pH also tended to reduce oxygen transfer.

The net effect of exercise on transient changes in placental oxygen exchange is shown by the broken line in Figure 12.11. Under the conditions described above, oxygen transfer is predicted to increase during exercise, reaching a maximum value at the end of the exercise period. During the recovery phase transient oxygen transfer declines but is still above control values 30 min after starting the experiment.

In the steady state, net oxygen transfer equals fetal oxygen consumption. Assuming fetal oxygen consumption remains constant, the umbilical arterial P_{O2} will rise, lowering placental oxygen exchange to control values. However, if the rise in fetal temperature increases fetal oxygen consumption according to van't Hoff Arrhenius' law (0.3°C rise in temperature results in a 4% increase in oxygen consumption), then net oxygen transfer under steady state conditions would be increased accordingly (Fig. 12.11).

The temperature effects on fetal metabolism theoretically would be greater during longer periods of exercise. For example, the temperature of the fetus rose 1.2°C after 40 min of maternal exercise at 70% maximum oxygen consumption as the maternal tem-

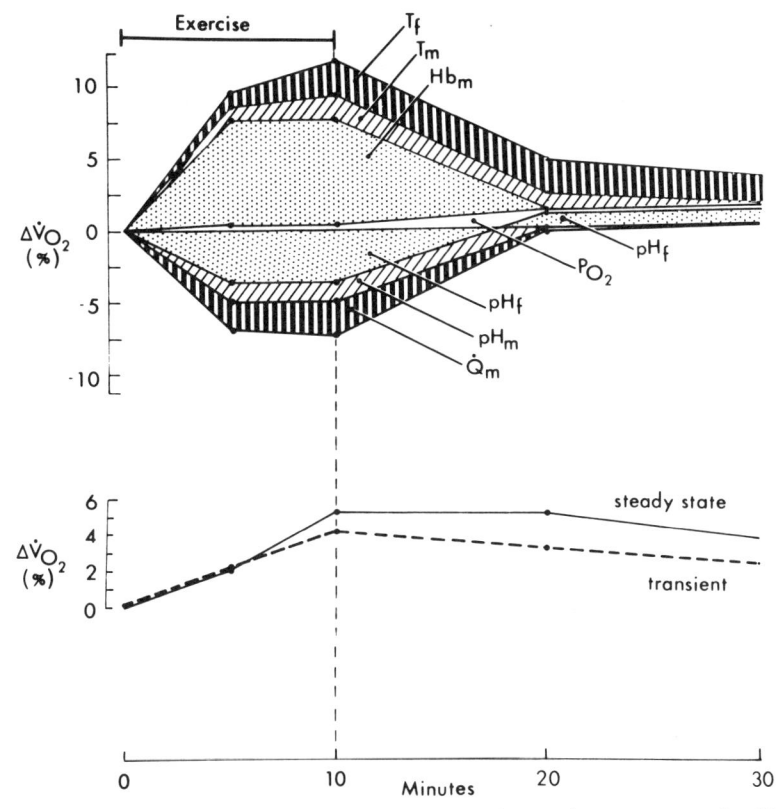

Figure 12.11. Theoretical effects of maternal exercise on placental oxygen transfer. The *top figure* shows the contribution of individual factors to the total increase or decrease in placental O_2 exchange. The *bottom figure* shows the net effect of these changes on the transient O_2 transfer rate, as compared to changes expected under steady state conditions (T_f = fetal temperature, T_m = maternal temperature, Hb_m = maternal hemoglobin concentration, Po_2 = maternal arterial O_2 tension, pH_f = fetal arterial pH, pH_m = maternal arterial pH, and $\dot{Q}_m$ = uteroplacental blood flow).

perature increased 1.4°C. This temperature rise in the fetus should have increased fetal metabolism by 16%. The physiologic changes accompanying exercise of this duration could account for about 6% of the increase in net oxygen transfer under steady state conditions. The remaining 10% could be provided by a 1.3 torr decrease in umbilical arterial Po_2. While it helps match placental oxygen delivery to fetal oxygen needs, such a decrease in fetal umbilical arterial Po_2 should result in a slightly lower umbilical venous Po_2. Such a mechanism might partly explain the slight decrease in fetal arterial Po_2 observed at the end of 40 min of exercise (97). However, a caveat must be emphasized in that no experimental data exist at the present time on the effect of temperature on metabolic rate in the fetal lamb.

Summarizing, exercise induces profound physiologic effects in the mother, some of which, interestingly, augment fetal oxygenation, whereas others depress it. Predominant among the favorable factors is hemoconcentration of maternal blood leading to increased oxygen-carrying capacity. Important negative factors include reduced uterine blood flow and increased pH of maternal and fetal blood. The net effect is predicted to be a balance with little change in oxygen transfer to the fetus. Whether these predictions can be confirmed in humans will require new technology and approaches.

Acknowledgments. The authors gratefully

acknowledge the assistance of Mr. P. S. Dale, who derived the algebraic equations used to calculate placental oxygen transfer, and to Mrs. S. Taylor who prepared the manuscript.

REFERENCES

1. Adamson JW, Parer JT, Stamatoyannopoulos G: Erythrocytosis associated with hemoglobin Ranier. Oxygen equilibria and marrow regulation. *J Clin Invest* 48:1376–1386, 1969.
2. Adamsons K, Beard RW, Myers RE: Comparison of the composition of arterial, venous, and capillary blood of the fetal monkey during labor. *Am J Obstet Gynecol* 107:435–440, 1970.
3. Adamsons K, James LS, Lucey JF, Towell ME: The effect of anemia upon cardiovascular performance and acid-base state of the fetal rhesus monkey. *Ann NY Acad Sci* 162:225–239, 1969.
4. Allen DW, Wyman Jr J, Smith CH: The oxygen equilibrium of fetal and adult human hemoglobin. *J Biol Chem* 203:81–87, 1953.
5. Anselmino KJ, Hoffmann F: Die Ursachen des Icterus neonatorum. *Arch Gynakol* 143:447–499, 1930.
6. Assali NS, Rauramo L, Peltonen T: Measurement of uterine blood flow and uterine metabolism; VIII. Uterine and fetal blood flow and oxygenation in early human pregnancy. *Am J Obstet Gynecol* 79:86–98, 1960.
7. Assali NS, Douglas Jr RA, Baird WW, Nicholson DB, Suyemoto R: Measurements of uterine blood flow and uterine metabolism; IV. Results in normal pregnancy. *Am J Obstet Gynecol* 66:248–253, 1953.
8. Barcroft J: The conditions of foetal respiration. *Lancet* 225:1021–1024, 1933.
9. Barcroft J: *Researches on Prenatal Life*. Oxford, Blackwell, 1946, vol 1.
10. Barron DH: The oxygen pressure gradient between the maternal and fetal blood in pregnant sheep. *Yale J Biol Med* 19:23–27, 1946.
11. Barron DH, Alexander G: Supplementary observations on the oxygen pressure gradient between the maternal and fetal bloods of sheep. *Yale J Biol Med* 25:61–66, 1952.
12. Barron DH, Battaglia FC: The oxygen concentration gradient between the plasmas in the maternal and fetal capillaries of the placenta of the rabbit. *Yale J Biol Med* 28:197–207, 1955–56.
13. Barron DH, Meschia G: A comparative study of the exchange of the respiratory gases across the placenta. *Cold Spring Harbor Symp Quant Biol* 39:93–103, 1954.
14. Bartels H: *Prenatal Respiration*. Amsterdam, North Holland, 1970.
15. Bartels H, Moll W: Passage of inert substances and oxygen in the human placenta. *Pflugers Arch Ges Physiol* 280:165–177, 1964.
16. Bartels H, Moll W, Metcalfe J: Physiology of gas exchange in the human placenta. *Am J Obstet Gynecol* 84:1714–1730, 1962.
17. Battaglia FC, Bowes W, McGaughey HR, Makowski EL, Meschia G: The effect of fetal exchange transfusions with adult blood upon fetal oxygenation. *Pediatr Res* 3:60–65, 1969.
18. Bauer C, Ludwig I, Ludwig M: Different effects of 2,3-diphosphoglycerate and adenosine triphosphate on the oxygen affinity of adult and foetal human haemoglobin. *Life Sci* 7:1339–1343, 1968.
19. Baumann R, Teischel F, Zoch R, Bartels H: Changes in red cell 2,3-diphosphoglycerate concentration as cause of the postnatal decrease of pig blood oxygen affinity. *Respir Physiol* 19:153–161, 1973.
20. Beer R, Bartels H, Raczkowski HA: Die Sauerstoffdissoziationskurve des fetalen Blutes und der Gasaustausch in der menschlichen Placenta. *Pflugers Arch Ges Physiol* 260:306–319, 1955.
21. Berman Jr W, Goodlin RC, Heymann MA, Rudolph AM: Relationships between pressure and flow in the umbilical and uterine circulations of the sheep. *Circ Res* 38:262–266, 1976.
22. Benesch R, Benesch RE: The effect of organic phosphate from the human erythrocyte on the allosteric properties of hemoglobin. *Biochem Biophys Res Commun* 26:162–167, 1967.
23. Bille-Brahe NE, Rorth M: Red cell 2,3-diphosphoglycerate in pregnancy. *Acta Obstet Gynecol Scand* 58:19–21, 1979.
24. Bissonnette JM: Control of vascular volume in the sheep umbilical circulation. *J Appl Physiol* 38:1057–1061, 1975.
25. Bissonnette JM, Farrell RC: Pressure-flow and pressure-volume relationships in the fetal placental circulation. *J Appl Physiol* 35:355–360, 1973.
26. Bissonnette JM, Longo LD, Novy MJ, Murata Y, Martin Jr CB: Placental diffusing capacity and its relation to fetal growth. *J Dev Physiol* 1:351–359, 1979.
27. Bissonnette JM, Wickham WK: Placental diffusing capacity for carbon monoxide in unanesthetized guinea pigs. *Respir Physiol* 31:161–168, 1977.
28. Blechner JN, Stenger VG, Prystowsky H: Uterine blood flow in women at term. *Am J Obstet Gynecol* 120:633–639, 1974.
29. Bøe F: Vascular morphology of the human placenta. *Cold Spring Harbor Symp Quant Biol* 19:29–35, 1954.
30. Bohr C, Hasselbalch K, Krogh A: Ueber einen in biologischer Beziehung wichtigen Einfluss, den die Kohlensaurespannung des Blutes auf dessen Sauerstoffbindung ubt. *Skand Arch Physiol* 16:402–417, 1904.
31. Born GVR, Dawes GS, Mott JC: Oxygen lack and autonomic nervous control of the foetal circulation in the lamb. *J Physiol (Lond)* 134:149–166, 1956.

32. Boyle JW, Lotgering FK, Longo LD: Acute embolization of the uteroplacental circulation: uterine blood flow and placental CO diffusing capacity. *J Dev Physiol* 6:377–386, 1984.
33. Brinkman R, Jonxis JHP: The occurrence of several kinds of haemoglobin in human blood. *J Physiol (Lond)* 85:117–127, 1935.
34. Brinkman R, Jonxis JHP: Alkaline resistance and spreading velocity of foetal and adult types of mammalian haemoglobin. *J Physiol (Lond)* 88:162–166, 1937.
35. Brinkman R, Wildschut A, Wittermans A: On the occurrence of two kinds of haemoglobin in normal human blood. *J Physiol (Lond)* 80:377–387, 1934.
36. Campbell AGM, Dawes GS, Fishman AP, Hyman AI, James GB: The oxygen consumption of the placenta and the foetal membranes in the sheep. *J Physiol (Lond)* 182:439–464, 1966.
37. Caton D, Crenshaw C, Wilcox CJ, Barron DH: O_2 delivery to the pregnant uterus: its relationship to O_2 consumption. *Am J Physiol* 23:R52–R57, 1979.
38. Capp GL, Rigas DA, Jones RT: Evidence for a new haemoglobin chain (ϵ-chain). *Nature* 228:278–280, 1970.
39. Capp GL, Rigas DA, Jones RT: Hemoglobim Portland 1: a new human hemoglobin unique in structure. *Science* 157:65–66, 1967.
40. Chanutin A, Curnish RR: Effect of organic and inorganic phosphates on the oxygen equilibrium of human erythrocytes. *Arch Biochem Biophys* 121:96–102, 1967.
41. Clapp III JF: The relationship between blood flow and oxygen uptake in the uterine and umbilical circulations. *Am J Obstet Gynecol* 132:410–413, 1978.
42. Comline RS, Silver M: A comparative study of blood gas tensions, oxygen affinity and red cell 2,3-DPG concentrations in foetal and maternal blood in the mare, cow and sow. *J Physiol (Lond)* 242:805–826, 1974.
43. Cornet A, Bard H: Changes in hemoglobin oxygen affinity in relation to gestational age (abstract). *Pediatr Res* 9:276, 1975.
44. Danesino V: Dispositivi di blocco ed anastomosi arter-venose nei vasi fetali della placenta umana. *Arch Obstet Ginecol* 55:251–272, 1959.
45. Darling RC, Smith CA, Asmussen E, Cohen FM: Some properties of human fetal and maternal blood. *J Clin Invest* 20:739–747, 1941.
46. Dawes GS: Oxygen supply and consumption in late fetal life, and the onset of breathing at birth. In Fenn WO, Rahn H (eds): *Handbook of Physiology; Sect. 3, Respiration; Vol. II*. Washington, D.C., American Physiology Society, 1965, pp 1313–1328.
47. Dawes GS, Mott JC: Changes in O_2 distribution and consumption in foetal lambs with variations in umbilical blood flow. *J Physiol (Lond)* 170:524–540, 1964.
48. Dawes GS, Lewis BV, Milligan JE, Roach MR, Tayner NS: Vasomotor responses in the hind limbs of foetal and new-born lambs to asphyxia and aortic chemoreceptors stimulation. *J Physiol (Lond)* 195:55–81, 1968.
49. De Verdier C-H, Garby L: Low binding of 2,3-diphosphoglycerate to haemoglobin F: a contribution to the knowledge of the binding site and an explanation for the high oxygen affinity of fetal blood. *Scand J Clin Lab Invest* 23:149–151, 1969.
50. Drescher H, Kunzer W: Der Blutfarbstoff des menschlichen Feten. *Klin Wochenschr* 32:92, 1954.
51. Eastman NJ, Geilling EMK, Delawdner AM: Foetal blood studies; IV. The oxygen and carbon-dioxide dissociation curves of foetal blood. *Johns Hopkins Hosp Bull* 53:246–254, 1933.
52. Faber JJ: Steady-state methods for the study of placental exchange. *Fed Proc* 36:2640–2646, 1977.
53. Faber JJ, Green TJ, Long LR: Permeability of the rabbit placenta to large molecules. *Am J Physiol* 220:688–693, 1971.
54. Faber JJ, Hart FM: The rabbit placenta as an organ of diffusional exchange. Comparison with other species by dimensional analysis. *Circ Res* 19:816–833, 1966.
55. Faber JJ, Hart FM: Transfer of charged and uncharged molecules in the placenta of the rabbit. *Am J Physiol* 213:890–894, 1967.
56. Fuller EO, Manning JW, Nutter DO, Galletti PM: A perfused uterine preparation for the study of uterine and fetal physiology. In Longo LD, Reneau DD (eds): *Fetal and Newborn Cardiovascular Physiology; Vol. 2, Fetal and Newborn Circulation*. New York, Garland Press, 1978, pp 421–435.
57. Gilbert RD, Cummings LA, Jachau MR, Longo LD: Placental diffusing capacity and fetal development in exercising or hypoxic guinea pigs. *Am J Physiol* 46:828–834, 1979.
58. Gratzer WB, Allison AC: Multiple haemoglobins. *Biol Rev* 35:459–506, 1960.
59. Halbrecht I, Klibanski C: Identification of a new normal embryonic haemoglobin. *Nature* 178:794–795, 1956.
60. Halbrecht I, Klibanski C, Bar Ilan F: Co-existence of the embryonic (third normal) haemoglobin fraction with erythroblastosis in the blood of two full-term newborn babies with multiple malformations. *Nature* 183:327–328, 1959.
61. Halbrecht I, Klibanski C, Brzoza H, Lahav M: Further studies on the various hemglobins and the serum protein fractions in early embryonic life. *Am J Clin Pathol* 29:340–344, 1958.
62. Hall FG: A spectroscopic method for the study of haemoglobin in dilute solutions. *J Physiol (Lond)* 80:502–507, 1934.
63. Hall FG: Haemoglobin function in the developing chick. *J Physiol (Lond)* 83:222–228, 1935.
64. Harding R, Sigger JN, Wickham PJD: Fetal and

maternal influences on arterial oxygen levels in the sheep fetus. *J Dev Physiol* 5:267–276, 1983.
65. Hellegers AE, Schruefer JJP: Nomograms and empirical equations relating oxygen tension, percentage saturation, and pH in maternal and fetal blood. *Am J Obstet Gynecol* 81:377–384, 1961.
66. Hill EP, Longo LD, Power GG: Kinetics of O_2 and CO_2 exchange. In West JB (ed): *Bioengineering Aspects of the Lung*. New York, Marcel Decker, 1975, pp 459–514.
67. Hill EP, Power GG, Longo LD: A mathematical model of carbon dioxide transfer in the placenta and its interaction with oxygen. *Am J Physiol* 224:283–299, 1973.
68. Hill EP, Power GG, Longo LD: A mathematical model of placental O_2 transfer with consideration of hemoglobin reaction rates. *Am J Physiol* 222:721–729, 1972.
69. Hlastala MP, Standaert TA, Franada RL, McKenna HP: Hemoglobin-ligand interaction in fetal and maternal sheep blood. *Respir Physiol* 34:185–194, 1978.
70. Hobel CJ: The influence of anemia on the acid-base state of the fetus and newborn. *Am J Obstet Gynecol* 106:303–308, 1970.
71. Huehns ER, Flynn FV, Butler EA, Beaven GH: Two new haemoglobin variants in a very young human embryo. *Nature* 189:496–497, 1961.
72. Hufner von CG: Neue Versuche zur Bestimmung der Sauerstoff-capacitat des Blutfarstoffs. Arch Anat Physiol Abt 130–176, 1894.
73. Huggett ASTG: Foetal blood-gas tensions and gas transfusion through the placenta of the goat. *J Physiol (Lond)* 62:373–384, 1927.
74. Hunt JA, Lehman H: Haemoglobin "Bart's": a foetal haemoglobin without α-chains. *Nature* 184:872–873, 1959.
75. Itskovitz J, Lagamma EF, Rudolph AM: The effect of reducing umbilical blood flow on fetal oxygenation. *Am J Obstet Gynecol* 145:813–818, 1983.
76. Jansen CAM, Krane EJ, Thomas AL, Beck NFG, Lowe KC, Joyce P, Parr M, Nathanielsz PW: Continuous variability of fetal P_{O_2} in the chronically catheterized fetal lamb. *Am J Obstet Gynecol* 134:776–783, 1979.
77. Jones RT, Osgood EE, Brimhall B, Koler RD: Hemoglobin Yakima; I. Clinical and biochemical studies. *J Clin Invest* 46:1840–1847, 1967.
78. Kaltsoya A, Fessas P, Stavropoulos A: Hemoglobins of early human embryonic development. *Science* 153:1417–1418, 1966.
79. Kirschbaum TH: Fetal hemoglobin composition as a parameter of the oxyhemoglobin dissociation curve of fetal blood. *Am J Obstet Gynecol* 84:477–485, 1962.
80. Kirschbaum TH, Brinkman III CR, Assali NS: Effects of maternal-fetal blood exchange transfusion in fetal lambs. *Am J Obstet Gynecol* 110:190–202, 1971.
81. Korber von E: Uber Differenzen des Blutfarbstoffes (Inaugural Dissertation), Dorpat, 1866.
82. Krogh A, Krogh M: On the rate of diffusion of carbonic oxide into the lungs of man. *Skand Arch Physiol* 23:236–247, 1910.
83. Krogh M: The diffusion of gases through the lungs of man. *J Physiol (Lond)* 49:271–300, 1915.
84. Kunzel W, Moll W: Uterine O_2 consumption and blood flow of the pregnant uterus. Experiments in pregnant guinea pigs. *Z Geburtshilfe Perinatol* 176:108–117, 1972.
85. Laga EM, Driscoll SG, Munro HN: Quantitative studies of human placenta; I. Morphometry. *Biol Neonate* 23:231–259, 1973.
86. Lamport H: The transport of oxygen in the sheep's placenta: the diffusion constant of the placenta. *Yale J Biol Med* 27:26–34, 1954–55.
87. Lecrone CN: Absence of special fetal hemoglobin in beagle dogs. *Blood* 35:451–452, 1970.
88. Liley AW: Intrauterine transfusion of foetus in haemolytic disease. *Br Med J* 2:1107–1109, 1963.
89. Longo LD, Ching KS: Placental diffusing capacity for carbon monoxide and oxygen in unanesthetized sheep. *J Appl Physiol* 43:885–893, 1977.
90. Longo LD, Delivoria-Papadopoulos M, Power GG, Hill EP, Forster II RE: Diffusion equilibration of inert gases between maternal and fetal placental capillaries. *Am J Physiol* 219:561–569, 1970.
91. Longo LD, Hardesty JS: Maternal blood volume: measurement, hypothesis of control, and clinical considerations. In Scarpelli EM, Cosmi V (eds): *Reviews in Perinatal Medicine*. New York, Raven Press, 1985, pp 35–59.
92. Longo LD, Hill EP, Power GG: Factors affecting placental oxygen transfer. In Reneau DD (ed): *Chemical Engineering in Medicine*. New York, Plenum, 1972, pp 88–129.
93. Longo LD, Hill EP, Power GG: Theoretical analysis of factors affecting placental O_2 transfer. *Am J Physiol* 222:730–739, 1972.
94. Longo LD, Power GG, Forster II RE: Placental diffusing capacity for carbon monoxide at varying partial pressures of oxygen. *J Appl Physiol* 26:360–370, 1969.
95. Longo LD, Power GG, Forster II RE: Respiratory function of the placenta as determined with carbon monoxide in sheep and dogs. *J Clin Invest* 46:812–828, 1967.
96. Lotgering FK, Gilbert RD, Longo LD: Exercise responses in pregnant sheep: oxygen consumption, uterine blood flow, and blood volume. *J Appl Physiol* 55:834–841, 1983.
97. Lotgering FK, Gilbert RD, Longo LD: Exercise responses in pregnant sheep: blood gases, temperatures, and fetal cardiovascular system. *J Appl Physiol* 55:842–850, 1983.
98. Lucius H, Gahlenbeck H, Kleine HO, Fabel H, Bartels H: Respiratory functions, buffer system, and electrolyte concentrations of blood during human pregnancy. *Respir Physiol* 9:311–317, 1970.

99. McCarthy EF: A comparison of foetal and maternal haemoglobins in the goat. *J Physiol (Lond)* 80:206–212, 1934.
100. McRoberts Jr WA: Postural shock in pregnancy. *Am J Obstet Gynecol* 62:627–632, 1951.
101. Mathers NP, James GB, Walker J: The oxygen affinity of the blood of infants treated by intrauterine transfusion. *J Obstet Gynaecol Brit Commonw* 77:648–653, 1970.
102. Meschia G, Battaglia FC, Bruns PD: Theoretical and experimental study of transplacental diffusion. *J Appl Physiol* 22:1171–1178, 1967.
103. Meschia G, Battaglia FC, Hay WW, Sparks JW: Utilization of substrate by the ovine placenta in vivo. *Fed Proc* 39:245–249, 1980.
104. Meschia G, Battaglia FC, Makowski EL, Droegemueller W: Effect of varying umbilical blood O_2 affinity on umbilical vein Po_2. *J Appl Physiol* 26:410–416, 1969.
105. Metcalfe J, Dhindsa DS, Novy MJ: General aspects of oxygen transport in maternal and fetal blood. In Longo LD, Bartles H (eds): *Respiratory Gas Exchange and Blood Flow in the Placenta.* Washington, D.C., U.S. Department of Health, Education and Welfare, DHEW Publication No. (NIH) 73-361, 1972, pp 63–74.
106. Metcalfe J, Moli W, Bartels H, Hilpert P, Parer JT: Transfer of carbon monoxide and nitrous oxide in the artificially perfused sheep placenta. *Circ Res* 16:95–101, 1965.
107. Metcalfe J, Romney SL, Ramsey LH, Burwell CS: Estimation of uterine blood flow in normal human pregnancy at term. *J Clin Invest* 34:1632–1638, 1955.
108. Mueggler PA, Jones G, Peterson JS, Bissonnette JM, Koler RD, Metcalfe J, Jones RT, Black JA: Postnatal regulation of canine oxygen delivery: erythrocyte components affecting Hb function. *Am J Physiol* 238:H73–H79, 1980.
109. Novy MJ, Frigoletto FD, Easterday CL, Umansky I, Nelson NM: Changes in umbilical-cord blood oxygen affinity after intrauterine transfusion for erythroblastosis. *N Engl J Med* 285:589–596, 1971.
110. Novy MJ, Parer JT: Absence of high blood oxygen affinity in the fetal cat. *Respir Physiol* 6:144–150, 1969.
111. Oski TA: Hematological problems. In Avery GB (ed): *Neonatology. Pathophysiology and Management of the Newborn.* Philadelphia, J.B. Lippincott, 1975, pp 379–422.
112. Parer JT: Oxygen transport in human subjects with hemoglobin variants having altered oxygen affinity. *Respir Physiol* 9:43–49, 1970.
113. Parer JT, de Lannoy CW, Hoversland AS, Metcalfe J: Effect of decreased uterine blood flow on uterine oxygen consumption in pregnant macaques. *Am J Obstet Gynecol* 100:813–820, 1968.
114. Permutt S, Riley RL: Hemodynamics of collapsible vessels with tone: the vascular waterfall. *J Appl Physiol* 18:924–932, 1963.
115. Power GG, Dale PS: Blood flow distribution within cotyledons of the sheep placenta. In Moawad AH (ed): *Uterine and Placental Blood Flow.* Masson, New York, 1982, pp 83–91.
116. Power GG, Dale PS, Nelson PS: Distribution of maternal and fetal blood flow within cotyledons of the sheep placenta. *Am J Physiol* 241:H486–H496, 1981.
117. Power GG, Gilbert RD: Umbilical vascular compliance in sheep. *Am J Physiol* 233:H660–H664, 1977.
118. Power GG, Hill EP, Longo LD: Combined diffusion and blood flow limitation in placental O_2 transfer. *Am J Physiol* 222:740–746, 1972.
119. Power GG, Jenkins F: Factors affecting O_2 transfer in sheep and rabbit placenta perfused in situ. *Am J Physiol* 229:1147–1153, 1975.
120. Power GG, Longo LD: Sluice flow in placenta: maternal vascular pressure effects on fetal circulation. *Am J Physiol* 225:1490–1496, 1973.
121. Power GG, Longo LD, Wagner Jr HN, Kuhl DE, Forster II RE: Uneven distribution of maternal and fetal placental blood flow, as demonstrated using macroaggregates, and its response to hypoxia. *J Clin Invest* 46:2053–2063, 1967.
122. Pritchard JA, Hunt CF: A comparison of the hematologic responses following the routine prenatal administration of intramuscular and oral iron. *Surg Gynecol Obstet* 106:516–518, 1958.
123. Prystowsky H: Fetal blood studies; VII. The oxygen pressure gradient between the maternal and fetal bloods of the human in normal and abnormal pregnancy. *Johns Hopkins Hosp Bull* 101:48–56, 1957.
124. Prystowsky H, Hellegers A, Bruns P: Fetal blood studies; XIV. A comparative study of the oxygen dissociation curve of nonpregnant, pregnant, and fetal human blood. *Am J Obstet Gynecol* 78:489–493, 1959.
125. Rankin J, Meschia G, Makowski EL, Battaglia FC: Relationship between uterine and umbilical venous Po_2 in sheep. *Am J Physiol* 220:1688–1692, 1971.
126. Rankin J, Meschia G, Makowski EL, Battaglia FC: Macroscopic distribution of blood flow in the sheep placenta. *Am J Physiol* 219:9–16, 1970.
127. Rankin JHG, Peterson EN: Application of the theory of heat exchangers to a physiological study of the goat placenta. *Circ Res* 24:235–250, 1969.
128. Riegel K, Bartels H, El Yassin D, Oufi J, Kleihauer E, Parer JT, Metcalfe J: Comparative studies of the respiratory functions of mammalian blood; III. Fetal and adult dromedary camel blood. *Respir Physiol* 2:173–181, 1967.
129. Rocco E, Bennett TR, Power GG: Placental diffusing capacity in unanesthetized rabbits. *Am J Physiol* 228:465–469, 1975.
130. Roos J, Romijn C: The oxygen dissociation curve of the cow's blood during pregnancy and the dissociation curve of the blood of the newborn

animal in the course of the first time after birth. *Proc Koninklijke Nederlandse Akademie van Wetenschappen* (Amsterdam) 40:803–812, 1937.
131. Roos J, Romijn C: Some conditions of foetal respiration in the cow. *J Physiol (Lond)* 92:249–267, 1938.
132. Scherrer M, Bachofen H: The oxygen-combining capacity of hemoglobin. *Anesthesiology* 36:190, 1972.
133. Schroder H, Leichtweiss HP: Perfusion rates and the transfer of water across the isolated guinea pig placenta. *Am J Physiol* 232:H666–H670, 1977.
134. Schroeder WA, Huisman THJ, Shelton JR, Shelton JB, Kleihauer EF, Dozy AM, Robberson B: Evidence for multiple structural genes for the α chain of human fetal hemoglobin. *Proc Natl Acad Sci USA* 60:537–544, 1968.
135. Schroeder WA, Shelton JR, Shelton JB, Cormick J, Jones RT: The amino acid sequence of the α chain of human fetal hemoglobin. *Biochemistry* 2:992–1008, 1963.
136. Seeds AE, Hellegers AE, Battaglia FC: Oxygen dissociation curves of lysed maternal and fetal erythrocytes. *Am J Obstet Gynecol* 103:68–70, 1969.
137. Smith AD, Gilbert RD, Lammers RJ, Longo LD: Placental exchange area in guinea pigs following long-term maternal exercise: a stereological analysis. *J Dev Physiol* 5:11–21, 1983.
138. Stockell A, Perutz MF, Muirhead H, Glauser SC: A comparison of adult and foetal horse haemoglobins. *J Mol Biol* 3:112–116, 1961.
139. Takenaka O, Morimoto H: Oxygen equilibrium characteristics of adult and fetal hemoglobin of Japanese monkey (Macaca Fuscata). *Biochim Biophys Acta* 446:457–462, 1976.
140. Tautz C, Kleihauer E: Gibt es ein fetales Hamoglobin beim Schwein? II. Analysen des Globins. *Res Exp Med* 159:44–49, 1972.
141. Torrance J, Jacobs P, Restrepo A, Eschbach J, Lenfant C, Finch CA: Intraerythrocytic adaptation to anemia. *N Engl J Med* 283:165–169, 1970.
142. Tweeddale PM: Blood oxygen affinities of the adult and foetal large white pig. *Respir Physiol* 19:145–152, 1973.
143. Tweeddale PM: DPG and the oxygen affinity of maternal and foetal pig blood and haemoglobins. *Respir Physiol* 19:12–18, 1973.
144. Tyuma I, Shimizu K: Different response to organic phosphates of human fetal and adult hemoglobins. *Arch Biochem Biophys* 129:404–405, 1969.
145. Walker J, Turnbull EPN: Haemoglobin and red cells in the human foetus and their relation to the oxygen content of the blood in the vessel of the umbilical cord. *Lancet* 2:312–318, 1953.
146. Wilkening RB, Meschia G: Fetal oxygen uptake, oxygenation, and acid-base balance as a function of uterine blood flow. *Am J Physiol* 244:H749–H755, 1983.
147. Winslow RM, Swenberg M-L, Gross E, Chervenick PA, Buchman RR, Anderson WF: Hemoglobin McKees Rocks ($\alpha_2\beta_2^{145\text{Tyr}\rightarrow\text{Term}}$). A human "nonsense" mutation leading to a shortened β-chain. *J Clin Invest* 57:772–781, 1976.
148. Wulf H: Der Gasaustausch in der reifen Plazenta des Menschen. *Z Geburtshilfe Gynaekol Beilageh* 158:117–134, 269–319, 1962.

13
Altered States of Fetal Circulation

FETAL CIRCULATION AND ITS REGULATION

In the adult, blood travels from the left ventricle to the systemic circulation and is returned to the right side of the heart. From there, it flows through the lungs for reoxygenation. This serial circulatory design is inappropriate for the fetus, because oxygenation occurs in the placenta, and a pair of parallel circulations is present. Fetal circulation is made possible by anatomic "shunts," which normally are closed rapidly at birth, when adult circulation is required (1).

The fetal circulation is illustrated in Figure 13.1 with approximate values of the percentage of saturation of blood with oxygen in various areas. Most of the physiological data presented in this section are taken from studies of chronically catheterized, unanesthetized sheep fetuses, because it is rarely possible to obtain such data from the human fetus. Although species differences may occur, it is likely that the same general trends and mechanisms apply to the human fetus as apply to the sheep fetus.

Well-oxygenated blood returns from the placenta by way of the umbilical vein. This vein enters the liver, where it joins with the portal venous system. Some of the blood is shunted directly to the inferior vena cava through the ductus venosus, and some traverses the hepatic parenchyma. An average of 50% takes the latter path, but the proportion is variable (2).

The saturation of blood in the inferior vena cava is lower than that in the ductus venosus, because it has mixed with poorly oxygenated blood returning from the lower body. The inferior vena caval blood enters the right atrium, and approximately 40% is diverted immediately by way of the foramen ovale (another temporary shunt) to the left atrium. Here it mixes with a relatively small quantity of pulmonary venous blood and enters the left ventricle and then the coronary circulation and the vessels that supply the head, neck, and upper extremities. Hence, the foramen ovale allows relatively well-oxygenated blood to supply two vital structures, the heart and the head.

Blood entering the right atrium from the superior vena cava joins with the remaining 60% of inferior vena caval blood and enters the right ventricle. From here, a small proportion enters the pulmonary circulation, but most is shunted from this bed by way of the ductus arteriosus, which joins the descending aorta. This blood supplies the gut, kidneys, and lower body and also the umbilical circulation.

Distribution of Blood Flows within the Fetus

The distribution of blood flows in the fetus generally is described as a percentage of the cardiac output. It is a simple concept in the adult who has two essentially equal serial circulations—systemic and pulmonary. In the fetus, with two unequal parallel circulations, distribution is described as the percentage of combined ventricular output,

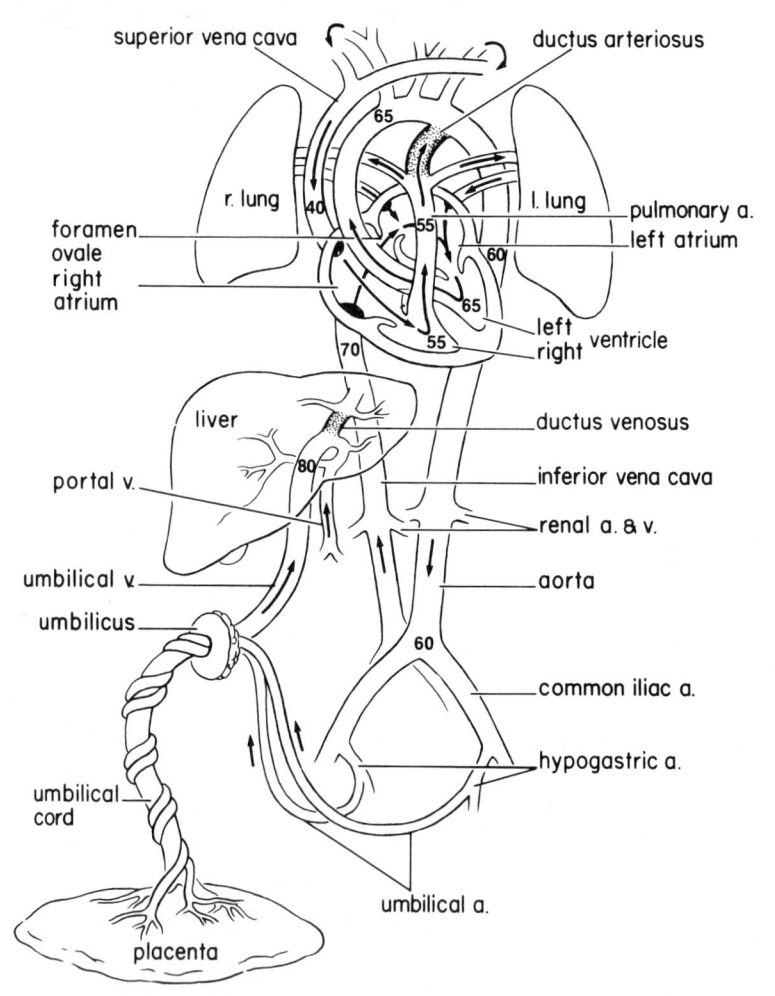

Figure 13.1. Diagram of the fetal circulation. *Arrows* show the direction of blood flow, and *numbers* represent the approximate values of the percentage of saturation of the blood with oxygen in the fetal sheep. (From J. T. Parer: *Handbook of Fetal Heart Rate Monitoring*, W. B. Saunders Co., Philadelphia, 1983.)

or CVO; that is, the combined output of the left and right ventricles.

The percentage of CVO in various areas of the heart and other vessels is shown in Figure 13.2. For obvious reasons, little of this information is available from human fetuses at term; the values depicted in the figure were obtained from unanesthetized chronically catheterized term sheep fetuses.

The sheep fetus at term is the same weight as the human fetus (approximately 3 kg), but species differences occur. For example, the proportion of blood flow to the brain is considerably greater in the human than in the sheep. In the term sheep fetus, the combined ventricular output is 450 ml per min per kg, with twice the quantity from the right as from the left ventricle. Approximately 45% of the CVO is umbilical blood flow, i.e., approximately 200 ml per min per kg (3).

Distribution of the cardiac output occurs in proportoin to the vascular resistance of each bed. These resistances are markedly changed during asphyxia, giving rise to preferential blood flow to certain vital organs, described under "Fetal Circulation during Asphyxial Stress."

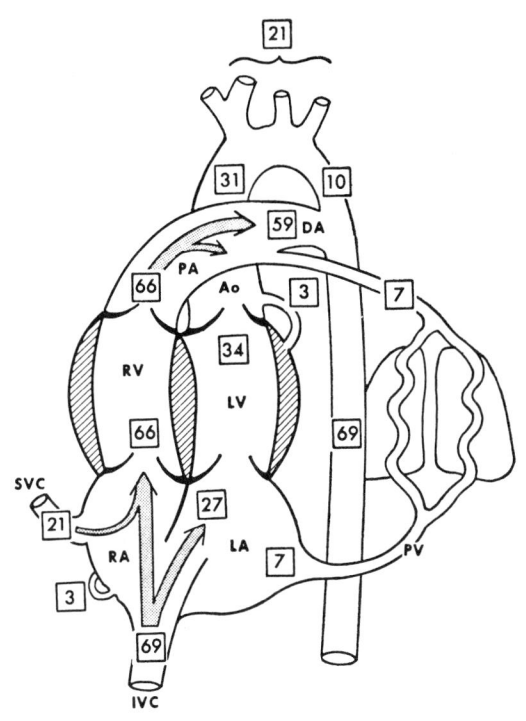

Figure 13.2. The distribution of blood flow in the heart and major blood vessels of the fetal sheep. *Numbers* represent the percentage of combined ventricular output in various areas. (From A. M. Rudolph: *Congenital Diseases of the Heart*, Year Book Medical Publishers, Chicago, 1974).

Fetal Blood Pressure

The fetus is surrounded by a fluid-filled amniotic cavity, so fetal blood pressures must be related to the pressure of amniotic fluid. In the absence of uterine contractions, this pressure is generally stable.

The systemic arterial blood pressure of the fetus is considerably lower than that of the adult, averaging 55 mm Hg (systolic/diastolic, approximately 70/45 mm Hg) at term. Right ventricular pressure, 70/4 mm Hg, is slightly greater (1–2 mm Hg) than left ventricular pressure. Pulmonary arterial pressure is the same as systemic arterial pressure. There is a slightly greater pressure in the right atrium (3 mm Hg) than in the left atrium (2 mm Hg), thus ensuring right-to-left blood flow across the foramen ovale (3).

Systemic blood pressures are somewhat lower earlier in gestation. This difference is reflected in the fact that premature newborns have a lower blood pressure than do term infants. Thus, at 30 weeks of gestation, the mean arterial blood pressure is only about 35 mm Hg (4).

Fetal Heart Rate and Its Variability

BASELINE RATE

The average heart rate in the nonmedicated term fetus before labor is 140 beats per minute (bpm). Earlier in pregnancy, the heart rate is greater, although the difference is not substantial. At 20 weeks, the average fetal heart rate is 155 bpm, and at 30 weeks of pregnancy, it is 144 bpm. Variations of 20 bpm above or below these values occur in normal fetuses (5).

The fetal heart is similar to that of the adult in that it has an intrinsic pacemaker function, which results in rhythmic contractions. The sinoatrial (SA) node, which is found in one wall of the right atrium, has the fastest rate of contraction and sets the rate in the normal heart. The next fastest pacemaking rate is found in the atrium. The ventricle has a slower rate of beating than either the SA node or the atrium. In cases of complete or partial heart block in the fetus, variations in the rate below normal can be seen. Typically, a fetus with complete heart block has a rate of approximately 50–60 bpm.

Bradycardia is defined as a heart rate below 120 bpm. To distinguish it from a deceleration the term is confined to such decreases in fetal heart rate (FHR) exceeding 2 min. A tachycardia is a baseline rate in excess of 160 bpm for at least 2 min. The mean FHR is a result of many physiological factors that modulate the intrinsic rate of the heart.

FETAL HEART RATE VARIABILITY

Fetal heart rate variability (FHRV) refers to the irregular fluctuations noted on a tracing from a cardiotachometer. The variability is due to differences in R-R intervals of the fetal electrocardiogram, and clinical FHR monitors are able to determine this to an accuracy of at least 4 msec, corresponding to a fetal heart rate difference of approximately 1 bpm at 120 bpm. Conventionally, the instantaneous FHR is displayed rather than the R-R interval. The cardiotachometer makes the calculation:

$$\text{FHR (bpm)} = \frac{60}{\text{R-R interval (sec)}}$$

and the FHR is displayed on a strip chart recorder with specific y-axis scaling (30 bpm/cm) and a paper speed of 3 cm/min. If each interval between heart beats were identical, the line would be smooth.

FHRV is clinically divided into several classes:

Short-term variability

Short-term variability (STV) is beat-to-beat variability, or differences between 2 adjacent or 3 serial beats. Recognition of STV requires the accurate detection of the cardiac event; only the R wave of the fetal ECG fulfills this requirement. A tracing from the Doppler ultrasound device usually contains artificial jitter; hence, this device cannot reliably be used to determine STV. Unlike the pattern presented by long-term variability the presence or absence of STV must be deliberately determined. STV is described as "present" or "absent."

Long-term Variability

Long-term variability (LTV) consists of irregular, crude sine waves with a cycle of approximately 3–6 per min. It can be detected by a direct electrode and also at times by the Doppler ultrasound method. It generally is described in terms of its approximate amplitude range in bpm.

Variability of the Oscillating Frequency

This term refers to the frequency of the sine wavelike patterns in a specific time period, generally 1 min. It is calculated by counting the number of times the heart rate tracing crosses an imaginary line drawn through the midpoint of each of the complexes.

Three basic classes of LTV are recognized:

Normal Variability

Variability in which the amplitude range of the variability is greater than 6 bpm.

Decreased Variability.

Variability in which the amplitude range is less than 6 bpm.

Absent Variability

Variability in which the amplitude range is less than 2 bpm, and looks "flat," or smooth.

A fourth pattern is FHRV of an amplitude greater than 25 bpm, called the saltatory pattern. This pattern consists of rapid variations in FHR with a frequency of 3–6 per min and an amplitude range greater than 25 bpm. It is qualitatively described as excessive variability and the excessive swings of heart rate have a strikingly bizarre appearance.

Regulation of the Fetal Circulation

This section will include a description of factors that regulate FHR, blood pressure, and distribution of blood flows. Factors causing major disturbance in the fetal circulation are described in a subsequent section.

PARASYMPATHETIC NERVOUS SYSTEM

The parasympathetic nervous system consists primarily of the vagus nerve (tenth cranial nerve), which originates in the medulla oblongata. Fibers from this nerve supply the SA node and also the atrioventricular (AV) node, the neuronal bridge between the atrium and the ventricle. Stimulation of the vagus nerve or injection of acetylcholine, the substance secreted at the nerve endings, produces a decrease in heart rate in the normal fetus as a result of vagal influence on the SA node, decreasing its rate of firing and decreasing the rate of transmission of impulses from atrium to ventricle. Similarly, blocking of this nerve in a normal fetus with a substance that competes with acetylcholine (e.g., atropine) causes an increase in the FHR of approximately 20 bpm at term (6). This effect shows that there is normally a constant vagal tone on the FHR that tends to decrease its intrinsic rate.

The vagus nerve apparently has another very important function: responsibility for transmission of impulses that cause beat-to-beat variability of the FHR. Blocking the vagus nerve with atropine results in the disappearance of this variability. Hence, it has been postulated that there are two vagal influences in the heart: a tonic influence that tends to decrease its rate and an oscillatory influence that results in fetal heart rate variability.

SYMPATHETIC NERVOUS SYSTEM

Sympathetic nerves are widely distributed in the muscle of the heart at term. Stimulation of the sympathetic nerves will release norepinephrine and will cause an increase in the FHR and an increase in the vigor of cardiac contractions. These effects result in an increase in cardiac output. The sympathetic nerves are a reserve mechanism to improve the pumping activity of the heart during intermittent stressful situations. There is normally a tonic sympathetic influence on the heart. Propranolol, a substance that blocks the action of these sympathetic nerves, causes a decrease of approximately 10–15 bpm in the FHR when it is administered to a normal fetus (7). There is, however, only a small decrease in FHRV after blockade of the sympathetic nerves in primates.

It is a commonly held theory that FHRV is a result of two neuronal inputs to the fetal heart, vagal and β-adrenergic, each with a different time constant. Because atropine almost abolishes visually determined FHRV, and propranolol decreases it by only a little, it is very unlikely that the theory holds true for the primate or sheep (8–10).

The responses mentioned previously refer primarily to β-adrenergic activity. α-Adrenergic activity also is important in altering the distribution of blood flow to specific organs during stress (11). Thus during hypoxia there is vasoconstriction of certain vascular beds (e.g., the gut, liver, and lung), which allows preferential flow of blood with the available oxygen to vital organs (e.g., the brain, heart, and adrenals), and blood flow to the placenta is maintained.

Several factors that cause parasympathetic and sympathetic nervous systems to increase their tonic activity will be described in the following sections.

CHEMORECEPTORS

Chemoreceptors are found both in the peripheral and in the central nervous systems. They have their most dramatic effects on the regulation of respiration, but they also are important in the control of the circulation. The peripheral chemoreceptors are found in the carotid and the aortic bodies, in the area of the carotid sinus and in the arch of the aorta. The central chemoreceptors are found in the medulla oblongata and respond to changes in the oxygen and carbon dioxide tensions in blood or cerebrospinal fluid perfusing this area.

In the adult, when oxygen in the arterial blood perfusing the central chemoreceptors is decreased or the carbon dioxide content is increased, there is ordinarily a reflex tachycardia. There is also a substantial increase in arterial blood pressure, which is extremely pronounced with increases in carbon dioxide concentration. Both of these effects, a tachycardia and an increase in blood pressure, are thought to be protective in attempting to circulate more blood through the affected areas in order to bring about a decrease in carbon dioxide tension or an increase in oxygen. Selective hypoxia or hypercapnia of the peripheral chemoreceptors by itself in the adult produces a bradycardia, in contrast to the tachycardia and hypertension seen with central hypoxia or hypercapnia. The interactions of the central and peripheral chemoreceptors are poorly understood in the fetus and are clearly different from adult responses. The net result of hypoxia or hypercapnia in the fetus is bradycardia and hypertension (12). Recently developed techniques allow the selective study of fetal chemoreceptors, and it has been shown that the chemoreflex can be elicited in utero (13). The chemoreflex is thought to be responsible for the "reflex late deceleration" seen clinically (14).

BARORECEPTORS

Small stretch receptors in the vessel walls that are sensitive to increases in blood pressure are found in the arch of the aorta and in the carotid sinus at the junction of the internal and external carotid arteries. When pressure rises, impulses are sent from these receptors by way of the vagus or the glossopharyngeal nerve to the midbrain, resulting in further impulses by way of the vagus nerve to the heart, which tend to slow cardiac activity. This response is extremely rapid, apparent with almost the first systolic rise of blood pressure. It is a protective, stabilizing function by the body in an attempt to lower blood pressure by decreasing heart rate and cardiac output when blood pressure is increasing. This mechanism is functional in the fetus although its degree of maturity is still controversial (15–17).

CENTRAL NERVOUS SYSTEM

In the adult there are influences on heart rate from the higher centers of the brain. Heart rate is increased by certain emotional stimuli such as fear or sexual arousal. Observations on fetal lambs and monkeys have shown that the electroencephalogram or the electro-oculogram shows increased activity at times in association with variability of the heart rate and body movements. At other times, apparently when the fetus is sleeping in utero, activity slows, and the FHRV decreases, suggesting an association between these two factors and central nervous system activity (18).

The hypothalamus is thought to be the area of dispatch of nerve impulses produced by physical expressions of emotion, including acceleration of the heart rate and elevation of the blood pressure. It has been shown in the fetal lamb that stimulating an electrode placed in the hypothalamus causes the fetal heart rate to increase, at least initially, and is followed by a decrease, probably because of the baroreflex mentioned earlier. The increases in blood pressure and heart rate appear to be mediated by the sympathetic nerves (19).

The medulla oblongata contains the vasomotor centers—integrative centers at which all the inputs result in either cardioacceleration or cardiodeceleration. This center is probably also where the net result of numerous cortical and peripheral inputs is processed to form irregular oscillatory vagal impulses, giving rise to FHRV.

HORMONAL REGULATION

Adrenal Medulla

The fetal adrenal medulla produces epinephrine and norepinephrine in response to stressful situations, e.g., asphyxia. Both of these substances act on the heart and the cardiovascular system in a way similar to sympathetic stimulation. That is they produce a faster heart rate, a greater force of contraction of the heart, and an increased arterial blood pressure.

Adrenal Cortex

The adrenal cortex produces aldosterone in response to decreases in blood pressure in the adult. This substance causes the kidney to decrease sodium output, thus tending to increase water retention and therefore causing a blood volume increase. The role of this substance in the fetus is as yet poorly understood.

Vasopressin

Vasopressin, like α-adrenergic activity, has been shown to affect the distribution of blood flow in the fetal sheep (20). It appears to be particularly important during hypoxia and possibly in other stressful situations (see later).

BLOOD VOLUME CONTROL

Capillary Fluid Shift

In the adult, when the blood pressure of the body is elevated by excessive blood volume, some fluid moves out of the capillaries into the interstitial spaces, thereby decreasing the blood volume back toward normal.

Conversely, if the adult loses blood through hemorrhage, some fluid shifts out of the interstitial spaces into the circulation, thereby increasing the blood volume back toward normal. There is normally a delicate balance between the pressures inside and outside the capillaries. This mechanism of regulating blood pressure is slower than the almost instantaneous regulation that occurs with the reflex mechanisms discussed previously. Its role in the fetus is not completely understood, although imbalances may be responsible for the hydrops seen in some cases of Rh isoimmunization and extreme fetal tachycardia.

Intraplacental Pressures

Fluid moves down hydrostatic pressure gradients; it also moves in response to osmotic pressure gradients. The actual values of these factors within the human placental site, where fetal and maternal blood closely approximate, is controversial. It seems likely, however, that there are some delicate balancing mechanisms within the placental site that prevent rapid fluid shifts between mother and fetus. As noted earlier, the arterial blood pressure of the mother is much higher (approximately 100 mm Hg) than that of the fetus (approximately 55 mm Hg), and osmotic pressures are not substantially different. Hence, some compensatory mechanism must be present to equalize the effective pressures at the exchange points.

Frank-Starling Mechanism

In the Frank-Starling mechanism, the amount of blood pumped by the heart is determined by the amount of blood returning to the heart. That is, the heart pumps all of the blood that flows into it without excessive damming of blood in the veins. When the cardiac muscle is stretched prior to contraction by an increased inflow of blood, it contracts with a greater force than before and is able to pump out more blood. This mechanism has been studied in the unanesthetized fetal lamb and has been shown to be less well developed than in the adult sheep (21). The imperfect mechanism in the fetus is probably caused by the fact that fetal heart muscle is not as well developed as adult heart muscle. It is likely that the same is true of the human fetus, because human neonates are generally more immature than are newborn lambs.

A consequence of the poor development of this mechanism is that in slowing of the FHR, the amount pumped per beat (stroke volume) does not increase substantially, and at values below normal, the output of the fetal heart is closely related to the heart rate. The same is true of modest increases in the heart rate above normal, but with greatly increased heart rates, the cardiac output is decreased because there is not sufficient time between contractions for the ventricles to fill. In other words, the cardiac output in the fetus is largely dependent on the heart rate, and the fetus can increase cardiac output markedly only by increasing heart rate, in contrast with the adult, who can increase cardiac output by increasing both heart rate and stroke volume.

This simple relationship does not apply to all fetal conditions (22). In particular, it appears that the fetus can in fact increase its stroke volume to a certain extent during hypoxic bradycardia (12).

Umbilical Blood Flow

The umbilical blood flow is approximately 300 ml per min immediately after delivery (23). This measurement, however, probably is decreased by the acute events occurring at this time and by the inevitable interference with umbilical blood flow. In comparison, the blood flow is 600 ml per min in the chronically instrumented term sheep fetus, which is approximately the same size as the human fetus at term. Recent noninvasive measurements of umbilical blood flow in term human fetuses still appear to be lower than this, i.e., about 120 ml per kg per min (24). This species difference can be explained by the greater oxygen carrying capacity of human fetal blood and the higher body temperature and therefore higher metabolic rate of the sheep (39°) compared with the human (37° C).

The umbilical blood flow in sheep is approximately 45% of the combined ventricular output, and roughly 20% of this blood flow is "shunted." That is, it does not exchange with maternal blood. It either is carried through actual vascular shunts within the fetal side of the placenta or does not approach closely enough to maternal blood to exchange substances with it.

Umbilical blood flow is not affected by acute moderate hypoxia but is decreased by severe hypoxia. The umbilical cord does not have direct innervation, although umbilical blood flow decreases with the administration of catecholamines. The flow is decreased by acute cord occlusion. There are no known means of increasing umbilical flow in cases in which it is decreased chronically. Certain fetal heart rate patterns, namely variable decelerations, however, have been ascribed to transient umbilical cord compression in the fetus during labor. Manipulation of maternal position either to the lateral or to the Trendelenburg position sometimes can abolish these patterns, the implication being that these maneuvers have removed the fetus from the cord, thus relieving the compression.

FETAL CIRCULATION DURING ASPHYXIAL STRESS

There are relatively few comprehensive studies of the fetal circulation under conditions of moderate to severe maternal exercise, although fetal heart rate has received some attention. Such studies are described in Chapter 9.

In sheep it has been shown that uterine blood flow decreased 24% after 40 min of exercise at 70% maximal oxygen consumption (25), but uterine oxygen uptake was maintained due to increased oxygen extraction and increased oxygen capacity due to hemoconcentration. Fetal arterial oygen pressure and content decreased moderately but heart rate and blood pressure did not change. Blood flow distribution was not altered in short-term (10 min) studies (26), nor was there stimulation of catecholamine release. It is likely that fetal oxygen uptake remained stable, and the authors concluded that maternal exercise of this degree in the sheep (presumably normally grown) did not represent a major stressful or hypoxic event to the fetus.

It is conceivable, however, that under conditions of more prolonged or intense exercise, or in the human, the reduction of uterine blood flow could result in fetal asphyxial stress. We will therefore review the fetal responses to hypoxia and asphyxia.

Causes of Fetal Asphyxia

Fetal asphyxia involves both hypoxia and acidosis which if progressive and uncorrected may lead to brain damage and fetal death. There are four basic mechanisms by which the fetus can become hypoxic: (*a*) insufficient blood flow to the maternal placenta (uterine blood flow), (*b*) insufficient blood flow to the fetal placenta (umbilical blood flow), (*c*) a decrease in maternal arterial oxygen tension and content (maternal hypoxia), or (*d*) a decrease in fetal oxygen carrying capacity (e.g., severe fetal anemia). Rarely the hypoxia may be secondary to increased fetal oxygen requirements, as in pyrexia. The associated acidosis may initially be "respiratory," that is, secondary to reduced fetomaternal CO_2 exchange across the placenta (*a*) or (*b*) above) but eventually a progressive metabolic acidosis can develop due to a change from aerobic to anaerobic metabolism in some fetal organs subsequent to inadequate tissue oxygenation.

Most experimental studies have been done using simply the imposition of hypoxia, and less information is available on the influence of deliberately imposed asphyxia. The former is achieved by giving the mother hypoxic gas mixtures to breathe, and the latter by placing adjustable occluders around the uterine artery or umbilical vessels. Hypoxia results simply in decreased O_2 tension with a metabolic acidosis that eventually develops because of the production of lactic acid as an end product of anaerobic metabolism. Asphyxia (e.g., produced by reduction of uterine blood flow by 50% or more) results in a decrease in O_2

tension and an increase in CO_2 tension (giving a respiratory acidosis), and eventually a lactic acidosis. The influence of asphyxia on the fetus appears to be more detrimental than equivalent degrees of hypoxia (12).

Blood Flow Distribution

From such studies in chronically prepared animals, a number of responses are known to occur during acute asphyxia or hypoxia in the previously normoxic fetus. There is a bradycardia caused by increased vagal activity with little change in cardiac output, and a redistribution of blood flow favoring the heart, brain, and adrenal gland (12, 27). These organs may therefore be considered the "priority organs." In addition, the placental blood flow is maintained. This initial response is presumed to be advantageous to the fetus in the same way as the diving reflex is in the adult seal, in that the blood containing the available oxygen and other nutrients is supplied preferentially to these organs. However, fetal adaptations to asphyxial stress can be sustained for a limited time only. This time depends on the degree of asphyxia suffered. Furthermore, there may be a point beyond which the fetus is not capable of sufficient physiologic adaptation and where the degree of asphyxia itself may abolish the compensatory response to hypoxia. These fetal adaptations to hypoxic and asphyxial stress will now be examined.

Distribution of the combined ventricular output has been previously described. It occurs in proportion to the vascular resistance of each vascular bed. The "resting" vascular resistances are markedly changed during asphyxia. Thus, although cardiac output changes little with asphyxia (11, 12, 27, 28) marked vasodilation in the priority organs increases their blood flow 2–5-fold. The vascular resistance of the placenta is essentially unchanged by asphyxia and umbilical blood flow is maintained. The preferential redistribution of blood flow to these organs requires simultaneous vasoconstriction in vascular beds less vital for survival, namely the splanchnic organs (liver, spleen, gut, and kidney), the lungs and peripheral structures (skin and musculoskeletal tissues) (11, 12, 27, 28).

Blood flow to the priority organs in the sheep fetus during normoxia represents less than 8% of cardiac output. During hypoxia combined flow to the priority organs may reach 20% of cardiac output, and umbilical flow remains unchanged at about 40% of cardiac output. Vasoconstriction in the nonpriority vascular beds reduces the combined blood flow to these organs from about 52% to 40%. Because cerebral blood flow is proportionately greater in human fetuses, the percentage of cardiac output to the priority organs is presumably greater during hypoxia than for the sheep fetus. This implies the need for an even greater vasoconstriction in nonpriority vascular beds of the human fetus. As these vascular beds represent the greater proportion of the total arterial tree of the fetal body, total peripheral resistance (and therefore arterial blood pressure) also rises (11).

Although this compensatory blood flow redistribution can occur for a prolonged period of time, it is not without metabolic consequences. Pyruvate and lactate accumulate from the vasoconstricted splanchnic and peripheral beds (29). The placenta may provide a pathway for clearance of excess lactate, but eventually metabolic acidosis (decreasing pH and base excess) becomes progressive unless the cause of the asphyxia is relieved.

Organ Oxygen Consumption

The oxygen consumption of an organ is proportional to its blood flow and its oxygen extraction (arteriovenous oxygen content difference). During asphyxia, arterial oxygen content is decreased. Total fetal oxygen consumption in sheep falls by up to 50–60% (30). This reduction can be maintained for up to 45 min and is completely reversible upon cessation of hypoxia. It is thought that the decrease in total oxygen consumption reflects a decrease in oxygen consumption in vascular beds which are constricted, as evidenced by the anaerobic metabolism which occurs in these organs during asphyxia. However, as an organ's oxygen consumption is proportional to its blood flow, oxygen consumption of the priority organs is largely protected by the increased flow to these organs that occurs during asphyxia.

The relationship between organ blood flow and oxygen consumption during asphyxia has been best studied in the brain and myocardium. As progressive hypoxia leads to a decreasing arteriovenous oxygen content difference across the cerebral circulation (ascending aorta minus sagittal sinus oxygen content), there is an almost exact matching of increased cerebral blood flow (31). This allows maintenance of cerebral oxygen consumption between the limits tested, repesenting an arterial O_2 content range from 4 ml·dl^{-1} to 1 ml·dl^{-1}, that is, from normoxia to moderately severe hypoxia.

A similar relationship was found between arteriovenous oxygen content difference across the myocardial circulation (ascending aortic minus coronary sinus oxygen content) in the unanesthetized fetal sheep during hypoxia (32). That is, the oxygen consumption of the myocardium remained constant because the increased blood flow exactly matched the decreased arteriovenous oxyen difference.

Whether this inverse proportionality between arteriovenous oxygen content difference and blood flow to the brain and myocardium holds during more severe hypoxia or asphyxia is not as yet known. The above studies involved hypoxia imposed by decreasing the ewe's inspired oxygen. As mentioned previously, a similar reduction of oxygen tension or content by an asphyxial method such as reduction of uterine blood flow may be more detrimental to the fetus. Reduction of uterine blood flow to 50% of normal for 10 min caused similar changes in blood flow redistribution to that obtained with moderately severe to severe hypoxia alone (33). However, when uterine blood flow was reduced to 25% of normal for 10 min, there was a reduction in the degree of increased cerebral and myocardial blood flow accompanied by a decrease in cardiac output. This was presumably due to a partial reversal or failure of the mechanisms regulating the compensatory blood flow responses to asphyxia in the face of overwhelming asphyxia. Although cerebral oxygen consumption has not been measured under these severe circumstances, it is likely that it would decrease since both the blood flow and arteriovenous oxygen content difference would be reduced. Thus a theoretical "critical point" exists; when arterial oxygen delivery falls below this point, the compensatory mechanisms would no longer be able to protect the brain against reduction of oxygen consumption, and asphyxial brain damage may result.

The possibility of a similar point of decompensation occurring for the myocardium is also unanswered. However, after 10 min of uterine occlusion to 25% of normal flow, cardiac output drops and there is reduction of myocardial blood flow similar to that of the brain (33). This suggests that a critical point does occur for the myocardium and at a similar severity of asphyxia. Presumably an inability to meet myocardial oxygen consumption needs at this critical severity of asphyxia would in time lead to myocardial failure and reduced cardiac output.

Metabolic Consequences of Hypoxia

The fetus depends partially on anaerobic metabolism for its energy requirements during hypoxia (29), in particular for maintaining metabolism in organs which are subjected to vasoconstriction during hypoxia/asphyxia. However only 4 moles of ATP are generated for each mole of glucose metabolized anaerobically and 2 moles of lactate are produced, whereas 36 moles of ATP are generated per mole of glucose metabolized aerobically, without lactate production. Thus the effects of prolonged anaerobic metabolism in the vasoconstricted beds include rapid exhaustion of carbohydrate stores and progressive metabolic (lactic) acidosis. In laboratory animals the newborn's ability to tolerate asphyxia depends upon its cardiac carbohydrate reserves (32).

Autonomic Changes during Asphyxia

Hypoxia leads to an increase in sympathetic and parasympathetic nervous system activity and an increase in the secretion of catecholamines, vasopressin, angiotensin, and other humoral agents. The cardiovascular responses to hypoxia are rapidly instituted (less than 30 sec) and are probably mediated by these neural and humoral mechanisms.

Hypoxia/asphyxia leads to a marked increase in activity in all three branches of the autonomic nervous system. For example, in studies involving total or selective autonomic blockade, it is estimated from FHR responses that parasympathetic activity is augmented 3–5-fold (34) and β-adrenergic activity about 2-fold (35). While the increased parasympathetic activity is all via the vagus nerve the increase in adrenergic activity arises from both sympathetic nerves (36) and adrenomedullary secretion of catecholamines (37).

The autonomically mediated cardiovascular responses to hypoxia represent a balance between vagal, α-adrenergic and β-adrenergic influences. This counterbalancing of influences appears vital for survival. For example, simultaneous blockade of both α-adrenergic and β-adrenergic activity during hypoxia rapidly leads to fetal demise (38). This may be due to the removal of the counter-vagal influences since total blockade of all postganglianic autonomic fibers (which includes the adrenal medulla) does not result in fetal demise (39). Therefore an important function of the increased β-adrenergic activity associated with hypoxia is limitation of the negative chronotropic effects of increased vagal activity. The aspects of the hypoxia-induced changes which are affected by the autonomic system have been determined by the use of autonomic blocking drugs such as atropine (parasympathetic blockade), phentolamine or phenoxybenzamine (α-adrenergic blockade) or propranolol (β-adrenergic blockade).

Parasympathetic blockade during hypoxia does not cause a change in the redistribution of cardiac output which occurs during hypoxia. α-Adrenergic blockade reverses both the hypoxia-induced hypertension and the vasoconstriction of the splanchnic organs (11). β-Adrenergic blockade during hypoxia does not affect blood pressure but causes a further drop in FHR and a proportionate drop in cardiac output (28). There is an increase in placental vascular resistance and therefore a drop in umbilical blood flow. The hypoxia-induced increase in myocardial blood flow is halved. The increased brain and adrenal blood flow associated with hypoxia is not significantly affected by any of the above manipulations.

From these experiments the following conclusions may be drawn: (a) The primary cardiovascular manifestation of the increased parasympathetic activity during hypoxia is a bradycardia. (b) The increased α-adrenergic activity causes systemic hypertension and vasoconstriction of the vascular beds of certain splanchnic organs (lungs, gut, liver, and spleen). This allows redistribution of blood to priority organs. (c) The umbilical circulation is spared the α-adrenergic influence because of its poor vasoconstrictive ability (40). Furthermore the increase in β-adrenergic activity during hypoxia maintains umbilical blood flow by maintaining placental vasodilatation (28, 35). (d) Active vasodilatation of the myocardial vascular bed appears to be partially mediated by β-adrenergic activity (28) but is probably also maintained in part by local metabolite production. (e) Although the factors controlling adrenal and cerebral vasodilatation remain unknown, blood flow to the brain is inversely proportional to the arteriovenous oxygen content difference (31), and directly proportional to increases in CO_2 pressure (41).

Humoral Changes during Asphyxia

Vasopressin levels are usually undetectable in normoxic sheep fetuses. However, vasopressin secretion increases with hypoxia, the levels reached correlate with the drop in arterial oxygen tension, the drop in pH and the hypertensive response to hypoxia (42). This vasopressin response is reduced but not eliminated by sectioning vagal and sympathetic nerve trunks. Carotid body and aortic chemoreceptors in the fetal lamb appear to be sensitive to hypoxia (43), and perfusion of the carotid sinus of the anesthetized dog with deoxygenated blood causes a rise in vasopressin secretion (44). When vasopressin is administered to normoxic fetal lambs, the cardiovascular response is similar to that seen with hypoxia (20). Included in this response is vasoconstriction in peripheral structures (musculoskeletal system and skin), which does not occur as an α-adrenergic effect. Other changes in blood flow are qualitatively similar to those which have been mentioned above as occurring in response to the increased α- and β-adrenergic activity during hypoxia. Thus the effect of vasopressin on blood flow redistribution is similar and presumably additive to that of the adrenergic system.

LaGamma et al. (45) demonstrated that endogenous opioids also modulate the hypoxic response. The opioid receptor antagonist naloxone, when administered during fetal hypoxemia, exaggerates the hypoxic response. Endogenous opioids may function in fetuses by modifying neurotransmission or humoral release. For example, endogenous opioids could inhibit or modify vasopressin release leading to a "push-pull" balancing mechanism.

The possibility that the renin-angiotensin system may be involved in the fetal hypoxic response has been studied by infusing angiotension II into normoxic sheep fetuses (6). However, the majority of the resultant cardiovascular responses are opposite to those which occur with hypoxia and it is therefore unlikely that angiotension II has a major role in the cardiovascular response to hypoxia.

In summary, the cardiovascular adaptation by hypoxia/asphyxia appears to be initiated by increased autonomic activity with subsequent humoral contributions. This increased activity includes the vagus nerve, sympathetic nerves and catecholamine secretion from the adrenal medulla and is modulated by endogenous opioid production. Vasopressin has an important additive effect to this response. Other agents may also be involved.

REFERENCES

1. Dawes GS: *Foetal and Neontal Physiology*. Chicago, Year Book, 1968.
2. Edelstone DI, Merick RE, Caritis SN, Mueller-Heubach E: Umbilical venous blood flow and its distribution before and during autonomic blockade in fetal lambs. *Am J Obstet Gynecol* 138:703–707, 1980.
3. Rudolph AM: *Congenital Diseases of The Heart*. Chicago, Year Book, 1974.
4. Kitterman JA, Phibbs RH, Tooley WH: Aortic blood pressure in normal newborn infants during the first 12 hours of life. *Pediatrics* 44:959–968, 1969.
5. Schifferli PY, Caldeyro-Barcia R: Effects of atropine and beta-adrenergic drugs on the heart rate of the human fetus. In Boreus L (ed): *Fetal Pharmacology*. New York, Raven Press, 1973, pp 259–279.
6. Mendez-Bauer C, Poseiro JJ, Arellano-Hernandez G, et al: Effects of atropine on the heart rate of the human fetus during labor. *Am J Obstet gynecol* 85:1033–1053, 1963.
7. Harris JL, Krueger TR, Parer JT: Effect of parasympathetic and β-adrenergic blockade on the umbilical circulation in the unanesthetized fetal sheep. *Gynecol Obstet Invest* 10:306–310, 1979.
8. Parer JT, Laros RK, Heilbron DC, Krueger TR: The roles of β-adrenergic activity in beat-to-beat fetal heart rate variability (FHRV). *Physiol Sci* 8:327–329.
9. Kovach AGB, Monose E, Rubanyi G (eds): *Cardiovascular Physiology*. New York, Pergamon Press, 1981.
10. Dalton KR, Dawes GS, Patrick JE: The autonomic nervous system and fetal heart rate variability. *Am J Obstet Gynecol* 146:456–462, 1983.
11. Reuss ML, Parer JT, Harris JL, Krueger JR: Hemodynamic effects of α-adrenergic blockade during hypoxia in fetal sheep. *Am J Obstet Gynecol* 142:410–415, 1982.
12. Cohn HE, Sacks EJ, Heymann MA, Rudolph AM: Cardiovascular responses to hypoxemia and acidemia in fetal lambs. *Am J Obstet Gynecol* 120:817–824, 1974.
13. Itskovitz J, Rudolph AM: Denervation of arterial chemoreceptors and baroreceptors in fetal lambs in utero. *Am J Physiol* 242:H916–H920, 1982.
14. Parer JT, Krueger TR, Harris JL: Fetal oxygen consumption and mechanisms of heart rate response during artificially produced late decelerations of fetal heart rate in sheep. *Am J Obstet Gynecol*

15. Shinebourne EA, Vapaavouri EK, Williams RL, et al: Development of baroreflex activity in unanesthetized fetal and neonatal lambs. *Circ Res* 31:710–718, 1972.
16. Faber JJ, Green TJ, Thornburg KL: Arterial blood pressure in the unanesthetized fetal lamb after changes in fetal blood volume and haematocrit. *Q J Exp Physiol* 59:241–255, 1974.
17. Itskovitz J, LaGamma EF, Rudolph AM: Baroreflex control of the circulation in chronically instrumented fetal lambs. *Circ Res* 52:589–596, 1983.
18. Nijhuis JG, Prechtl HFR, Martin CB Jr., Bots RSGM: Are there behavioural states in the human fetus? *Early Hum Dev* 6:177–195, 1982.
19. Williams RL, Hof RP, Heymann MA, Rudolph AM: Cardiovascular effects of electrical stimulation of the forebrain in the fetal lamb. *Pediatr Res* 10:40–45, 1976.
20. Iwamoto HS, Rudolph AM, Keil LC, Heymann MA: Hemodynamic responses of the sheep fetus to vasopressin infusion. *Circ Res* 44:430–436, 1979.
21. Rudolph AM, Heymann MA: Cardiac output in the fetal lamb: the effects of spontaneous and induced changes of heart rate on right and left ventricular output. *Am J Obstet Gynecol* 124:183–192, 1976.
22. Kirkpatrick SE, Pitlick PT, Naliboff J, Friedman WF: Frank-Starling relationship as an important determinant of fetal cardiac output. *Am J Physiol* 231:495–500, 1976.
23. McCallum WD: Thermodilution measurement of human umbilical blood flow at delivery. *Am J Obstet Gynecol* 127:491–496, 1977.
24. Gill RW, Trudinger BJ, Garret WT, et al: Fetal umbilical venous flow measured in utero by pulsed Doppler and β-mode ultrasound; I. Normal pregnancies. *Am J Obstet Gynecol* 139:720–725, 1981.
25. Lotgering FK, Gilbert RD, Longo LD: Exercise responses in pregnant sheep: oxygen consumption, uterine blood flow and blood volume. *J Appl Physiol* 55:834–841, 1983.
26. Lotgering FK, Gilbert RD, Longo LD: Exercise responses in pregnant sheep: blood gases, temperatures, and fetal cardiovascular system. *J Appl Physiol* 55:842–850, 1983.
27. Peeters LLH, Sheldon RE, Jones MD, et al: Blood flow to fetal organs as a function of arterial oxygen content. *Am J Obstet Gynecol* 135:637–646, 1979.
28. Court DJ, Parer JT, Block BSB, Llanos AJ: Effects of beta-adrenergic blockade on blood flow distribution during hypoxemia in fetal sheep. *J Dev Physiol* 6:349–358, 1984.
29. Mann LI: Effects in sheep of hypoxia on levels of lactate, pyruvate and glucose in blood of mothers and fetuses. *Pediatr Res.* 4:46–54, 1970.
30. Parer JT: The effect of acute maternal hypoxia on fetal oxygenation and the umbilical circulation in the sheep. *Eur J Obstet Gynaecol Reprod Biol* 10:125–136, 1980.
31. Jones MD Jr, Sheldon RE, Peeters LL, et al: Fetal cerebral oxygen consumption at different levels of oxygenation. *J Appl Physiol* 43:1080–1084, 1977.
32. Fisher DJ, Heymann MA, Rudolph AM: Fetal myocardial oxygen and carbohydrate consumption during acutely induced hypoxemia. *Am J Physiol* 242:H657–H661, 1982.
33. Yaffe H, Parer JT, Llanos A, Block B: Fetal hemodynamic responses to graded reductions of uterine blood flow in sheep. Proceedings of the Society for Gynecologic Investigation, Dallas, 1982, p 113.
34. Parer JT: The effect of atropine on heart rate and oxygen consumption of the hypoxic fetus. *Am J Obstet Gynecol* 148:1118–1122, 1984.
35. Parer JT: The influence of β-adrenergic activity on fetal heart rate and the umbilical circulation during hypoxia in fetal sheep. *Am J Obstet Gynecol* 147:592–597, 1983.
36. Iwamoto HS, Rudolph Am, Mirkin BL, Keil LC: Circulatory and humoral responses of the sympathectomized fetal sheep to hypoxemia. *Am J Physiol* 245:H767–H772, 1983.
37. Comline RS, Silver M: The release of adrenaline and noradrenaline from the adrenal glands of the foetal sheep. *J Physiol (Lond)* 156:424–444, 1961.
38. Parer JT, Krueger TR, Harris JL and Reuss ML: Autonomic influences in umbilical circulation during hypoxia in fetal sheep. Proceedings of the Society for Gynecologic Investigation, San Diego, Calif. 1978.
39. Court DJ, Parer JT: Unpublished observations.
40. Berman W, Goodlin RC, Heymann MA, Rudolph AM: Relationships between pressure and flow in the umbilical and uterine circulations of the sheep. *Circ Res* 38:262–266, 1976.
41. Rosenberg AA, Jones MD, Traystman RJ, Simmons MA, Molteni RA: Response of cerebral blood flow to changes in Pco_2 in fetal, newborn and adult sheep. *Am J Physiol* 242:H862–H866, 1982.
42. Rurak DW: Vasopressin levels during hypoxaemia and the cardiovascular effects of exogenous vasopressin in fetal and adult sheep. *J Physiol (Lond)* 277:341–357, 1978.
43. Itskovitz J, LaGamma EF, Bristow J, Rudolph AM: Role of arterial chemoreflex in fetal circulatory response to acute hypoxemia. Proceedings of the Society for Gynecologic Investigation, Washington, D.C., 1983, p 126.
44. Share L, Levy MN: Effect of carotid chemoreceptor stimulation on plasma antidiuretic hormone titer. *Am J Physiol* 210:157–161, 1966.
45. LaGamma EF, Itskovitz J, Rudolph AM: Effects of naloxone on fetal circulatory responses to hypoxemia. *Am J Obstet Gynecol* 143:933–940, 1982.
46. Iwamoto HS, Rudolph AM: Effects of angiotension II on the blood flow and its distribution in fetal lambs. *Circ Res* 48:183–189, 1981.

14

Fetal Responses to Maternal Exercise

Over recent years, recognition of various fetal heart rate (FHR) patterns has provided the obstetrician with a most valuable tool in assessing fetal well being. Typical changes in FHR patterns are known to reflect hypoxic and nonhypoxic stress, hypoxia or asphyxia, and sympathetic and parasympathetic activity. The significance and the pathophysiology of such changes are described at length in the previous chapter.

Exercise induces significant cardiovascular changes of which the selective redistribution of blood flow to the working muscles away from the splanchnic organs has the most potential adverse effects on the fetus. It is recognized that uterine blood flow could be compromised during exercise as reported in both human being and animal studies, though reports to the contrary have also been published (1–5). Reduction of blood flow to the uterus could potentially lead to fetal asphyxia and to induce hypoxia; to cause such changes, the reduction in uterine blood flow should be in excess of 50%. Such circumstances may result in decreased O_2 tension and an increase in CO_2 tension (respiratory acidosis) (6). In the normal healthy pregnant woman, such occurrences should be only rarely encountered during mild and moderate exercise, but they are more likely to occur during strenuous and prolonged exercise.

It appears that the healthy fetus can tolerate brief periods of asphyxia, such as those that may occur during limited periods of maternal exercise.

Initially, the fetus will respond to such events with tachycardia and an increase in blood pressure. This appears to be a protective mechanism for the fetus to facilitate circulation of more blood, that will increase the O_2 and decrease the CO_2 tension.

As discussed in Chapter 10, maternal exercise is associated with a significant increase in circulating catecholamines. Due to a high concentration of enzymes (COMT and MAO), the placenta metabolizes the catecholamines very efficiently and, under normal conditions, only 10–15% of the catecholamines in maternal circulation reach the fetus. Elevated catecholamines could have an additional constrictive effect on the umbilical blood flow. The combined effect of reduced blood flow to the uterus and vasoconstriction secondary to elevated catecholamines could lead to fetal asphyxia and bradycardia. Such a possibility is more than a theoretical consideration, but it is not currently known how often it occurs.

In Table 14.1 we have summarized the published literature on FHR responses to maternal exercise. Because of the different methodology utilized in these studies, comparison and interpretation of data must be done with great caution. Nevertheless, it appears that, by and large, the FHR response to maternal exercise is associated with an increase of approximately 10–30 beats per minute. Our own studies (19) indicate that such changes are consistent and are independent of either gestational age or intensity of maternal exercise. Figures 14.1–14.3 illustrate schematically the changes in fetal heart rates following mild maternal

Table 14.1. Fetal Heart Rate (FHR) Responses to Maternal Exercise[a]

Author	Sample Size	Population	GA	Monitoring Device	Type of Exercise	Intensity of Exercise	FHR during exercise	FHR after exercise
Hon and Wohlgemuth (7)	26	Mixed	34–41	Abdominal ECG	Master step test	Moderate	—	=↑
Soiva et al. (8)	24	Mixed	28–40	Phonocardiograph	Bicycle ergometer	Mild, moderate, strenuous	—	=↑
Hodr and Brotanek (9)	56	Mixed	29–36	Phonocardiograph	Master step test	Moderate	—	=↑
Stembera and Hodr (10)	67	Mixed	38–40	Phonocardiograph	Master step test	Moderate	—	=↑
Pokorny and Rous (11)	14	Mixed	36–40	Phonocardiograph	Bicycle ergometer	Mild	=↑	=→
Pomerance et al. (12)	54	Normal	35–37	Auscultation	Bicycle ergometer	Moderate	—	≡→
Eisenberg de Smoler et al. (13)	22	Mixed	28–40	Abdominal ECG	Master step test; treadmill	Moderate	—	=→
Pernoll et al. (14)	16	Mixed	24–40	Doppler ultrasound	Bicycle ergometer	Mild	—	↑↓
Sibley et al. (15)	7	Normal	17–40	Doppler ultrasound	Swimming	Strenuous	↑	=
Dale et al. (16)	4	Normal	31–37.5	Doppler ultrasound	Treadmill	Strenuous	→	=
Hauth et al. (17)	7	Normal	28–38	Doppler ultrasound	Jogging	Moderate	—	↑
Collings et al. (18)	20	Normal	22–34±	Doppler ultrasound	Bicycle ergometer	Strenuous	↑	↑
Artal et al. (19)	15	Normal	35.1 ± 5.65[b]	Doppler ultrasound	Treadmill	Mild	↑	↑
Artal et al. (19)	11	Normal	34.7 ± 4.31	Doppler ultrasound	Treadmill	Moderate	↑↓	↑↓
Artal et al. (19)	11	Normal	34.1 ± 6.85	Doppler ultrasound	Treadmill	$\dot{V}_{O_2 max}$	↑↓	↑↓

[a] ↑, increase in FHR baseline; ≡, minimum or no change in FHR; ↓, bradycardia; GA, gestational age; PIH, pregnancy-induced hypertension.
(7) 10 healthy pregnant, 5 PIH, 2 essential hypertension, 2 diabetes mellitus.
(8) 13 healthy pregnant, 5 postdates, 11 PIH.
(9) 50 healthy pregnant, 6 premature labor.
(10) 15 healthy pregnant, 52 (unspecified number of PIH, postdates pregnancy, diabetes mellitus, poor obstetrical history).
(11) 12 healthy pregnant, 1 PIH, 1 diabetes mellitus.
(12) 54 healthy pregnant.
(13) 18 healthy pregnant, 2 severe PIH, 2 fetal CNS anomalies.
(14) 8 healthy pregnant, 1 twins, 1 heart disease, 1 drug addict, 5 obese.
(15) 7 healthy pregnant.
(16) 4 healthy pregnant athletes.
(17) 7 healthy pregnant athletes.
(18) 20 healthy pregnant.
[b] Mean ± 1 s.d.

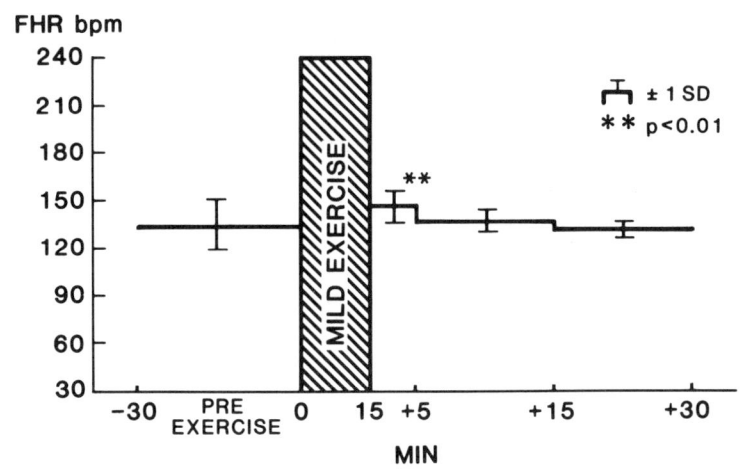

Figure 14.1. Fetal heart rate responses to mild maternal exercise. (From R. Artal et al. (19).)

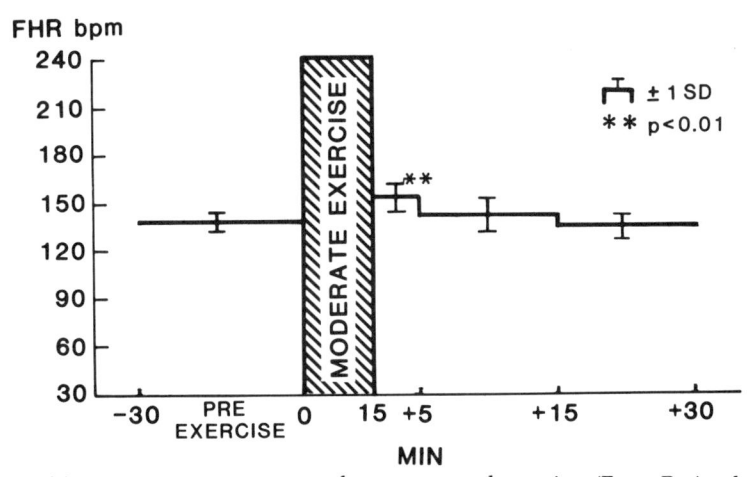

Figure 14.2. Fetal heart rate responses to moderate maternal exercise. (From R. Artal et al. (19).)

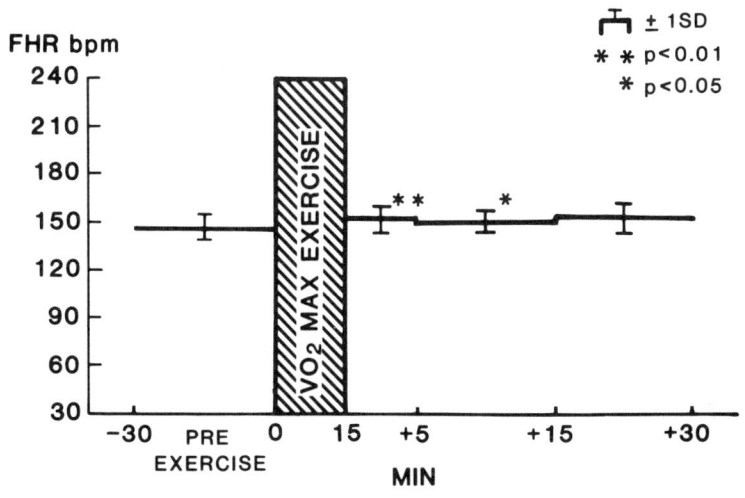

Figure 14.3. Fetal heart rate responses to strenous (V_{O_2}) maternal exercise. (From R. Artal et al. (19).)

exercise (approximately 2.5 METs), moderate exercise (approximately 5 METs), and strenuous exercise (approximately 8 METs) as observed in 37 patients. Immediately after and within 5 min of exercise, the FHR remained significantly elevated with every type of exercise. Within 15 min, the FHR returned to pre-exercise values in the subjects enrolled in the mild and moderate exercise studies, while, in the strenuous exercise ($\dot{V}_{O_2max}$) group, the FHR remained elevated for at least 30 min.

To date, published data on FHR responses to maternal exercise include 354 subjects. In 22 subjects, fetal bradycardia was reported to occur during or after exercise, an incidence of 6.2%. While half of the subjects who experienced bradycardia had an abnormal pregnancy (pregnancy-induced hypertension and premature labor), the other 11 subjects were normal.

Recording of FHR during exercise is technically very difficult. Nevertheless, there are a few reports of such recordings (11, 15, 16, 18, 20). By and large, the recordings obtained during exercise indicate an increase in FHR baseline over the preexercise values. In 82 recorded cases during exercise, fetal bradycardia was observed in only 7 cases (an incidence of 8.5%). Six of the 7 cases were normal patients and completed successfully their pregnancy.

Figures 14.4–14.6 illustrate FHR recordings with episodes of bradycardia during and immediately after maternal exercise (20). These recordings, although not continuous during the exercise testing, have been chosen for publication because they illustrate unique and confirmatory information obtained in our laboratory, such as fetal bradycardia emerging from the exercise period and continuing into the recovery period (20). The FHR tracing in these cases remained identical during and after exercise. It is not yet clear whether brief episodes of fetal bradycardia are common during maternal exercise and the mechanism by which they are triggered can only be speculated upon.

It appears very likely that a reduction in uterine blood flow, accompanied by elevated catecholamines, leads to brief periods of fetal asphyxia which are generally well tolerated by the majority of fetuses. The initial response is tahycardia, but with prolonged hypoxia and vagal stimulation, it results in bradycardia.

Another possibility is that such occurrences are within the realm of normal fetal reflex responses to major maternal hemodynamic and hormonal events. This later explanation could explain those cases in which fetal bradycardia occurs as soon as the subject begins to exercise.

Further such interactions between fetus and mother are discussed in the next section.

FETAL ACTIVITY AND MATERNAL EXERCISE

The interactions between the fetus and mother compose a fascinating, but often poorly understood, relationship. The introduction of additional indexes to assess fetal well being constitutes a further refinement of this process.

Fetal behavior, movements, and breathing have been extensively researched in recent years. Such parameters have been incorporated into a fetal biophysical profile, that appears to accurately identify more than 85% of anomalous factors leading to fetal asphyxia, distress, and death (21).

Hypoxia appears to significantly affect and reduce the frequency of fetal breathing and body movements. Fetal breathing movements (FBM) are episodic and occur approximately 30% of the time during the last trimester of pregnancy. FBM occurrence appears to be related to the stage in gestation, time of day, and maternal plasma glucose and catecholamine levels. Some investigators have suggested that measurements of FBM may be a more sensitive indicator of fetal state than is FHR (22). Furthermore, it has been suggested that irregular FBM occur during increased long-term FHR variability and regular FBM occur during lower long-term FHR variability (23).

Another component of the fetal biophys-

Fetal Responses to Maternal Exercise 199

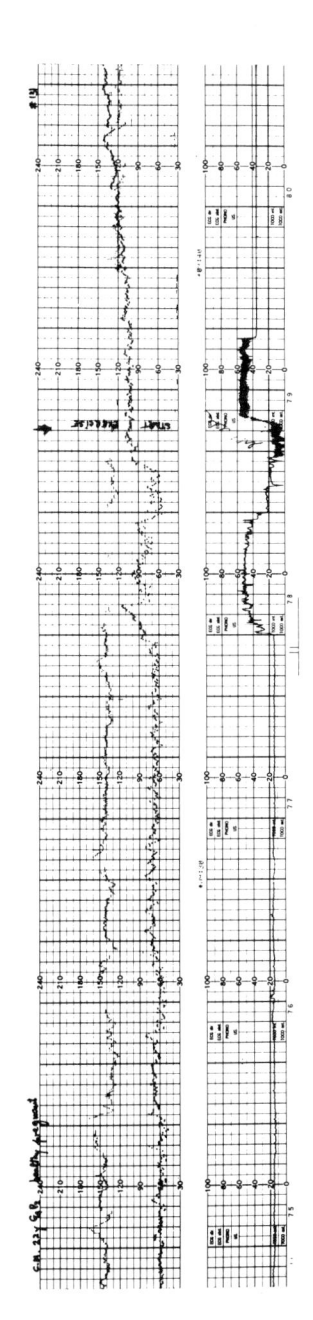

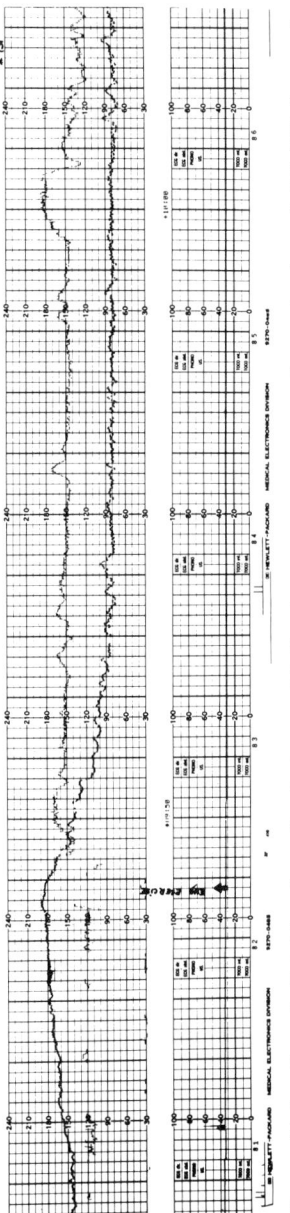

Figure 14.4. Case 1: Fetal bradycardia during and following strenuous maternal exercise (panels 79–82). In panels 75–77 and 83–86, the upper tracings are fetal heart rates and the lower tracings are maternal heart rates. In panels 79–82, the upper tracings are maternal heart rates, the lower tracings are fetal heart rates.

Figure 14.5. Case 2: Fetal bradycardia during and following strenuous maternal exercise (panels 109–113). In panels 106–109 and 115–117, the upper tracings are fetal heart rates and the lower tracings are maternal heart rates. In panels 110–113, the upper tracings are maternal heart rates, the lower tracings are fetal heart rates.

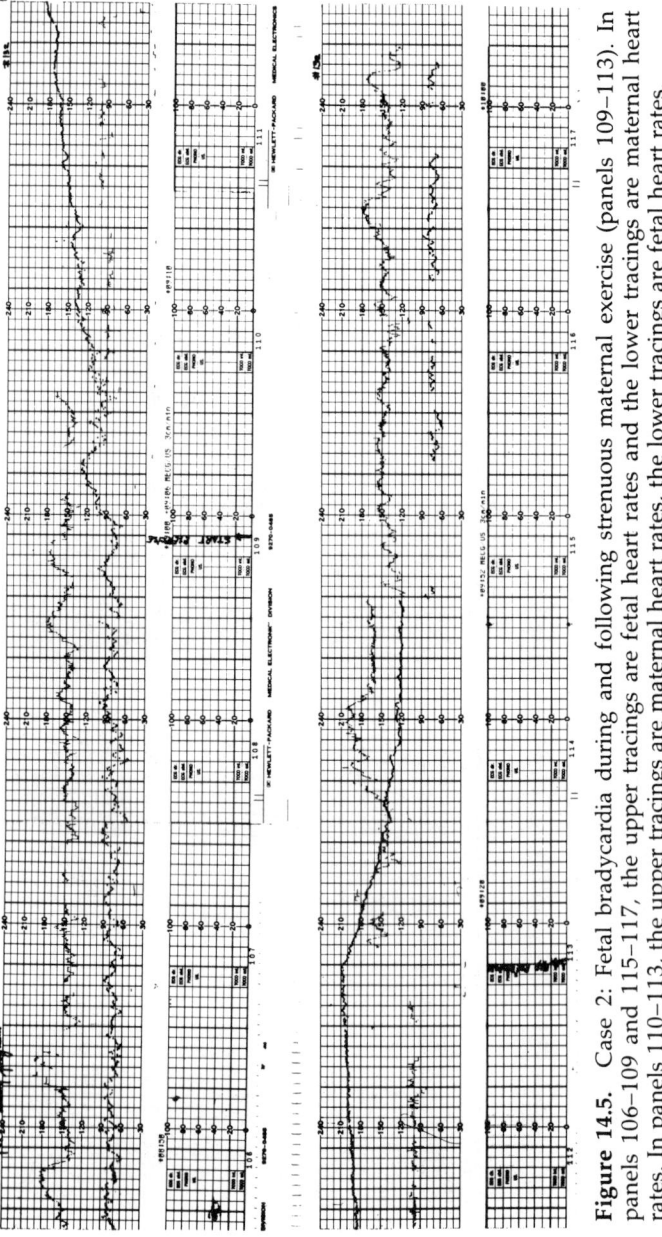

Figure 14.6. Case 3: Fetal bradycardia following strenuous maternal exercise (panels 137–139). In panels 133–136 and 141–145, the *upper tracings* are fetal heart rates, *lower tracings* are maternal heart rates. In panels 137–139, the *upper tracings* are maternal heart rates, the *lower tracings* are fetal heart rates.

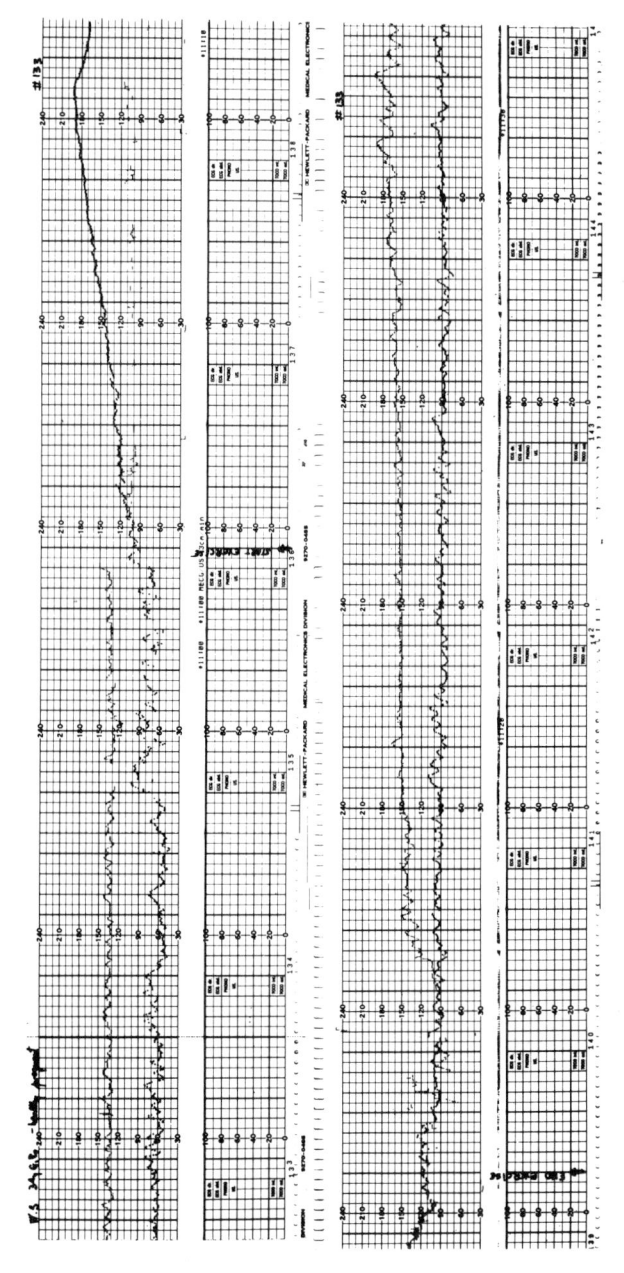

ical profile is fetal movements (FM). FM also appear to closely reflect fetal conditions and, as such, are utilized for both research and clinical surveillance (25, 26). FM occur on an average of 5–20% of each hour.

Fetal activity during and after maternal exercise has been studied very little. One study reported a transient increase in the incidence of FBM after brief moderate maternal exercise. In addition, the same study demonstrated a greater responsiveness of FBM to exercise when compared with FHR (24).

Recognizing the existence of significant responses by the maternal sympathoadrenal system to exercise in pregnancy (27) we have studied its interactions with FBM and FM (28). The results of this study are illustrated in Figure 14.7. In this particular study, we have demonstrated a direct relationship between the level of sympathetic activity in the mother and the incidence of FBM and FM following maternal exercise. The results suggest that catecholamine levels may alter glucose levels and, as such, lead to an increase or decrease in FBM; such correlations have been previously recognized (29). In addition, the data also suggest fetal well being, and as such, could be readily utilized to confirm such status. Fetuses of hypertensive mothers suspected to be distressed have a decrease in FBM following maternal exercise and so do hypoxic fetuses and fetuses monitorerd immediately prior to and during labor.

LONG-TERM EFFECTS OF MATERNAL EXERCISE ON THE FETUS

The existing published data suggests that maternal exercise may have brief or lasting effects on the fetus. While most of the interactions between maternal exercise and the fetus may be transitory, questions remain as to the long lasting effects on the fetus.

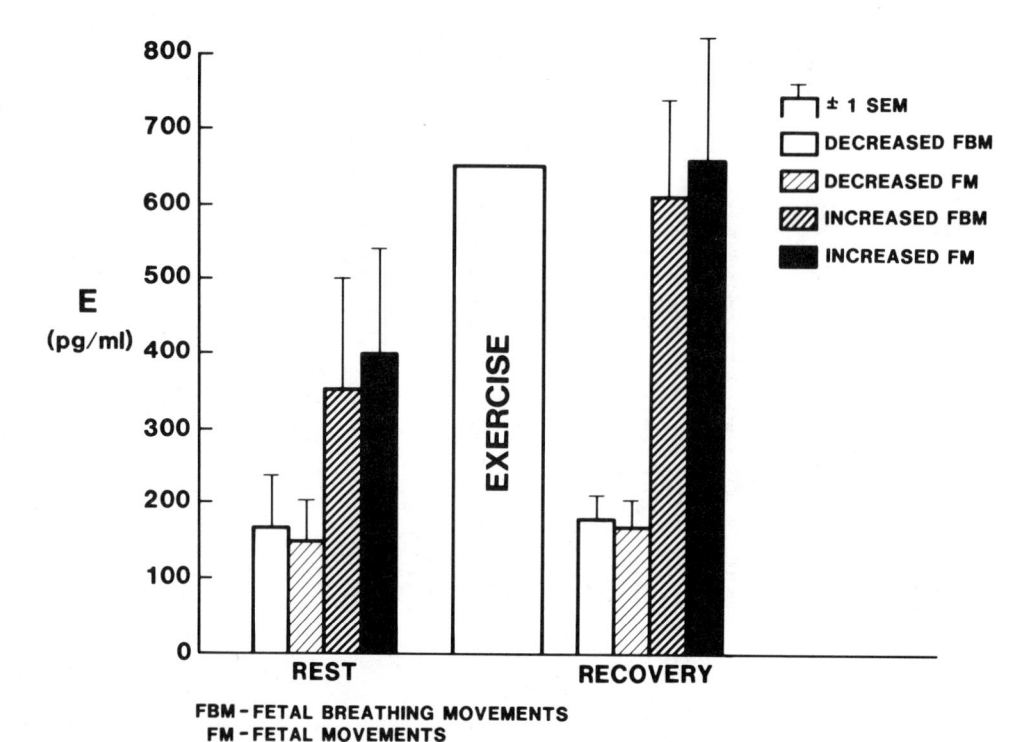

Figure 14.7. Fetal breathing movements and fetal movements in relation to maternal plasma epinephrine (*E*) prior to and after exercise.

Of much relevance and concern is the fact that with exercise the body core temperature may increase to levels that could have teratogenic effects. Such effects have to be evaluated with extreme caution since it appears that maternal body temperature is modulating the fetal temperature (31) and most of the fetal heat is transferred across the placenta to the mother (32) and, as such, could reach significant elevations in the fetus. The data derived from studies conducted in research animals strongly indicate that exposure in early gestation to temperatures in excess of 39°C is teratogenic and frequently results in neurotubal defects (33–35). The published information in the human is less convincing since it has been collected among individuals at risk for malformations (36–38) and an only prospective study conducted among 165 women exposed to first trimester fever has failed to confirm such findings (39). Nevertheless, until a well confirmatory study is done, we must exercise caution and limit exposure to hyperthermia in the first trimester of pregnancy. One other aspect of hyperthermia is dehydration and it should be considered for latter stages in pregnancy when it could precipitate premature labor.

Though most of the time it is very difficult to distinguish between the various parameters leading to reduced birthweight and intrauterine growth retardation (IUGR), strenuous exercise in pregnancy could have such an adverse effect on the fetus. It has been recognized for a long time that infants of working mothers do have decreased birth weight by as much as 400 g (41–43). It also appears that pregnant laboratory animals that are forced to exercise strenuously also deliver smaller offspring (44, 45).

Anecdotal reports of similar effects have been reported in the human, and recently a larger study has determined that women who continued strenuous exercise through pregnancy gained less weight, delivered earlier (by 8 days), and their infants had a consistently reduced birthweight (by approximately 500 g) (40). These reports must be interpreted with caution, but nevertheless, alert us to the possible complications.

Consequently, pregnant women who do engage in strenuous exercise should be carefully monitored for developing complications and exercise under medical supervision alone.

Monitoring the interactions between mother and fetus during and after exercise could serve not only as a research tool but also be incorporated as a clinical aid for fetal surveillance.

REFERENCES

1. Lotering KR, Gilbert RD, Longo LD: Exercise responses in pregnant sheep: oxygen consumption uterine blood flow and blood volume. *J Appl Physiol* 55:834, 1983.
2. Chandler JCD, Bell AW: Effects of maternal exercise on fetal and maternal respiration and nutrient metabolism in the pregnant ewe. *J Dev Physiol* 31:161, 1981.
3. Clapp JF: Acute exercise stress in the pregnant ewe. *Am J Obstet Gynecol* 136:489, 1980.
4. Curret LB, Ott JA, Rankin JHG, Ungerer T: Effect of exercise on cardiac output and distribution of uterine blood flow in pregnant ewes. *J Appl Physiol* 40:725, 1976.
5. Morris N, Osborn SB, Wright HP, Hart A: Effective uterine blood flow during exercise and normal and pre-eclamptic pregnancies. *Lancet* 2:481, 1956.
6. Wilkening RB, Meschia G: Fetal oxygen uptake, oxygenation and acid-base balance as a function of uterine blood flow. *Am J Physiol* 244:H749, 1983.
7. Hon EH, Wohlgemuth R: The electronic evaluation of fetal heart rate. *Am J Obstet Gynecol* 81:361, 1961.
8. Soiva K, Salmi A, Gronroos M, Peltonen T: Physical working capacity during pregnancy and effect of physical tests on foetal heart rate. *Ann Chir Gynaecol* 53:187, 1963.
9. Hodr J, Brotanek Y: Changes of actography and foetal heart rates in premature deliveries. In Horsky J, Stembera ZK (eds): *Intra-Uterine Dangers to the Foetus*. Amsterdam, Excerpta Medica Foundation, 1967, p 343.
10. Stembera ZK, Hodr J: The exercise test as an early diagnostic aid for foetal distress. In Horsky J, Stembera ZK (eds): *Intra-Uterine Dangers to the Foetus*. Amsterdam, Excerpta Medica Foundation, 1967, p 349.
11. Porkorny J, Rous J: The effect of mother's work on foetal heart sounds. In Horsky J, Stembera ZK (eds): *Intra-Uterine Dangers to the Foetus*. Amsterdam, Excerpta Medica Foundation, 1967, p 359.

12. Pomerance JJ, Gluck L, Lynch VA: Maternal exercise as a screening test for uteroplacental insufficiency. *Obstet Gynecol* 44:383, 1974.
13. Eisenberg de Smoler P, Karchmer SK, Ayala LC, Dominguez JA: El electrocardiograma fetal durante el ejercicio materno. *Ginecol Obstet Mex* 35:521, 1974
14. Pernoll ML, Metcalfe J, Paul M: Fetal cardiac response to maternal exercise. In Longo LD, Reneau DD (eds): *Fetal and Newborn Cardiovascular Physiology*,. New York, Garland Press, 1978, vol 2, p 389.
15. Sibley L, Ruhling RO, Cameron-Foster J, Christensen C, Bolen T: Swimnming and physical fitness during pregnancy. *J Nurse-Midwifery* 26:3, 1981.
16. Dale E, Mullinax KM, Bryan DH: Exercise during pregnancy: Exercise during pregnancy: effects on the fetus. *Can J Appl Sport Sci* 7:98, 1982.
17. Hauth JC, Gilstrap LC, Widmer K: Fetal heart rate reactivity before and after maternal jogging during the third trimester. *Am J Obstet Gynecol* 142:545, 1982.
18. Collings CA, Curet LB, Mullin JP: Maternal and fetal responses to a maternal aerobic exercise program. *Am J Obstet Gynecol* 145:702, 1983.
19. Artal R, Romem Y, Wiswell R: Fetal heart responses to mild, moderate and $\dot{V}_{O_2max}$ maternal exercise (submitted for publication).
20. Artal R, Romem Y, Paul RH, Wiswell R: Fetal bradycardia induced by maternal exercise. *Lancet* 2:258, 1984.
21. Manning FA, Morrison I, Lange IR: Antepartum determination of fetal health: composite biophysical profile scoring. *Clin Perinatol* 9:285, 1982.
22. Boddy K, Dawes GS: Fetal breathing. *Br Med Bull* 31:3, 1975.
23. Timor-Tritsh J, Zador I, Hertz RH, Rosen MG: Human fetal respiratory arrhythmia. *Am J Obstet Gynecol* 127:662, 1977.
24. Marsal K, Lofgren O, Gewnser G: Fetal breathing movements and maternal exercise. *Acta Obstet Gynecol Scand* 58:197, 1979.
25. Manning FA, Platt LD, Sipos L: Fetal movements in humans in the third trimester. *Obstet Gynecol* 54:699, 1977.
26. Sadovsky E, Yaffe H: Daily fetal movement recording and fetal diagnosis. *Obstet Gynecol* 41:845, 1973.
27. Artal R, Platt LD, Sperling M, Kammula R, Jilek J, Nakamura RM: Maternal exercise: cardiovascular and metabolic responses in normal pregnancy. *Am J Obstet Gynecol* 140:123, 1981.
28. Platt LD, Artal R, Semel J, Sipos L, Kammula RK: Exercise in pregnancy; II. Fetal responses. *Am J Obstet Gynecol* 147:487, 1983.
29. Lewis PJ, Trudinger BJ, Mangez J: Effect of maternal glucose on fetal breathing and body movements in late pregnancy. *Br J Obstet Gynaecol* 85:586, 1979.
30. Bousfield P: The fetal response to maternal exercise. In: Proceedings of the Seventh International Workshop on Fetal Breathing and Other Measurements, Oxford, England, June 1980.
31. Schroder H, Gilbert RD, Power GG: Fetal heat dissipation: a computer model and some preliminary experimental results from fetal sheep. Proceedings of the Society for Gynecology Investigation, Dallas, Texas, 1982, p 113.
32. Abrams R, Caton D, Clapp J, Barron DH: Thermal and metabolic features of life in utero. *Clin Obstet Gynecol* 13:549, 1970.
33. Edwards MJ: Congenital defects in guinea pigs: fetal resorptions, abortions and malformations following induced hyperthermia during early gestation. *Teratology* 2:313, 1969.
34. Skreb N, Frank Z: Developmental abnormalities in the rat induced by heat shock. *J Embryol Exp Morphol* 11:445, 1983.
35. Kilham L, Ferm VH: Exencephaly in fetal hamsters exposed to hyperthermia. *Teratology* 14:323, 1976.
36. Miller P, Smith DW, Shepard TH: Maternal hyperthermia as a possible cause of anencephaly. *Lancet* 1:519, 1978.
37. Smith DW, Clarren SK, Harvey MAS: Hyperthermia as a possible teratogenic agent. *J Pediatr* 92:878, 1978.
38. Fraser FC, Skelton J: Possible teratogenicity of maternal fever. *Lancet* 2:634, 1978.
39. Clarren SK, Smith DW, Harvey MAS, Ward RH, Myrianthopoulos NC: Hyperthermia—a prospective evaluation of a possible teratogenic agent in man. *J Pediatr* 95:81, 1979.
40. Clapp JF, Dickstein S: Endurance exercise and pregnancy outcome. *Med Sci Sports Exerc* 16:556, 1984.
41. Fox ME, Harris RE, Brekken AL: The active-duty military pregnancy: a new high-risk category. *Am J Obstet Gynecol* 129:705, 1984.
42. Taferi N, Naey RL, Gobzie A: Effects of maternal under-nutrition and heavy physical physical work during pregnancy on birth weight. *Br J Obstet Gynaecol* 87:222, 1980.
43. Naeye RL, Peters E. Working during pregnancy, effects on the fetus. *Pediatrics* 69:721, 1982.
44. Terada M: Effect of physical activity before pregnancy on fetuses of mice exercised forcibly during pregnancy. *Teratology* 10:141, 1974.
45. Nelson PS, Gilbert RD, Longo L: Fetal growth and placental diffusing capacity in guinea pigs following long-term maternal exercise. *J Dev Physiol* 5:1, 1983.

15
Sports Activities and Aerobic Exercise during Pregnancy

During the Victorian era pregnant women were cloistered throughout their pregnancy and not allowed to work or take part in any physical exercise. Currently, obstetricians and their patients have a different attitude and they include physical activity as a regular and acceptable part of the prenatal period. During this transition of thought many theories evolved on what type of exercise is good for the mother and/or the baby and whether the exercises did in fact ease the actual pregnancy or facilitate labor, birth, and the postpartum return of fitness. Unfortunately, early prescriptions often had no basis in fact.

Around the turn of the century obstetricians noted that the lower, working class mothers in England had easier labors and it was decided that this was due to their physical activity. Thus in several of the early antenatal books, "gentle exercises" such as croquet were recommended (1, 2). These thoughts continued to affect prenatal preparation until the 1950s when controlled research found no significant differences in the length of labor or the incidence of complications between women who exercised and women who did not (3, 4).

Earlier exercise prescription emphasized mobility or flexibility exercise and avoided those exercises that stimulated the cardiovascular system. This was based on the accepted assumption that the maintenance of good posture during pregnancy was important. An exercise that was often recommended as beneficial was the squat. Since it was known that primitive people squatted during labor, squatting was suggested to be the natural way to an easy labor. While these prescriptions were being put forth, concurrent research demonstrated that the squat exercise did not in fact change the dimensions of the pelvis (5), nor was there distension or separation of the public symphysis during the actual labor (6). Even though the literature does not support the contention that squatting exercise has a significant anatomical effect, there were still two proposed benefits of proper squatting with the back straight. One is good balance, which keeps strain off the lower back when lifting. The other is the prevention of heartburn later in pregnancy when bending over too far can cause regurgitation (7).

Pelvic floor exercises (the Kegel or elevator exercises) were originally prescribed to increase the elasticity and tonicity of the perineum and to prevent tears during labor. However, there has been no hard evidence to support this and, in fact, once an episiotomy is performed these muscle activities are completely abolished. The trend today is to perform an episiotomy and suture rather than to overstretch the perineum and cause lacerations. The suggested benefit of pelvic floor exercises is for the postpartum period when they may help the muscle return to its prestretched condition (7, 8).

Since the fitness increased awareness of the 1960s there has been a shift in emphasis from calisthenics to sports or aerobic exercises (jogging, swimming, bicycling, or aerobics). These activities are generally done in conjunction with prenatal exercises or prepatory childbirth exercises of relaxation, breathing, and toning. Many proposed but not proven benefits of aerobics and sports have been suggested. These include shorter labors, fewer complications during pregnancy, faster recovery from labor and delivery, prevention of varicose veins, thrombosis and leg cramps, and improved mental outlook of the patients (7–11).

REDUCED AEROBIC EXERCISE CAPACITY DURING PREGNANCY

Pregnancy has a known influence on cardiorespiratory dynamics such as increased cardiac output, increased resting heart rate, increased vital and inspiratory capacity, decreased expiratory reserve volume, and decreased functional reserve capacity (12–14). There is still a great deal of controversy about energy costs and the basal metabolic costs of pregnancy. It has been suggested that there is an increased caloric need of up to 80,000 kcal due to building tissue, increased basal metabolic rate (BMR), and the work of carrying a heavier body (15, 16). This assumes that the pregnant woman continues at the same activity pattern as prior to the pregnancy. Blackburn and Calloway (15, 16) found that in actuality the BMR increased more than the body weight and that this was the largest part of the increased energy demand. The activity level is reduced to compensate for the increased weight and, therefore, the energy demand is probably closer to 27,000 kcal or about 100 kcal per day (15, 16).

There have been several longitudinal studies of the physical work capacity (PWC) and oxygen consumption ($\dot{V}O_2$) of pregnant women during exercise. Pregnant women show an increase in steady state oxygen consumption, due primarily to an increased BMR. During weight-bearing exercise, pregnant women will have higher $\dot{V}O_2$ because the additional weight alters the amount of work performed (12), but in non-weight-bearing exercise, such as bicycling or swimming, the higher $\dot{V}O_2$ is due almost exclusively to the increased BMR and only slightly to hyperventilation (12, 17, 18).

Knuttgen and Emerson (12) found with bicycling and treadmill walking that hyperventilation was caused by an increased tidal volume and that the ventilatory equivalent ($\dot{V}_E/\dot{V}O_2$) was elevated as well, indicating either increased ventilatory efficiency or a decreased metabolic oxygen utilization efficiency. This change in $\dot{V}_E/\dot{V}O_2$ began early in pregnancy and continued until delivery, varying slightly with the changes in $\dot{V}O_2$ (12). Even with the hyperventilation there was no evidence of ventilatory impairment or dyspnea, suggesting that low levels of exercise, i.e., treadmill walking or bicycling at 60 watts (W) (367 kg-min^{-1}) at 60 rpm, can be tolerated and do not elicit severe stress. These early investigations were not controlled but simply longitudinal descriptive studies.

As more women continued to exercise through pregnancy, investigators changed to experimental studies comparing exercise and control groups rather than comparing just pregnant and nonpregnant groups. An early study by Ihrman (19) tested subjects trained in the laboratory versus subjects trained on their own and found no difference in PWC. Because of the inconvenience of having to train in the laboratory and because of the lack of significant differences in Ihrman's study, subjects have been allowed to train at their own convenience following the suggestions of the investigator (13) or use recall of activities of their own choosing when they come in to be tested (20, 21, 23). Our own findings do not support Ihrman's results and we suggest that caution be used when allowing patients to exercise on their own as part of any research project.

Results of another study, using bicycle ergometers in an aerobics class, indicated that pregnant subjects have a spontaneous increase in PWC of approximately 10%. This increase for women in their 38th week of pregnancy brings them to a level only slightly lower than the norm for nonpregnant women. The exercising women had an increase in work capacity of 17.6% more than women in the control group. This may indicate a training effect of exercise for the pregnant woman in addition to the increased PWC due to weight gain and the concomitant work of moving a heavier body (13). For the women in the aerobics class, there was an 18% improvement in $\dot{V}O_{2max}$ (L·min^{-1}) compared to a 4% decline for their controls. These results were based on submaximal exercise tests. The above study also reported an increase of 8% in $\dot{V}O_{2max}$ (ml·kg^{-1}·min^{-1}) for the exercisers and a decrease of 10% for the controls, suggesting that another benefit of exercise may be controlled weight gain during the pregnancy (22).

In the recall studies where there was limited control over the activity pattern of the subjects, the investigators were more interested in the pregnancy outcome or fetal response to the exercise rather than in the maternal benefits. One study where $\dot{V}O_2$ was measured used a step test to monitor heart rate (HR) and blood pressure (BP) response. These readings were used to determine $\dot{V}O_2$ (ml·kg^{-1}·min^{-1}) with a regression equation. The subjects were declared fit or unfit on the basis of the submaximal test given when they were seen initially. As a group, the fit women maintained a higher $\dot{V}O_2$ throughout the pregnancy (20). None of the studies showed a greater incidence of maternal or fetal complications before, during, or after delivery. HRs and diastolic BPs were generally lower in the active subjects, but this finding was not always significant (13, 20, 22). In the studies where fetal HR was observed, one study during exercise (22) and one with a nonstress test (NST) immediately after exercise (21), all subjects showed an increase in fetal HR, with reactive pattern. Each subject was tested only once some time during the third trimester. Thus the results cannot conclusively show that a subject could not have an abnormal test at some other time during the pregnancy. In our own study 3 out of 19 subjects experienced a decrease in fetal HR during and immediately after exercise with rapid postexercise recovery. The significance of these findings is still being studied (24). (See Chapter 14 for additional information).

Two complications associated with continued employment on the mother and her fetus have been investigated. One was preterm delivery and the second lower birth weight (25, 26). For 488 case studies (175 preterm and 313 term infants) there was no correlation between work or physical activity and preterm births (25). In the above study physical activity had a significant effect on the decreased risk of preterm delivery. When evaluating the effect of exercise on fetal weight there has been conflicting information. The only strong evidence showed several possible causes of lower fetal weight, low weight gain, low weight at the time of conception, and jobs requiring standing during the third trimester. The suggested cause for low birth weight with stand-up jobs is decreased uteroplacental blood flow, known to cause growth retardation in the fetus (26).

AEROBIC PROGRAMS

Since the current research is corroborating the descriptive and anecdotal studies on high level athletes having no increased incidence of complications in pregnancy and delivery while continuing to train (27–29), it will be the purpose in the remainder of this chapter to describe the types of activities that can be performed by pregnant women who want to remain active throughout their participation are not without risk even in a nonpregnant population. Table 15.1 presents the number of sports emergencies in sents the number of sports emergencies in the general population that are related to just strains and sprains. The number of untreated or self-treated injuries is most likely considerably greater than the treated injuries. Whether or not the risk of strains and sprains in pregnant women is significantly greater than in the general population is not known. Nevertheless, it should be obvious that there is an orthopaedic risk associated

Table 15.1 Estimated Numbers of Hospital Emergency Department-treated Strains and Sprains[a]

Sports Activity	No. of Strains and Sprains, 1980
Track and field	17,373
Squash and racquetball	14,514
Tennis	15,187
Bicycling	47,633
Cross-country skiing	1,023
Football	159,388
Basketball	225,566

[a] From the Consumer Product Safety Commission, National Electronic Surveillance System, December 1981.

with these activities and continuance during pregnancy may provide limited benefit.

Exercise programs should be modified during the pregnancy to allow for the physical and mental changes taking place and finally resumed following delivery to facilitate recovery to prepregnancy conditions (30). We recommend that pregnant women engaged in fitness programs be tested periodically to assess the effect of their exercise program on the developing fetus and readjusted to their level of tolerance.

Each activity should be begun with a 10–15-min warm-up period and ended with a 10–15-min cool-down period. During exercise maternal HR should not exceed 140 beats per minute (bpm). We believe that, due to changes in cardiac functions (increased cardiac output and HR, HRs in excess of 140 bpm could precipitate emergencies in unfit individuals. The cardiorespiratory changes as well as changes in the ligaments and joints require special care to be taken to exercise safely. (See Chapters 9 and 16 in this text).

CARDIORESPIRATORY ENDURANCE ACTIVITIES

Jogging

Many women have found jogging to be an adequate form of exercise and want to continue for as long as possible into the pregnancy. This activity is not one which should be initiated after the pregnancy has begun. For those that continue their jogging programs, during the first trimester special precautions should be taken if certain common complications occur, e.g., nausea, vomiting, or poor weight gain. Ketosis and hypoglycemia may occur during strenuous exercise. Because of morning sickness and/or the feeling of fatigue that is prevalent at this time, women may be unable to run any long distances. In the first 12 weeks of pregnancy we advise to reduce mileage to no more than 2 miles per day if the ambient temperature is high. There is a known teratogenic effect of increased body core temperature during this time. The mother dissipates the fetal heat which usually runs approximately one degree higher than her own; but if, due to higher temperature or humidity during jogging, the mother experiences dizziness, syncope, heat stress or heat exhaustion, this could be detrimental to the fetus during a critical stage of development (30).

In published longitudinal studies through pregnancy women averaged from 1.5 to 2.5 miles per day with no apparent deleterious effects. The number of birth abnormalities or problem pregnancies was no higher in the running population than in the general population (21, 23). During the second and third trimesters increased body weight may interfere and running may become difficult. During this period other factors may affect performance, such as lower limb edema, varicose veins, or joint laxity secondary to hormonal changes and connective tissue changes. Thus there could be added strain or even damage during pregnancy where there would be only limited damage in the fit, nonpregnant runner. In fact, it is thought that coordination of the gross motor movements may be impaired as a result of the joint laxity, suggesting that pregnant women need to be especially alert to their running path (8).

Animal studies have shown uteroplacental circulatory deficiences as well as a rise in maternal temperature when the animal is exercised to exhaustion (31, 32). Though as a result of this acute exercise, there does not seem to be any fetal compromise. In the studies where jogging distances were reported by the subjects rather than assigned by the investigator, there was a voluntary reduction from 2.5 miles per day on an average during the first trimester to approximately 1.75 miles per day in the second and 1 mile per day in the third trimester (23). In the study of Hauth and Gilstrap (21) the subjects continued at 1.5 miles per day throughout. These distances were all well tolerated by the mothers and by the fetuses; so, the recommendation for the distances will reflect these results. The mothers should be running to maintain fitness rather than engage in competitive activities so the shorter distances will suffice. During the first trimester, if subjects would like to exceed 2 miles per day, such activity should be coordinated with the obstetrician.

Jogging

1. Do not begin a jogging program while pregnant.
2. Reduce mileage to less than 2 miles per day.
3. If temperature and/or humidity is high, do not exercise.
4. Special attention should be given to terrain and running surface due to connective tissue changes associated with pregnancy.

"Aerobics" Programs

In the last 5–10 years, women who wanted to get the benefit of the aerobic workout associated with jogging but did not like running by themselves looked for another way to exercise. This spawned the aerobics enthusiasm. Aerobics combined dance with an aerobic workout allowing women to work out in groups using a form of exercise they enjoyed and thus kept them exercising long enough to improve their aerobic capacity. As in jogging the number of women who wanted to continue an aerobic activity during their pregnancy has led to a proliferation of aerobic classes specifically for pregnant women. There have not been any studies to base such programs on. Studies to be conducted will have to evaluate whether these programs can be called aerobic, i.e. do they fulfill the requirements of aerobic activity, raising HR to a training level and maintaining the HR at that level for 15–20 min, which is necesssary to stress the cardiovascular system sufficiently to effect training. Because aerobics is a weight-bearing exercise, the same problems that are associated with jogging should be considered by the mother, i.e., heat stress, fetal stress, and joint and ligament problems, during the progress of her pregnancy; and, if necessary, the programs should be modified. Accordingly, until prospective well-controlled studies have been conducted, we are reluctant to endorse such programs for pregnant women. If one should engage in such programs, we recommend testing the mother during each trimester to determine how she and the fetus are responding to the exercise. We strongly believe that such programs should be created and supervised by an exercise physiologist, physical therapist, and obstetrician.

Aerobics

1. Programs should have a scientific basis.
2. Specific exercises that should be avoided include:
   a. Over extension
   b. Exercises performed on the back
3. Avoid hard surfaces when exercising.
4. Warm-up and cool down gradually.

Bicycling

There are several aerobic exercises that do not involve weight bearing—bicycling is one of them. In a study comparing bicycling with treadmill walking to evaluate whether weight bearing affects the oxygen cost of exercise, Knuttgen and Emerson (12) found the difference of 13% increased O_2 cost for treadmill walking correlated with the 15% weight gain of the subjects. Also of interest in the study was the measurement of cardiac output (Q). It is accepted that at rest during pregnancy Q is increased, and there is a significant decrease postpartum (14). During cycling exercise there is no significant difference between prepartum to postpartum. The above was not a training study, but it was evident that bicycling at 60 W for 10–15 min had no acute deleterious effect on the mother or fetus (12).

In another training study the work load was determined by the use of submaximum $\dot{V}O_2$ results to predict a maximum value and then using a training intensity of 65–70% $\dot{V}O_{2max}$. Training HRs averaged 152 bpm. The program initiated in the second trimester continued, into the third trimester and ended at approximately 34 weeks. A training effect was observed so that one could assume that a woman may begin a bicycle training program even after the pregnancy has begun. This suggestion will have to be confirmed by other studies.

Bicycling is not without risk; with a stationary bicycle heat dissipation may become a problem, and exercising out of doors in traffic and smog, may have unknown negative effects on both mother and fetus. Bicycling may potentially strain the lower back in the aerodynamic position while riding a 10-speed, as the weight of the stomach accents the lordosis; but this can be reduced by using a more upright position and/or exercising to strengthen the abdominal wall. Also, the extra weight and especially its distribution could make the woman less stable so this should be a concern of the rider to prevent falls.

Bicycling

1. Program can be started during pregnancy.
2. Stationary bicycle preferable to standard cycling due to weight and balance changes during pregnancy.
3. Bicycling may cause low backstress.
4. Bicycling should be avoided out of doors during high temperatures and high pollution.

Swimming

Swimming is another non-weight-bearing aerobic exercise. Many consider swimming to be the perfect aerobic exercise, especially well suited for the pregnant woman (33). We tend to agree because of the changing body composition, the mother becomes more bouyant, making swimming easier. Also, being in a swimming pool, as long as the temperature of the water is not too high (above 85–90° F), thermoregulation is not a problem (34). The problem arises when the mother is not a competent swimmer and thus is not able to work sufficiently hard to create a training effect. When this is the case a water calisthenic and walking-in-water program can replace the actual swimming program.

With a change in weight distribution during the second and third trimesters, breathing may be more difficult with strokes on the stomach. Since distance swimming is the only means of increasing aerobic capacity, the swim program, where the majority of the workout is repeat, short distances, can only be considered anaerobic.

Another benefit professed by swim programs for the pregnant woman is being able to do childbirth preparatory exercises in the water, where water resistance is encountered; and the individual is bouyed up at the same time for ease of exercising (33).

Through the pregnancy the mother may be able to maintain a given distance but take longer to complete it (35). This may suffice as long as the original time is long enough to permit a training effect. This will maintain the training effect through the pregnancy or possibly even allow for some improvement.

Swimming

1. Respiratory changes may make swimming difficult in late pregnancy.
2. Calisthenic exercise in water is encouraged for maintenance of strength and flexibility.
3. Swimming in water that is either too cold or too hot should be avoided.
4. Jacuzzi temperatures above 38.5° C may cause fetal damage.

MUSCULAR STRENGTH AND ENDURANCE ACTIVITIES

Weight Lifting

For many years, weight lifting was not recommended for women in general; for pregnant women it was unheard of. As more and more health clubs began opening, weight lifting became a complimentary exercise for whatever form of aerobic exercise was being undertaken. As a result, as women become pregnant they do not want to give up any part of their routine; and they need to know how to weight lift safely. As weight machines are used frequently rather than free weights, the fear of damage to the baby by dropping a weight is alleviated. This is not to say that free weights cannot be used, but rather that spotting is more adequate at this time. The fetus is well protected by the maternal anatomical structures, but there is evidence that a blow to the abdomen could damage the uterus or disturb the placental attachment (30). The only such available program in print is the Nautilus program outlined in *Making Mama Fit: The Ultimate Game Plan* (38); but though a scientific basis for the program is claimed, none is cited. Any program which works the entire body, promoting toning and flexibility, can be recommended only within certain limits. One possible problem that could arise for the inexperienced weight lifter is transient hypertension caused by the Valsalva maneuver, with significant diversion of blood from the splanchnic organs to the working muscle. Breathing properly, i.e., exhaling while straining during a lift, will keep this from happening. Low weights and high repetitions should make up the program to maintain flexibility while toning the muscles. Using very light weights as the pregnancy progresses is recommended to prevent injuries to ligaments (8). Exercises should not be performed while in a supine position. If possible, such activities should be limited or avoided in pregnancy and, when done, only under strict prescription and supervision.

Weight Training

1. Lifting light weight for maintenance of strength can be cautiously continued throughout pregnancy.
2. Heavy weights should be avoided.
3. The use of free weights should be avoided.
4. Proper breathing is necessary to avoid the Valsalva maneuver.

Sports Activities

All sporting events include some inherent danger to the participants. When a pregnant woman desires to engage in such activities she must be advised and consider these dangers and decide whether she can modify her activities accordingly, or whether the activity must be avoided altogether. Contact sports such as basketball, football, or hockey are probably better avoided not just for fear of potential trauma to the abdomen, but also because of the unpredictability of the opponent's movements and/or equipment unreliability. Volleyball, gymnastics, and English horesback riding follow close behind on the dangerous sports list (8, 30), while western horseback riding may be less strenuous and/or dangerous.

Racket sports such as tennis, racquetball, and squash are considered, within certain limits, fairly safe sports. The intensity should be reduced as the pregnancy progresses to prevent injuries due to impaired coordination secondary to the new weight distribution and change in center of gravity. Especially in racquetball and squash, heat stress should be considered since they are played in a confined area with little air circulation (30). In addition, overstretching could be traumatic to joints and ligaments.

Water sports other than distance swimming also should be engaged in with caution. Scuba diving, because of the pressure and compressed air environment, can be dangerous to both mother and fetus. The mother may develop decompression sickness and the fetus, intravascular air embolism (30). It is not clear at this time if the maternal diving reflex is reproduced by the fetus with lasting deleterious effects. In a survey of pregnant women divers the number of complications and birth defects was significantly higher than in the normal population, suggesting that scuba diving especially to depths greater than 33 feet should be totally avoided (39).

Two sporting activities which can be safely continued through the pregnancy with little inherent danger are golf and slow pitch softball, sports which women are taking up in increasing numbers and again do not want to stop during pregnancy. The golf swing may have to be modified, but the walk around the golf course could provide a nice diversion from the usual walk around the neighborhood for the woman who is using walking as her form of exercise. Slow pitch softball, if the game is not too competitive, can also be continued through the pregnancy. The pregnant woman should be advised that her balance is compromised by additional weight and not to take unnecessary risks (8, 30). Actions such as sliding into bases and blocking bases should be avoided.

Winter activities can also be enjoyed if care is taken to protect against the cold. The cardiopulmonary system is compromised by the pregnancy, and exercise in the cold can put an additional strain on it. Exposure to extreme cold must be avoided. If the pregnant woman is skiing (either downhill or cross-country) or skating, she is probably already expert in the sport; and therefore an activity which could be inherently dangerous to an unskilled person would not be considered dangerous. Therefore it is recommended that these sports not be taken up during pregnancy and for the competent athlete they should not be undertaken competitively during pregnancy, i.e., fatigue and strain should be avoided. Because of the possibility of injuries caused by poor balance during pregnancy, probably downhill skiing and skating would be given up sooner than cross-country skiing (30). For the mother who lives in a climate where snow and cold weather are common for much of the winter, cross-country skiing can be a very good activity for maintaining cardiovascular fitness. Such activities should be interrupted with frequent periods of rest and adequate hydration. Cross-country skiing stresses the cardiovascular system to a higher degree than either of the other activities because all the large muscle groups are being used, and therefore cross-country skiing at a moderate pace will promote a higher fitness level. The muscle and joint injuries associated with running may be avoided if properly fit (35). Precautions should be taken to prevent cold exposure.

NONAEROBIC ACTIVITIES

Yoga

Yoga has experienced a popularity with pregnant women for two reasons: one, the relaxation effect which many women seek during their pregnancy, and second the desire to maintain muscle tone and flexibility throughout the 9 months (36, 37). These are both good reasons; and as long as yoga is accompanied by some form of aerobic work, it can be an adequate form of workout. Yoga postures may have to be modified as the pregnancy progresses, i.e., using chairs, or pillows, or another person for better balance or posture. Yoga can be done alone or in a class, depending on the expertise of the mother; but as with every other form of exercise, consistency is the most important component of the program. Supine and prolonged standing exercises should be eliminated since they may induce hypotension.

Preparatory Childbirth Exercises

With the popularity of "natural childbirth," mothers and fathers are increasingly encouraged to attend classes to learn how to prepare for labor and delivery. Undoubtedly these classes fulfill an important educational role and have a major psychological impact on both parents and increase the fetal-maternal bonds. In general, classes include a section on the anatomy, physiology, and psychology of labor and birth. These classes include instruction in relaxation and breathing techniques to be utilized in labor and delivery. As was stated earlier, there is no scientific evidence that any of these exercises result in shorter labors, easier labors, less complications, or benefit the baby (7). The toning and stretching exercises that are used may have some benefit after the birth to speed recovery. Some of the stretching routine may have to be modified to prevent injuries.

The exercises are generally divided into areas of the body, first emphasising the upper body, next the legs, and finally the stomach area. They combine yoga, dance, and calisthenic routines. There are no standard exercises employed in these programs (40-42). Moderation should be advised and there is no reason not to modify such activities if they are too difficult to perform correctly, i.e., a sit-up is a good exercise for the abdomen, but as the abdomen begins protruding, perhaps a half sit-up or a sit-back, where the mother begins in the up position and slowly lies down, would be of more benefit. Supine exercises should not be performed under any circumstances. It is very important to remember that there is already major stress on the lower back in pregnancy because of the extra weight in the stomach area, so all exercises that require the mother to be on her back need to be done in a semirecumbent position with the legs bent and the knees up. If unable to mobilize both legs, exercise may include one leg at a time in something like a leg lift since the subject may not be able to keep the lower back on the floor otherwise.

Consistency is the most important part of the above exercises; if the individual is not willing to exercise regularly, she would probably be better off not exercising at all, and by doing so prevent injuries.

REFERENCES

1. Johnstone RW: *A Textbook of Midwifery.* London, Adams, Charles & Black, 1913, p 101.
2. Haultan WFT, Fahmy ECF: *Antenatal Care.* Edinburgh, Livingston, 1929, p 13.
3. Burnett C: Value of antenatal exercise. *J Obstet Gynaecol Br Emp* 63:40, 1956.
4. Roberts H, Wooton IDP, Kane KM, Burnett WE: The value of antenatal preparation. *J Obstet Gynaecol Br Emp* 60:404, 1953.
5. Young J: Relaxation of pelvic joints in pregnancy. *J Obstet Gynaecol Br Emp* 47:49, 1940.
6. Heyman J, Lundquist A: The symphysis pubis in pregnancy and parturition. *Acta Obstet Gynecol Scand* 12:191, 1932.
7. Blankfield A: Is exercise necessary for the obstetric patient? *Med J Aust* 1:163-165, 1967.
8. Danforth DN: Pregnancy and labor from the vantage point of the physical therapist. *Am J Phys Med* 46:653-658, 1967.
9. Jarrett II JC, Spellacy WN: Jogging during pregnancy: an improved outcome? *Obstet Gynecol* 61:705-709, 1983.
10. Pomerance JJ, Gluck L, Lynch VA: Physical fitness in pregnancy: its effect on pregnancy outcome. *Am J Obstet Gynecol* 119:867-876, 1974.
11. Speroff L: Can exercise cause problems in pregnancy and menstruation? *Contemp Ob/Gyn* 16:57-63, 1980.
12. Knuttgen HG, Emerson K: Physiological response to pregnancy at rest and during exercise. *J Appl Physiol* 36:549-553, 1974.
13. Erkkola R: The influence of physical training during pregnancy on pnysical work capacity and circulatory parameters. *Scand J Clin Lab Invest* 36:747-754, 1976.
14. Ueland K, Navy MJ, Metcalfe J: Cardiorespiratory responses to pregnancy and exercise in normal women and patients with heart disease. *Am J Obstet Gynecol* 115:4-10, 1973.
15. Blackburn MW, Calloway DH: Energy expenditure and consumption of mature, pregnant, and lactating women. *J Am Diet Assoc* 69:29-37, 1976.
16. Blackburn MW, Calloway DH: Basal metabolic rate and work energy expenditure of mature pregnant women. *J Am Diet Assoc* 69:24-28, 1976.
17. Pernoll ML, Metcalfe J, Schlenker TL, Welch JE, Matsumoto JA: Oxygen consumption at rest and during exercise in pregnancy. *Respir Physiol* 25:285-293, 1975.
18. Seitchik J: Body composition and energy expenditure during rest and work in pregnancy. *Am J Obstet Gynecol* 94:701-713, 1967.
19. Ihrman K: A clinical and physiological study of pregnancy. The effect of physical training during pregnancy on the circulatory adjustment. *Acta Soc Med Upsal* 65:3, 1960.
20. Dibblee L, Graham TE: A longitudinal study of changes in aerobic fitness, body composition, and energy intake in primigravid patients. *Am J Obstet Gynecol* 147:908-914, 1983.
21. Hauth JO, Gilstrap LC, Widmer K: Fetal heart rate reactivity before and after maternal jogging during the third trimester. *Am J Obstet Gynecol* 142:545-547, 1982.
22. Collings CA, Curet LB, Mullin JP: Maternal and fetal responses to a maternal aerobic exercise program. *Am J Obstet Gynecol* 145:702-707, 1983.
23. Jarrett JC, Spellacy WN: Jogging during pregnancy: an improved outcome? *Obstet Gynecol* 61:705-709, 1983.
24. Artal R, Romem Y, Paul RH, Wiswell RA: Fetal bradycardia induced by maternal exercise. *Lancet* 2:258-260, 1984.
25. Berkowitz BS, Kelsey JL, Holford TR, Berkowitz

RL: Physical activity and the risk of spontaneous preterm delivery. *J Reprod Med* 28:581–588, 1983.
26. Naeye RL, Peters EC: Working during pregnancy: effects on the fetus. *Pediatrics* 69:724–727, 1982.
27. Erdelyi GJ: Gynecological survey of female athletes. *J Sports Med Phys Fitness* 2:174–179, 1975.
28. Higdon H: Running through pregnancy. *The Runner* p 46, 1981.
29. Korcok M: Pregnant jogger: what a record! *JAMA* 246:201, 1981.
30. Bullard JA: Exercise and pregnancy. *Can Fam Physician* 27:977–982, 1981.
31. Clapp JF: Acute exercise in the pregnant ewe. *Am J Obstet Gynecol* 136:489, 1980.
32. Emmanouilides GC, Hobel CJ, Yashiro K, Klyman G: Fetal responses to maternal exercise in the sheep. *Am J Obstet Gynecol* 112:130, 1972.
33. Katz J: *Swimming through Your Pregnancy, the Perfect Exercise for Pregnant Women.* New York, Dolphin Books, Doubleday, 1983, pp 1–159.
34. St. John W. Body composition of female college Age swimmers. Master's thesis, University of Cincinnati, 1978, p 15.
35. Astrand PO, Rodahl K: *Textbook of Work Physiology,* ed 2. New York, McGraw-Hill, 1977.
36. Thompson J: *Healthy Pregnancy the Yoga Way.* New York, Dolphin Books, Doubleday, 1977.
37. Leboyer F: *Inner Beauty Inner Light Yoga for Pregnant Women.* New York, Bolzoi Book, Alfred A. Knopf, 1978.
38. Hall DC, Geinl GK: *Making Mama Fit: The Ultimate Game.* New York, Leisure Press, 1982, pp 177–192.
39. Kizer KW: Women and diving. *Phys Sports Med* 9:84–92, 1981.
40. Simkin D: *The Complete Pregnancy Exercise Program.* New York, New American Library, Mosby Times Mirror, 1980.
41. Harris NF: *Controlled Childbirth.* Palm Springs, Calif., Harris Industries, 1976.
42. Bing E: *Six Practical Lessons for an Easier Childbirth.* New York, Grosset & Dunlap, 1978.

16
Orthopaedic Problems in Pregnancy

Edema during pregnancy is commonly regarded as an abnormal sign and a possible precursor of hypertension proteinuria. Some studies have questioned this theory (11). Robertson systemically evaluated the incidence of edema in 83 women observed during pregnancy: 77 of them were primigravidae. Each was seen at 4-week intervals from the 12th to the 24th week of pregnancy, then fortnightly until the 34th week and then weekly until delivery. Each patient was weighed with minimal clothing on an accurate scale, blood pressure measured and urine tested for protein and glucose. Of the 83 subjects, 11 developed some hypertension during late pregnancy and 2 of these also had proteinuria. Most of the remainder had perfectly normal pregnancies. Lower limb volume was measured by modification of the techniques used by White (12) and Hytten and Taggart (4). In essence, the amount of water displaced from a tub was measured.

Ankle girth was measured with a flexible steel tape at a level 10 cm above the internal malleolus. Finger size was judged by changes in the size of the 3rd ring finger with a jeweler's ring.

The incidence of swelling noted by the patient rose from 6% at 12 weeks to 68% at 38 weeks but 83% of the women reported swelling at some stage. The majority had continued swelling only during the last 8 weeks of pregnancy.

Edema was observed by the clinician less often than swelling was noted by the patient; 56 (67%) were found to have detectable edema at some stage in pregnancy. The incidence rose from 2% at 12 weeks to 59% at 38 weeks.

This "physiologic" edema is thought to be responsible for various orthopaedic nerve compression syndromes as outlined below.

NERVE COMPRESSION SYNDROMES

Carpal Tunnel Syndrome

The median nerve travels through the carpal tunnel, a space at the wrist. This is a space bounded by bony tunnel below and fibrous ligament on the top (Fig. 16.1). Its space is somewhat limited and with any significant swelling the nerve can be compressed. The nerve functions to innervate the thenar muscles of the thumb which allows the thumb to become opposed to the fingers (Fig. 16.2). In addition, there are sensory branches that provide enervation to the thumb and index and middle finger.

The patient complains of numbness and tingling of the thumb and index and middle finger and may be aware of weakness of the thumb. Patients often note that this is bothersome at night and they are awakened from sleep. These symptoms can be relieved only by shaking their hands.

Examination reveals a tenderness at the median nerve over the wrist with a positive Tinel's sign on palpation of the median nerve with pain radiating to the thumb and index and middle finger. Careful evaluation of the thenar muscle strength and any sign

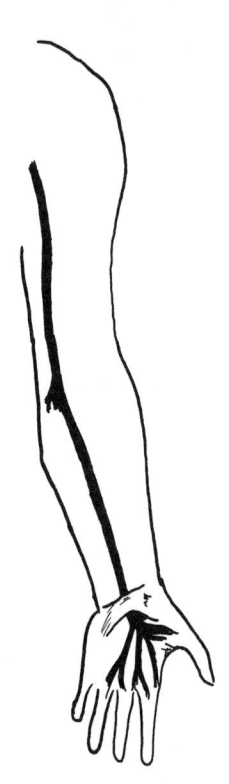

Figure 16.1. Median nerve through carpal tunnel at wrist.

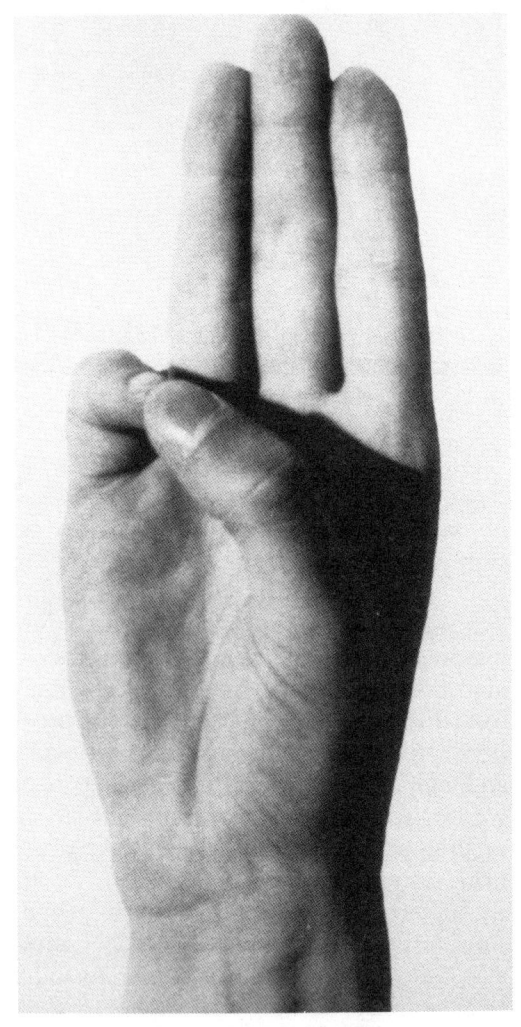

Figure 16.2. Opposing thumb.

of atrophy must be made. Phalen's test is performed by hyperflexing the wrist, holding for a period of 30–45 sec, and noting any reproducibility of the symptoms of numbness of the thumb and index and middle finger.

Treatment involves placing the patient in a neutral wrist extension splint (Fig. 16.3) for sleeping at night and avoiding hyperflexion posture, and ice packs 2–3 times a day to decrease inflammation. Obviously during pregnancy, anti-inflammatory medication is not indicated. In some cases, should the above measures fail to relieve symptoms, one or two injections of Xylocaine steroid preparation in the perineural space can dramatically relieve symptomatology.

Gould and Wissinger (2) studied the overall incidence of median nerve compromise in 100 consecutive obstetric admissions in 1978. Twenty-one patients reported paresthesias or hypesthesias in the median nerve distribution during pregnancy. Of the 21, 18 became asymptomatic before or shortly after delivery and remained asymptomatic 3 months after delivery. Should symptoms persist for more than 2 months after pregnancy, EMG with nerve conduction studies and orthopaedic evaluation is indicated.

Ulnar Nerve

The ulnar nerve travels to the hand through Guyon's canal at the wrist and may also be compressed, similar to the compression of the median nerve. The patient complains of numbness and tingling of the 4th and 5th fingers and may have inner osseous weakness (Fig. 16.4).

Treatment is as outlined for median nerve

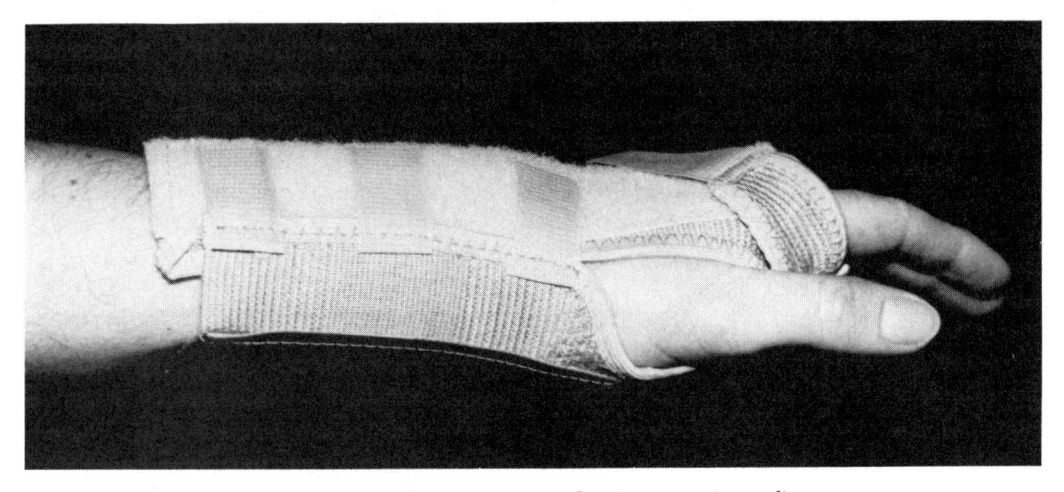

Figure 16.3. Patient in neutral wrist extension splint.

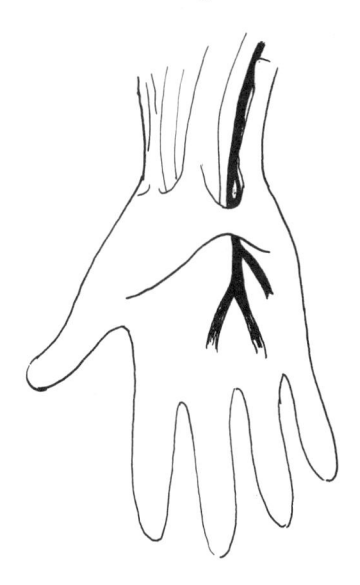

Figure 16.4. Ulnar nerve passing through Guyon's canal at wrist.

compression, although its overall incidence in pregnancy is much less.

The ulnar nerve may also be compressed at the medial aspect of the elbow posterior to the medial epicondyle (Fig. 16.5). This is often due to incorrect sleeping posture with sleeping with the hands behind the head. Symptoms consist of numbness and tingling in the 4th and 5th fingers with weakness inner ossei. In this case treatment at times involves posterior splint immobilization of the elbow, ice packs, and/or possible injection.

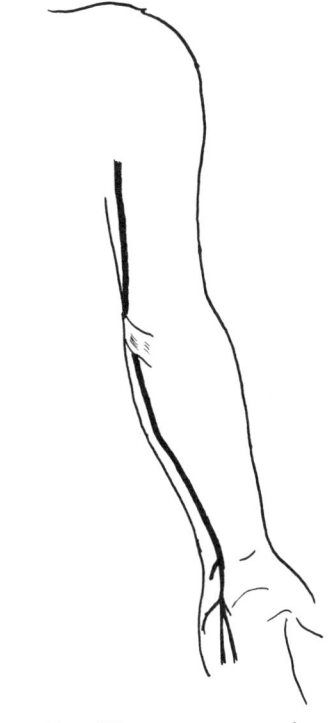

Figure 16.5. Ulnar nerve can become compressed where it passes behind medial epicondyle.

Posterior Tibial Nerve

The posterior tibial nerve travels to the foot posterior to the medial malleolus (Fig. 16.6). There is a tarsal tunnel consisting of a thick fibrous layer of tissue holding the flexor tendons to the foot and the posterior tibial nerve, artery and vein, posterior to the

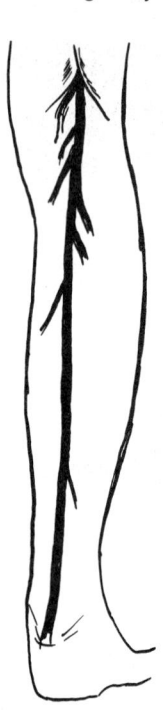

Figure 16.6. Posterior tibial nerve.

medial malleolus. In some cases with edema and/or trauma, the tibial nerve can be compressed and produce numbness and tingling of the medial aspect of the foot with some weakness of the flexors of the toes.

Examination reveals a positive Tinel's sign over the posterior tibial nerve immediately posterior to the medial malleolus and decreased sensation medial arch and foot with questionable weakness of the toe flexors.

Treatment is designed to minimize ankle motion, with ice packs to the area with possible injections in the paraneural space taking care to avoid either the artery or vein at this level (anatomically, coming from anterior to posterior). The posterior tibial artery may be palpated, then the vein, and then the nerve.

KNEE PAIN

Chondromalacia Patella

Many women are afflicted with patellofemoral or chondromalacia of the patella secondary to increased ligamentous laxity, increased femoral torsion and wider pelvis,

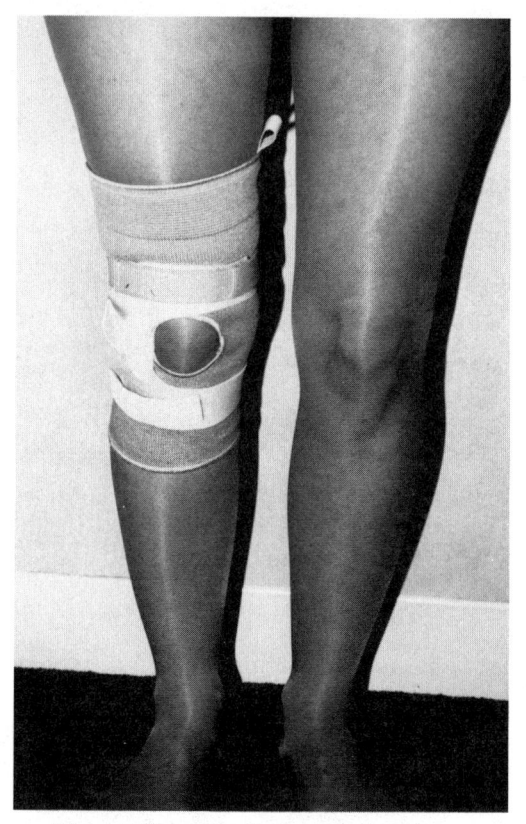

Figure 16.7. Patellar restraining brace.

all of which combine to produce increased lateral vectors about the kneecap during flexion-extension maneuvers. This symptom complex manifests itself as an ache about the anterior knee, increasing on flexion-extension, or prolonged sitting. Patients often complain of discomfort when sitting in a theater with their knees flexed. During pregnancy, these symptoms often increase secondary to swelling and congestion with possible decreased activity.

Treatment involves strengthening the quadriceps mechanism so as to allow the kneecap to track correctly. This involves performing straight leg lifts and quadsetting exercises. In addition, ice packs about the anterior knee 2–3 times per day can be very rewarding. A patellar restraining brace (Fig. 16.7), may also prove helpful.

If these measures fail, one or two intraarticular Xylocaine steroid preparation injections immediately beneath the patella can dramatically relieve symptomatology. In most instances, if this is an entirely new symptom complex associated with pregnancy, it goes into remission after pregnancy. Patients are asymptomatic until the children start crawling at which time the women start squatting and kneeling to pick the children up, thus exacerbating their preexisting condition.

HIP PAIN

Avascular Necrosis

Hip pain in a pregnant patient may be related to low back strain with sciatic radiation. However, if this is persistent and is not in conjunction with localized back pain, the possibility of avascular necrosis of the femoral head must be considered. This situation arises secondary to a number of causes (e.g., alcoholism, Cushing syndrome, chronic steroid use, decompression, trauma, etc.). Cheng et al. (1) reported 7 cases in a series of patients with avascular necrosis of the femoral head related to pregnancy. They postulated higher adrenal cortical activity during pregnancy with probable increased mechanical stress due to weight gain. X-ray findings show early lucency with segmental collapse of the femoral head (Fig. 16.8). Obviously, if the patient continues to complain of hip pain postpartum, orthopaedic evaluation is mandatory with appropriate x-rays and evaluation.

BACK PAIN

It is estimated that 50–75% of the general population will experience significant back pain in their life to require medical attention.

In England, Mantel et al. (7) performed an analysis of 180 women during pregnancy and found 48% experienced backache. In ⅓ of those it was severe. The prevalence of back pain increased with both increasing age and increasing parity and it was difficult to separate the relative contributions of these two factors. No evidence was found of association from backache during pregnancy and height and weight, obesity index, weight gain, or the baby's weight. Analysis of the aggravating and relieving factors indicates some difference between bachache in the pregnant and mechanical back pain in the nonpregnant; however, this was not stastically significant. Slightly less backache was reported among patients attending antinatal physiotherapy classes, but the figures do not provide clear evidence of any protective effect of this attendance.

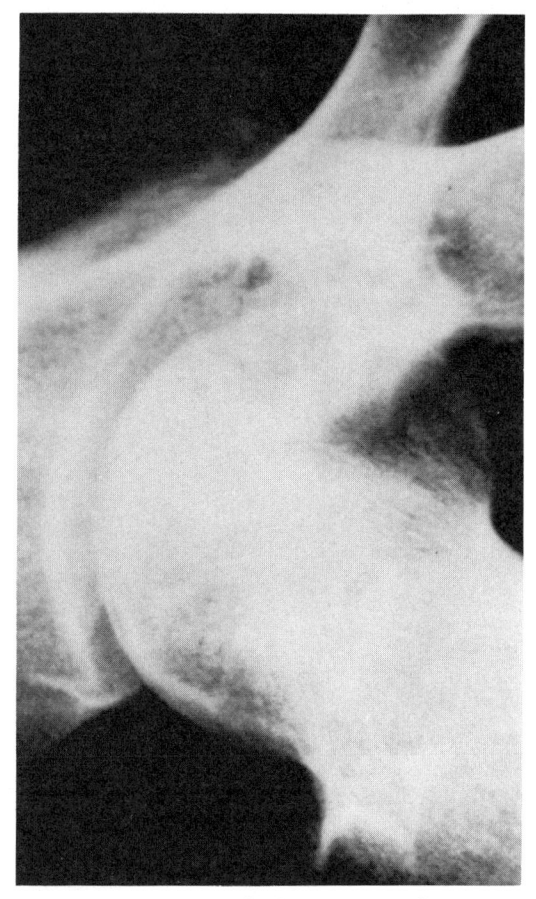

Figure 16.8. X-ray findings—avascular necrosis—femoral head.

Standard back postural exercises should be prescribed during pregnancy including pelvic tilt, hip flexion without abdominal sit-ups. The importance of proper chair sitting (Fig. 16.9) and the use of a car seat may also be considered.

CONNECTIVE TISSUE DISEASE

Rheumatoid Arthritis

Rheumatoid arthritis is defined as an autoimmune disease of the synovial tissues in

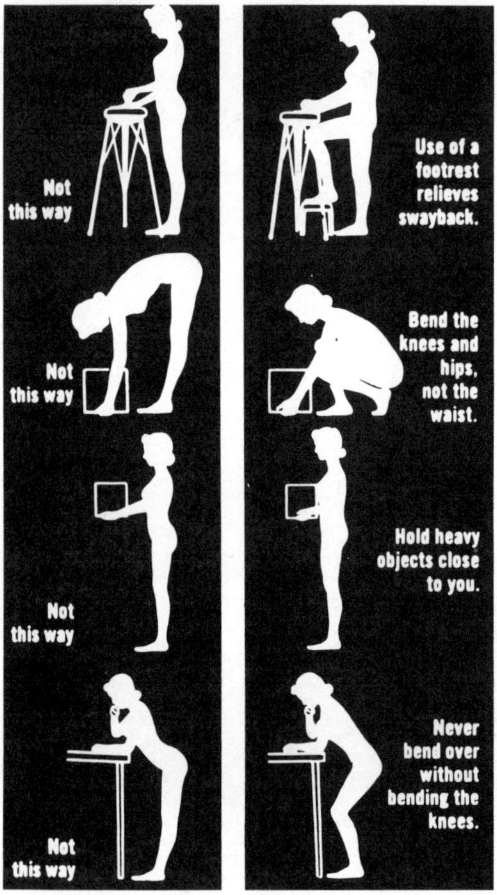

Figure 16.9. Postural exercises.

which there is proliferation and inflammation of the synovium with a tendency toward invasion of subchondral bone, articular cartilage, and surrounding structures leading to arthritis and subsequent destructive arthritic processes (5). Associated with this are often systemic manifestations such as morning stiffness, motion pain or tenderness in at least one joint, swelling of joints, subcutaneous nodules, fever, and typical findings such as positive "rheumatoid factor", poor mucin precipitate of synovial fluid, and characteristic histologic changes of synovium and nodules. The etiology of rheumatoid arthritis is unknown, although there is some speculation as to possible infectious etiology.

The disease's course is characterized by spontaneous exacerbations and remissions, although in a certain percentage of patients it is an inexorably progressive one, leading to joint destruction and crippling. Rheumatoid arthritis is considered to be one of the major cripplers of young people (9).

Early in the study of rheumatoid arthritis, it was recognized that pregnancy would frequently induce remission (3, 6). Why remissions occur during pregnancy is still not clear, but there is some thought that it may be related to increased concentration of blood cortisol. This observation led to the use of cortisone for the treatment of rheumatoid arthritis (8). There have been patients who have improved during pregnancy whose cortisol levels were not increased. Other patients with active rheumatoid arthritis who did have increased cortisol levels did not remit. Furthermore, though plasma and cortisol levels returned to normal within 48 hours after delivery, the remission that occurs usually lasts about 6 weeks after delivery.

Unfortunately, there are no solid data that explain remissions in rheumatoid arthritis during pregnancy. The incidence of improvement in rheumatoid arthritis in pregnancy is approximately 70%. Improvement seems to begin the first trimester and continues into the second and third trimester. In 90% of the patients, however, symptoms recur within 2 months after delivery (8).

Systemic Lupus Erythematosus

Systemic lupus erythematosus affects women primarily in the childbearing age. Symptoms include arthralgias, arthritis, pleuritis, pericarditis, nephritis, nephrosis, thrombocytopenic purpura, and anemia with neurologic symptoms as well as personality changes (10).

Most feel that lupus patients with active renal disease should not become pregnant. If, on the other hand, the illness has been under control with relatively small amounts of prednisone (10 mg per day or less), and they were willing to accept the risks associated with pregnancy, they are not advised against it. Patients on antimalarial therapy or immunosuppresive therapy are advised against getting pregnant because of the possible teratogenic effects of these drugs. When the patients do become pregnant, they are followed closely both clinically and in terms of their serologic abnormalities. With any hint of a flareup, their corticosteroids are increased.

In summary, systemic lupus can be exacerbated by pregnancy, especially when there is active renal disease present. The patients with active renal disease or serious central nervous system disease are advised against getting pregnant.

OSTEITIS PUBIS

Osteitis pubis is a painful condition in the region of the symphysis pubis which may develop after surgical trauma and is characterized by bony reaborption about the symphysis and spontaneous reossification with subsidence of symptoms.

The actual cause is unknown. Infection has been blamed but local inflammatory signs are absent. A softening of the pelvic ligaments, such as occurs during pregnancy, suggests a predisposing factor.

Gradually over a period of a few days, excruciating pain develops about the symphysis pubis and pubic rami and radiates along the adductor aspects of both thighs. The pain is increased by any movement of the extremities, especially abduction which puts the abductor muscles on a stretch. The sites of attachment of the adductors are particularly tender, although the bodies and the rami of both pubes are diffusely tender. The area lacks the swelling, redness, and warmth of inflammation and the temperature is normal. Injection of a local anesthetic into the points of attachment of the adductors frequently relieves the pain.

The patient is often disabled and bedridden. She often seeks a position of maximum comfort which is one of flexion and adduction. The pain is intense for a period varying from days to weeks and then gradually subsides over an indefinite period from a few months to several years.

X-rays in the early days or weeks are negative. As the disease progresses, the bone adjacent to the symphysis undergoes spotty demineralization which intensifies until the symphyseal gap appears to be widened (Fig. 16.10). Characteristically the opposing aspects of the pubic bodies are moth-eaten, rarefied and cup-shaped. The rami are diffusely osteoporotic. Gradually, over many months, reossification occurs with restoration of bony architecture. The patient is usually placed at absolute bed rest with lower extremities close together and flexed over a pillow, maximum relief of pain is obtained by ice bags, but narcotics are sometimes necessary.

OSTEITIS CONDENSANS ILII

Osteitis condensans ilii is a disturbance of the normal architecture of the ilium in which increased condensations of bone occur in the articular portion of the ilium without a correspondence change in the sacroiliac joint or the sacrum.

The actual cause is unknown. Mechanical strain may be responsible for the situation. The sacrum tends to rotate about a fulcrum situated at the 2nd sacral segment. The strong sacroiliac ligaments become taut and resist this rotation. When tendency to rotation is increased because of an acute lumbosacral angle or during pregnancy when the pelvic ligaments soften, additional strain is thrown upon the ligaments at their attachment to the ilium. The auricular process of the ilium responds by bony thickening.

Patients complain of low back pain which is persistent, never severe, and radiates to one or both buttocks, never into the sciatic distribution. Symptoms are aggravated by activity and relieved by rest. There is no night pain. The condition occurs in females of childbearing age, frequently having its onset in the final trimester of pregnancy or immediately after delivery. Symptoms recur or exacerbate during subsequent pregnancies.

On examination spasm of the paraspinal muscles is present. Lumbar lordosis is often increased. Erthryocyte sedimentation rate is within normal limits.

X-ray reveals condensations of the auric-

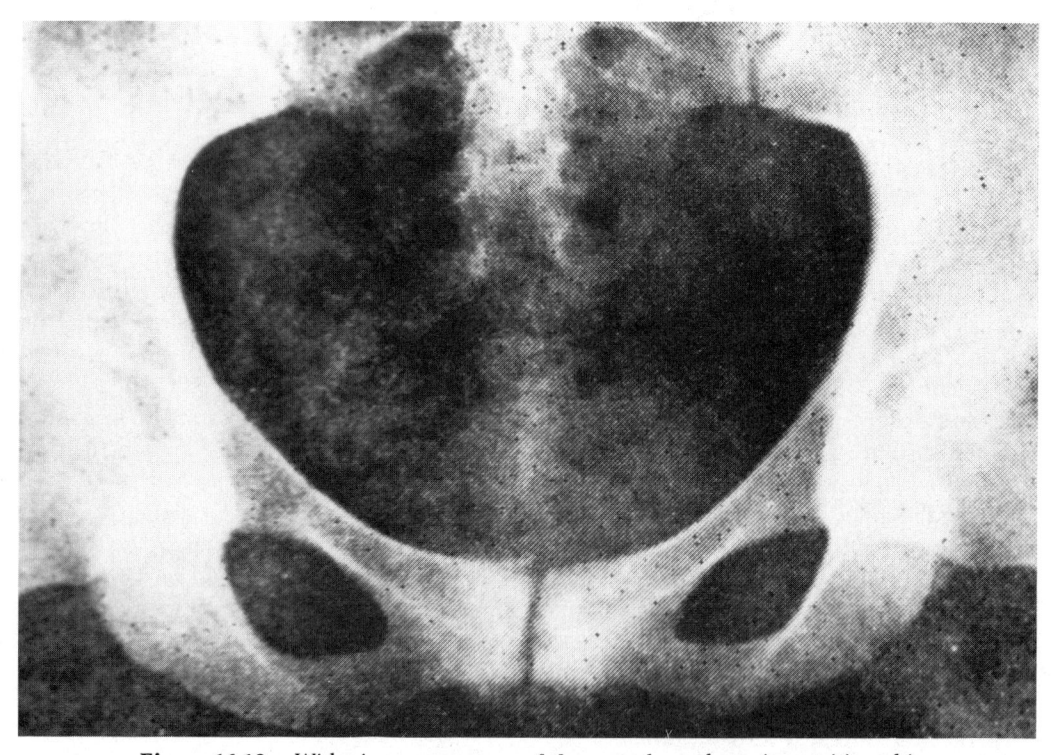

Figure 16.10. Widening appearance of the symphyseal gap in osteitis pubis.

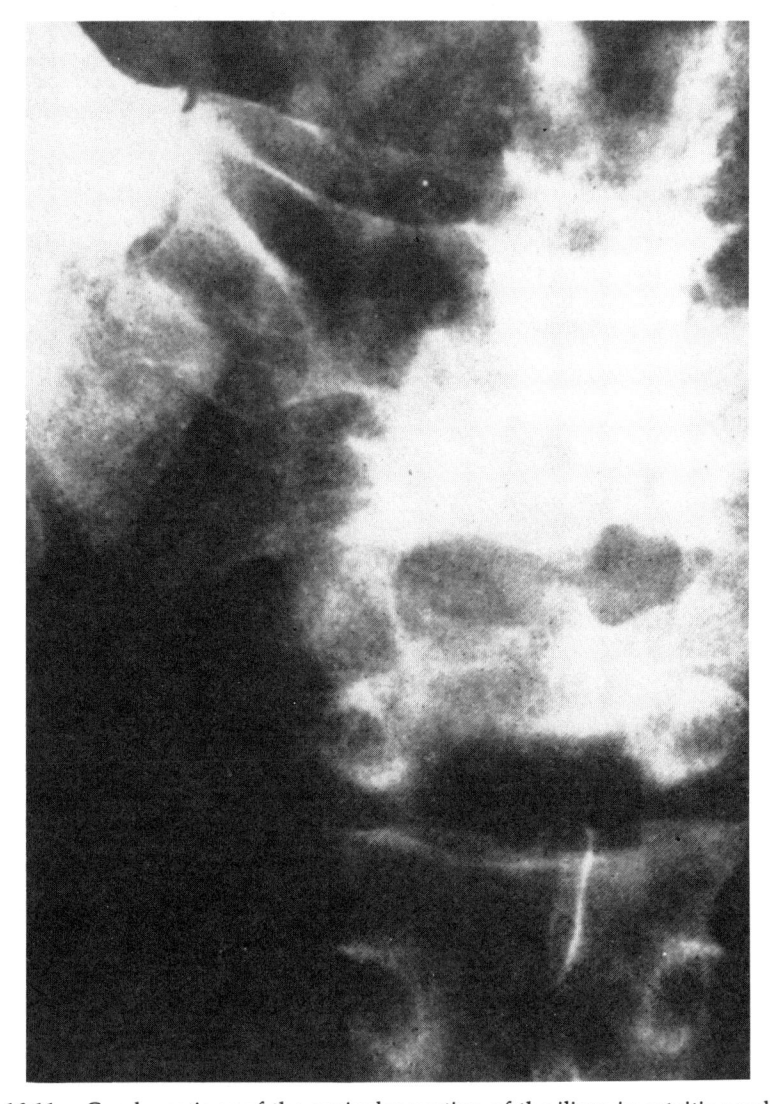

Figure 16.11. Condensations of the auricular portion of the ilium in osteitis condensans.

ular portion of the ilium (Fig. 16.11). This area is localized behind the anterior margin of the sacroiliac joint. The roentgenographic picture is not proportionate to the severity of symptoms.

Ankylosing spondolitis or Marie-Strümpell arthritis must be considered in a diagnosis; however, this involves changes on both sides of the joint, the male is more commonly involved and the sacroiliac tests are positive.

The sedimentation rate is also elevated.

In terms of treating osteitis condensans ilii, attempts should be made at reducing lumbosacral angulation by postural exercise, weight reduction, and a bed board, a hard mattress, and a lumbosacral corset are sometimes prescribed. Rarely surgical arthrodesis may be indicated postpartum.

REFERENCES

1. Cheng N, Burssens A, Mulier JC: Pregnancy and post pregnancy avascular necrosis of the femoral head. *Arch Orthop Trauma Surg* 100:199–210, 1981.
2. Gould JS, Wissinger HA: Carpal tunnel syndrome in pregnancy. UC South Medical Journal 71/72:144–145, 1978.
3. Hench PS: The beneficial effect of pregnancy on

chronic atrophy (infectious, rheumatoid) arthritis and intermittent hydroarthrosis. *Mayo Clin Proc* 13:161–167, 1983.
4. Hytten FE, Taggart N: Limb volumes in pregnancy. *J Obstet Gynaecol Br Commonw* 74:663, 1967.
5. Katz WA: *Rheumatic Diseases: Diagnosis and Management.* Philadelphia, J. B. Lippincott, 1977, p 385.
6. Kendall EC: The adrenal cortex in rheumatoid arthritis. *Lancet* 2:586–587, 1951.
7. Mantel NJ, Greenwood RN, Currey HLF: Backache in pregnancy. *Rheumatol Rehabil* 16:95, 1977.
8. Persellin RH: The effect of pregnancy on rheumatoid arthritis. *Bull Rheum Dis* 27:922–927, 1977.
9. Reynolds MD: Prevalence of rheumatic diseases on causes of disability and complains by ambulatory patients. *Arthritis Rheum* 21:377, 1978.
10. Rothfield NF: Systemic lupus erythematosus. In Katz WA (ed): *Rheumatic Diseases: Diagnosis and Management.* Philadelphia, W. B. Saunders, 1977.
11. Thompson AN, Hytten FE. Billewicz WC: The epidemiology of oedema during pregnancy. *J Obstet Gynecol Br Commonw* 74:1, 1967.
12. White R: Transactions of the Edinberg Obstetrical Society. *Edinburgh Med J* 57:20, 1950.

17

Exercise Prescription in Pregnancy

Regular exercise is becoming a way of life, and more individuals are continuing such activities while pregnant. Though exercise in pregnancy provides primarily psychological benefits, it appears that it might offer some physical benefits as well. With so many women conducting such activities, there is a need for proper guidelines for exercise prescription in pregnancy.

Pregnancy is characterized by a multitude of "normal" anatomical and physiological alterations, that have been detailed in this text. As such, recommendations have to be made against this background.

Of all the subgroups in the general population, pregnant women are the only ones who have no exercise standards. At present, recommendations for pregnant and postpartum women are based on "common sense." Many highly specific programs for exercise in pregnancy can be found that have based their routines on this principle alone. A recent review of such programs revealed medical content that was in many cases inappropriate, inaccurate or incomplete (1). Few such programs imply that exercise may affect and shorten labor and delivery while others are based on motivational arguments that push mentally prepared individuals beyond their physical capabilities.

There is no organization that presently regulates exercise activities in pregnancy, but it is the opinion of these authors that such a forum should be created to regulate these activities, monitor qualifications for instructors, and maintain guidelines and standards as they become available. Ideally, a multidisciplinary medical advisory committee should be created to guide such exercise programs and provide medical clearance for the participants. Such a committee should include obstetricians, exercise physiologists, and sports medicine experts.

By and large, pregnant women who engage in exercise programs are healthy but very few are aware of the anatomical and physiological changes that might predispose them for injuries. In addition, the short- and long-term effects of maternal exercise on the fetus should always be considered.

OBSTETRICAL AND MEDICAL SCREENING

The American College of Sports Medicine (2) guidelines indicate that, if an individual is asymptomatic, less than 35 years of age, has no evidence or history of cardiovascular disease, has no risk factors for coronary heart disease, and has had a medical evaluation during the previous year, no medical clearance is necessary prior to an increase in physical activity level. No mention is made with regard to pregnancy. Guidelines for exercise should be safe and include standards for normal physiological responses to various types of activity, their intensity, duration, and frequency.

Contraindications

The absolute and relative contraindications to exercise in pregnancy are listed in Table 17.1. Before approving an exercise program a careful history of the cardiovas-

Table 17.1. Contraindication to Exercise in Pregnancy

Absolute
1. Active myocardial disease
2. Congestive heart failure
3. Rheumatic heart disease (Class II and above)
4. Thrombophlebitis
5. Recent pulmonary embolism
6. Acute infectious disease
7. At risk for premature labor, incompetent cervix, multiple gestations
8. Uterine bleeding, ruptured membranes
9. Intrauterine growth retardation or macrosomia
10. Severe isoimmunization
11. Severe hypertensive disease
12. No prenatal care
13. Suspected fetal distress

Relative Contraindications
1. Essential hypertension
2. Anemia or other blood disorders
3. Thyroid disease
4. Diabetes mellitus
5. Breech presentations in the last trimester
6. Excessive obesity or extreme underweight
7. History of sedentary life-style

Additional contradications should be left for the physician to individualize

cular, pulmonary, metabolic, and musculoskeletal system should be taken.

Physicians will have to individualize exercise programs in individuals with relative contraindications. Some of these individuals may actually benefit from a medically supervised exercise program (e.g., diabetic patients).

The following symptoms and signs should signal the patient to stop exercise and contact her physician: (*a*) pain of any kind, chest pain, headache; (*b*) uterine contractions (frequent at 20-min intervals); (*c*) vaginal bleeding, leaking amniotic fluid; (*d*) dizziness, faintness; (*e*) shortness of breath; (*f*) palpitations, tachycardia; (*g*) persistent nausea and vomiting; (*h*) back pain; (*i*) pubic or hip pain; (*j*) difficulty in walking; (*k*) generalized edema; and (*l*) decreased fetal activity. Patients should be educated to recognize and be alert to the above signs and symptoms.

Applications for Exercise Stress Testing

Ideally, every individual planning to undertake an exercise program should have a graded exercise stress test. Though a variety of stress tests are available for the nonpregnant, none have been yet developed for use in pregnancy. When developed, such a test should recommend an exercise routine that is both possible and safe. Based on our preliminary observations we believe that maximal exercise capacity is reduced by approximately 20–25% in pregnant patients.

Exercise testing in pregnancy could also be utilized to test placental reserve capacity. By and large, exercise testing provides a unique opportunity to test all body functional reserves, and as such exposing conditions that otherwise would not have been uncovered. If exercise testing is undertaken in pregnancy every effort should be made to test the fetus prior and after the procedure. A reactive fetal heart rate pattern with no obvious signs for fetal distress should be reassuring. In addition, monitoring the frequency of fetal movements should become a useful tool for long-term monitoring of individuals engaged in exercise programs.

EXERCISE PRESCRIPTION IN PREGNANCY

The creation of exercise programs during pregnancy should specify the type of activity, the intensity, duration, and frequency. Safety for both mother and fetus should be a primary concern. Table 17.2 lists a few of the potential risks for exercise in pregnancy.

Table 17.2. Risks of Exercise in Pregnancy

Maternal
1. Increased risk of musculoskeletal injuries
2. Cardiovascular complications
3. Premature labor
4. Hypoglycemia

Fetal
1. Fetal distress
2. Intrauterine growth retardation
3. Fetal malformations
4. Prematurity

Though some of the listed risks may be only theoretical, caution should be exercised to prevent such complications. Given such constraints, the intensity, duration, and frequency of exercise routines utilized outside pregnancy have to be altered. Under unsupervised conditions the intensity of the exercise should be reduced by approximately 25%, maximum maternal heart rate should not exceed 140 beats/min, and peak activity should not be maintained for more than 15 min. We believe that by maintaining such constraints the incidence for the above listed risks can be reduced significantly.

A clear distinction has to be made between the different exercise programs in pregnancy:

1. Childbirth preparatory exercise
2. Recreational and sports activities
3. Postpartum exercise.

Special consideration has to be given to changes that occur in the first, second and third trimester of pregnancy.

To recapitulate, the following anatomical and physiological changes can affect the ability to engage in exercise activities in pregnancy: First trimester: nausea, vomiting, tachycardia; second and third trimester; change in center of gravity, increased connective tissue laxity with resulting joint instability, lordosis and kyphosis, edema with resulting nerve compression syndrome, increase in blood volume, tachycardia, and hyperventilation (these changes reduce the cardiac reserve and the residual lung capacity).

By and large, exercise programs in pregnancy should be directed toward muscle strengthening to minimize the risk of joint and ligament injuries and toward correcting postural changes, carefully avoiding strain or point of fatigue, and with rest and relaxation interspersed. The goal should be to maintain physical fitness within the physiological limitation of pregnancy. The following instruction have been developed by a task force of the American College for Obstetricians and Gynecologists (1).

INSTRUCTIONS FOR PREGNANT WOMEN WHO WISH TO EXERCISE

The following guidelines are based on the unique physical and physiological conditions that exist during pregnancy and the postpartum period. They can be used by patients to select physical activities that are most safe at these times.

During Pregnancy and the Postpartum Period

1. Regular exercise (at least 3 times per week) is preferable to intermittent activity. Competitive activities should be discouraged.
2. Vigorous exercise should not be performed in hot, humid weather or during a period of febrile illness.
3. Ballistic movements (jerky, bouncy motions) should be avoided. Exercise should be done on a wooden or a tightly carpeted surface to reduce shock and provide a sure footing.
4. Deep flexion or extension of joints should be avoided because of connective tissue laxity. Avoid activities that require jumping, jarring motions or rapid changes in direction because of joint instability.
5. Vigorous exercise should be preceded by a 5-min period of muscular warm-up. This can be accomplished by slow walking or stationary cycling with low resistance.
6. Vigorous exercise should be followed by a period of gradually declining activity that includes gentle static stretching. Stretches should not be taken to the point of maximum resistance, as connective tissue laxity increases the risk of injury.
7. Heart rate should be measured at times of peak activity. Target heart rates and limits established in consultation with the physician should not be exceeded.
8. Care should be taken to gradually rise up from the floor to avoid orthostatic hypotension. Some form of activity

involving the legs should be continued for a brief period.
9. Liquids should be taken liberally before, during, and after exercise to prevent dehydration. If necessary, activity should be interrupted to replenish fluids.
10. Women who have led sedentary life-styles should begin with physical activity of very low intensity and advance activity levels very gradually.
11. Activity should be stopped and the physician consulted if any unusual symptoms appear.

During Pregnancy Only

1. Maternal heart rate should not exceed 140 beats/min.
2. Strenuous activities should not exceed 15 min in duration.
3. No exercises should be performed in the supine position after the fourth month of gestation is completed.
4. Exercises that employ the Valsalva maneuver should be avoided.
5. Caloric intake should be adequate to meet not only the extra energy needs of pregnancy, but also of the exercise performed.
6. Maternal core temperature should not exceed 38.5°C.

The type of activity should be prescribed on the basis of limitations imposed by pregnancy. Some exercises may be easily performed and tolerated in pregnancy: brisk walking, swimming, stationary cycling, and modified forms of calisthenics. It is important to point out to patients that a sedentary life-style in pregnancy does not in any way affect the outcome of that pregnancy.

Pregnancy should not be a state of confinement and women should be encouraged to live a normal life and continue their pre-pregnancy activities. Recognizing limitations and following guidelines can limit the risk for injuries.

The guidelines outlined in this text are an attempt to interpret and apply the available literature. Certainly, much work remains to be done to systematically research and establish normative data and standards for exercise in pregnancy.

REFERENCES

1. American College of Obstetricians and Gynecologists (ACOG) Technical Bulletin on Exercise in Pregnancy, 1985.
2. American College of Sports Medicine: *Guidelines for Graded Exercise Testing and Exercise Prescription.* Philadelphia, Lea & Febiger, 1980.

Index

Page numbers in *italics* denote figures; those followed by "*t*" or "*f*" denote tables or footnotes, respectively.

Acetate
  metabolism, exercise effects on, 23
  uterine uptake, 33, 38
Acetylcoenzyme A, 84
Acid base status, maintenance, 147
Acidosis
  metabolic, 188
  respiratory, 188, 195
ACTH (corticotrophin)
  DOC levels and, 77
  levels in pregnancy, 74, 76, 77, 86
  release, 52
  stress effects on, 86
Actinomyosin, degradation, 83
Adrenal gland
  hormonal regulation of fetal circulation, 186
  water metabolism and, 76–77
α-Adrenergic activity, fetal heart regulation and, 185
β-Adrenergic activity
  associated with hypoxia, 191
  fetal heart rate regulation and, 185
α-Adrenergic blockade, during hypoxia, 191
β-Adrenergic blockade, during hypoxia, 191
Advice to Women in the Care of their Health before, during and after Confinement, 1–2
Aerobic exercise
  benefits, 206
  capacity standards for women, 10*t*
  programs during pregnancy, 207–208, 209
  reduced capacity during pregnancy, 206–207
Aerobic fitness, measurement
    by energy expenditure, 10–12*t*
    by exercise metabolism, 8
    by maximal oxygen uptake, 9–*10*
    by mechanical efficiency, 12–14*t*
    by relative vs absolute work, 10, *11*
    exercise protocol, 14–15*t*
Aerobic metabolism, 190

Afterload, importance in stroke volume change, 115–116
Aldosterone
  levels during pregnancy and postpartum, 77, *78*
  production in response to decreased blood pressure, 186
Alkalosis, resipratory, 147, 152
Alveolar ventilation, increased, 147
Amenorrhea
  etiology, 53–56
  management, 56
  relationship to strenuous training, 51
American College for Obstetricians and Gynecologists, instructions for exercise during pregnancy, 227–228
American College of Sports Medicine, guidelines for exercise in pregnancy, 225
Amino acid(s)
  fasting blood levels, 88, *90*
  transport across placenta, 33, 38
  tubular reabsorbtion, 69
Anaerobic metabolism, 190
Androgen production
  adrenal, 51
  corpus luteum, 70
Androstenedione, 70
Anemia
  in athletes, 107
  fetal, 188
  physiologic, 67
Angiotensin
  hypoxia and, 191
  uterine blood flow and, 121
Angiotensin II, 78
Angiotensinogen, 78
Animals, laboratory
  experimental methods, 39–40
    blood and plasma volume, 42
    cardiac output and VO$_2$ measurement, 40

Index

Animals (*continued*)
    fetal cardiac output and blood flow distribution, 43
    fetal heart rate and arterial pressure, 43
    placental diffusing capacity for carbon monoxide, 42–43
    principles, 40
    respiratory gases, 42
    surgery, 40, *41*
    temperatures, 42
    uterine blood flow and vascular resistance, 40–42
  fetal outcome, 38–39
  fetal responses, 31, 36*t*
    body temperature, 33–34
    circulation, 35–36
    metabolism and endocrinology, 32–33
    oxygen consumption, 31–32
    respiration and blood gases, 34–35
  maternal responses, 21, 31*t*
    body temperature, 23–24
    cardiac output distribution, 26–30
    circulation, 25–26
    oxygen consumption, 21–22
    metabolism, 22–23
    physical working capacity, 22
    respiration and blood gases, 24–25
    uterine oxygen consumption, 30–31
  placental responses, 36–38
  rationale for usage, 21
  studies, on uterine blood flow during exercise, 121
Ankylosing spondolitis, 223
Aorta, and positioning of electomagnetic flow probe, 41
Aortic capacitance, 115
Aortic diastolic dimension, 116
Apgar scores, 136
Appetite, total energy needs and, 110–111
Appetite-satiety center, progesterone and, 74
Asphyxia, fetal
  adrenal medulla and, 186
  autonomic changes during, 191
  blood flow distribution, 188
  fetal circulation during, 188
  humoral changes during, 191–192
  organ oxygen consumption, 189–190
ATP production, anaerobic vs aerobic, 190
Atropine
  effect on fetal heart rate variability, 185
  hypoxia-induced change and, 191
Autonomic nervous system, activity during fetal asphyxia, 191

Back pain, 219, *220*
Baroreceptors, in regulation of fetal circulation, 186
Basal body temperature
  changes during pregnancy, 23
  effects of exercise on, 23–24
Basal metabolic rate (BMR), 74, 206
Beta cell, artificial implantable, 94–95*f*
Bicarbonate, serum, 147
Bicycle
  recumbant, 14*t*
  with treadmill testing, 14*t*
Bicycle ergometers
  evaluation of exercise effect in pregnancy, 14*t*
  mechanical efficiency determinations, 13*t*
  physical working capacity study, 206–207
Bicycling
  during pregnancy, 209–210
  hyperventilation and, 206
  mechanical efficiency, 13
  risk, 210
Birth weight
  heavy maternal physical activity and, 99
  low, 203
    related to employment, 207
  maternal diet reduction and, 99
    social class and, 2
    working women and, 2
Blood, fetal (*see also* specific determinants)
  hemoglobin, 157
  oxygen affinity, 157–158
  oxygen capacity, 158
Blood flow (*see also* Uterine blood flow)
  distribution, measurement in animals, 43
  fetal
    distribution, 181–182, 183*f*
    countercurrent, 161
    crosscurrent, 161
    effect on transplacental oxygen transfer, 168–170*f*
  maternal
    breast, 120
    countercurrent, 161
    crosscurrent, 161
    effect on transplacental oxygen transfer, 166–168*f*
    to kidney, 127
  placental
    effect on fetal temperature, 33
    effect on transplacental oxygen transfer, 166–170*f*
  redistribution, 142
Blood gases (*see also* specific gases)
  correction for exercise-induced temperature changes, 24
  fetal, 34–35
  inability to transfer, 147
  maternal responses after exercise, 24–25
  measurement techniques in animals, 42
  respiratory exchange, effects of, 159
Blood, maternal (*see also* specific determinants)
  hemoglobin, 155
  oxygen affinity, 155, 157
  oxygen capacity, 157
  redistribution, 127, *128*
Blood pressure, arterial
  fetal, 36, 183
    increase, 185
    increased, as protective mechanism, 195
    measurement technique in animals, 43
  maternal, 31*t*
    changes during exercise, 25–26
    mean (MAP), changes during pregnancy, 67, *68*

Index   231

Blood volume
    fetal control
        by capillary fluid shift, 186–187
        Frank-Starling mechanism and, 187
        by intraplacental pressures, 187
        umbilical blood flow and, 187–188
    maternal
        central, increased during pregnancy, 64
        changes in animals, 26, 27
        changes throughout pregnancy, 66–67
        exercise and, 23
        placental, 170
        measurement technique in animals, 42
Body temperature
    basal, 23–24
    core temperature, maternal, 228
    fetal, 33–34, 38
        oxygen consumption and, 31–32
    maternal responses in animals, 23–24
    measurement in animals, 42
Body weight
    amenorrhea and, 51
    gain during pregnancy, 83–84
        chart, 110
        constituents of, 84
        excessive, 101
        for obese pregnant women, 100
        indication of caloric intake, 62
        monitoring of physically active woman, 111
        rate, 101, 111
Bohr effect, 159
Bone density, in postmenopausal exercising women, 107
Bradycardia, fetal
    defined, 183
    fetal distress and, 35
    maternal hypoxia or hypercapnia and, 185, 189, 191
Breast(s)
    blood flow, 120
    effects of estrogen and progesterone on, 73
    preparation for lactation, 74

Calcitonin, 74, 75
Calcium
    excretion, increased dietary protein and, 106
    mean levels during pregnancy, 75f
    metabolism during pregnancy, 74–76
    requirements
        in active nonpregnant women, 107
        of pregnant sedentary women, 103–104
Caloric intake, total, 100
Caloric need, 206
Capacitance, aortic, 115
Carbohydrate(s)
    complex, 106
    metabolism, maternal responses in animals, 22
    storage, 83
Carbon dioxide
    production during mild, moderate and VO_2 max exercise, 152
    tension
        fetal, 36t
        increased, maternal, 195
        during exercise, 24
Carbon monoxide placental diffusing capacity
    in human, 162–163t
    measurement techniques in animals, 42–43
Cardiac output (see also specific determinants)
    determinants of changes, 114–120
    distribution, exercise and, 26–30
    effects
        of estrogens on, 120
        of exercise intensity on distribution, 129
        of pregnancy on, 130, 131
    fetal, 35, 36t
        distribution of blood flow and, 181–183
        measurement technique in animals, 43
    maternal, 31t
        during exercise, 117–120, 130, 154
        during pregnancy, 14, 65–68, 147
        during bicycling, 209–210
        factors involved, 113
        magnitude, 113–114
        strenuous exercise and, 7
    measurement
        in animals, 40
        validity of, 114
    redistribution, 127, 128
    time course, 113
Cardiovascular system
    adaptations to pregnancy, 116–117
    adjustments in pregnancy, 65–68f
    autonomically mediated responses to hypoxia, 191
    conditioning during pregnancy, 131, 134
    endurance activities, 208–210
    response to exercise during pregnancy, 130–131
        studies, summary of, 132t–133t
    response to maternal exercise, 127–131
Carpal tunnel syndrome, 61, 215–216
Catecholamine(s), (see also Epinephrine; Norepinephrine)
    blood flow redistribution and, 142
    effects
        on fetal heart rate, 35
        on umbilical blood flow, 35–36
        on uterine blood flow, 29
    fetal cardiac output and, 35
    fetal concentrations
        after maternal exercise, 36t
    functions, 141
    maternal hypoxia and, 191
    placenta metabolism of, 195
    uterine blood flow and, 27
Center of gravity, in pregnancy, 60
Central nervous system
    dysfunction and amenorrhea, 51
    in regulation of fetal circulation, 186
Chemoreceptors, in regulation of fetal circulation, 185–186
Chemoreflex, in utero, 186
Childbirth preparation
    cardiovascular conditioning and, 131, 134, 135t
    exercises, preparatory, 212–213, 227

Childbirth preparation (*continued*)
    psychoprophylactic, 3, 131, 136
Chondromalacia patella, *218–219*
Circulatory system
    adaptations in pregnancy, 127
        that influence exercise capacity, 128*t*
    fetal responses to maternal exercise, 35–36
    maternal responses in animals, 25–26
    reserve, 130
Collagen, degradation, 83
Combined ventricular output (CVO), 181–182, *183*
Complications of pregnancy, exercise and, 8
Connective tissue
    change in ground substance by progesterone, 74
    disease, 219–223
Contractility, myocardial, 115, 116
Controlled stress concept, 85–86, *87*, 88
Corpus luteum
    hormone production, 69
    hormone production by, 69–70
    maintenance during pregnancy, 71
Corticosteroid, fetal, 32
Corticotrophin (ACTH)
    DOC levels and, 77
    levels in pregnancy, 74, 76, 77, 86
    release, 52
    stress effects on, 86
Cortisol
    effects of exercise on menstrual cycle, 55
    improvement of rheumatoid arthritis and, 220
    levels in pregnancy, 86
    plasma levels, 76, *77*
        during exercise, *144–145*
    preexercise vs postexercise concentrations, *140*
    stress effects on, 86
Cortisone-binding globulin, 86
Cotyledon, maternal-fetal blood flow ratio, 162, *163*
Counseling, nutritional, 105
Creatinine clearance, 69

Dehydroepiandrosterone, 70
Dehydroepiandrosterone (DHEA), 76
11-Deoxycorticosterone (DOC), 77, *78*
Deoxyhemoglobin, 159
Diabetes
    effect of exercise on, 92
    hormonal effects on fuel supply, *89*
    hormonal responses to mild exercise, *142*
    metabolic considerations during pregnancy, 92–95
Diabetic ketoacidosis, 91
Diaphragm, adaption to pregnancy, *64*, 147
Diet, of mother and effect on fetal growth, 99
Dihydrotestosterone, 76
2,3-Diphosphoglycerate (2,3DPG), 155, 157
Disabilities, pregnancy-related
    in employee benefit plans, 5
Disposal systems, adjustments during pregnancy, 68–69
Diuretics, use during pregnancy, 104, 110
Dyspnea, in pregnancy, 65

Echocardiography, M-mode of myocardial contractile response, 118–*120*
Edema, relationship to hypertension proteinuria, 215
Electomagnetic flowmeter, 41
Electrolyte(s)
    balance, during exercise, 7
    composition of sweat, 107*t*
Elevator exercises, 205
Employement of pregnant women
    continued, complications of, 207
    legislation prohibiting, 2
End-diastolic dimension (EDD), 118, 119*f*
Endocrine system
    activity, exercise and, 7
    adjustments during pregnancy, 69–78
        adrenal gland, 76–77
        mineralocorticoids, 77–78
        parathyroid and calcium metabolism, 74–76
        placenta, 70–71, *72*
        placental steroids and, 71–74
        pituitary, 74
        thyroid, 74
        water metabolism, 76–78
    responses to pregnancy, 146
b-Endorphin, release in response to physical exertion, *52*
End-systolic dimension (ESD), 118, *119*
Endurance activities, during pregnancy, 210–212
Energy
    cumulative cost of pregnancy, *63*
    expenditure
        measurement, 10–12*t*
    expenditure during pregnancy, 134
    fetal requirements
        anaerobic metabolism and, 190
    generating systems, adjustments to pregnancy, 61–68
    output, 7
    requirements
        fetal, 92
        methods of classifying, 12*t*
        of active nonpregnant women, 105–106
        of active pregnant woman, 109
        of active pregnant women, 110–111
        of pregnant sedentary women, 100–101
met-Enkephalin, release, 52
Epinephrine
    changes related to exercise intensity, 142, *144*
    concentrations during exercise, 139, *142*
    effects
        on blood chemistry, 85*t*
        on uterine blood flow, 121
    levels in pregnancy, 76, 86
    maternal plasma, and fetal movement, 202
    modulation of glucagon and FFA, 141
    production in response to stress, 186
    responses to exercise, *140*
    stress and, 86
Estetrol, 71
Estradiol (E2)
    corpus luteum secretion, 70
    estrogen replacement therapy and, 56

levels during submaximal exercise in pregnancy, *145*
in relation to symptom-limited incremental exercise, 53, *54*
Estriol, 71
Estrogen(s) (*see also* specific estrogens)
  effects
    on peripheral vascular resistance, 120
    on uterine blood flow, 27
    on uterine muscle, 73
  evaluation of status in amenorrhea, 56
  inhibition of PTH, 75
  mean plasma concentrations, 73*f*
  placental, 71
  production by corpus luteum, 70
  protection of maternal skeleton, 75
  release in early pregnancy, 60
  replacement therapy, for amenorrhea, 56
  respiratory alkalosis and, 147
  role in fuel metabolism, 86–87
Estrone
  corpus luteum secretion, 70
  in relation to symptom-limited incremental exercise, 53, *54*
Exercise
  acute metabolic response to, *15–18*
  adjustment to, 7
  animal studies
    on placental oxygen transfer, 172, *173*
  benefits of, 8
  complications of pregnancy and, 8
  contraindications in pregnancy, 225–226*t*
  early attitudes regarding pregnancy, 205
  early publications regarding, 3–5
  effects
    on fetus, long-term, 202–203
    on neurotransmitter-hypothalamic function, 51–53
    on pituitary function, 53, *54*, 55
    on placental oxygen transfer, 172, 174–175
    on steroid hormones, 53, 55–56
    on uterine blood flow, 28–29
  fetal responses to, 195–203*f*
  goals, 227
  injuries from, 5
  instructions during pregnancy, 227–228
  intolerance, 147
  limiting of, 6
  maternal hemodynamics of, 117–*120*
  menstrual dysfunction and, 7–8
  metabolic maternal responses in animals, 22–23
  metabolism, 8
  moderation in, 2
  of unaccustomed severity, 123
  physical benefits, 225
  physiological changes affecting pregnancy, 227
  psychological benefits, 225
  physiology, defined, 7
  prenatal classes, 4
  prescription, 17–18*t*, 226–227
  recommendations for pregnant and postpartum women, 225
  response
    acute response, 130–131
    studies, summary of, 132*t*–133*t*
  risks of, 226*t*, 227
  role in maturation process, 7–8
  steady-level, 15
  submaximal, 15
  symptoms indicating discontinuance, 226
  tolerance and capacity, ventilatory function and, 9
  types, 205
    gentle, 205
    mobility and flexibility, 205
Exercise Plus Pregnancy Program, 4
Exercise protocol(s) (*see also* specific protocols)
  commonly used, *15*
  in evaluation of exercise on pregnant women, 14–15*t*
Exercise stress testing, applications for, 226
Exercise training studies, during pregnancy, 134, 135*t*
Exercises before Childbirth, 4
Exercises for Increased Awareness in Education and Counseling in Childbirth, 4
Expectant Motherhood, 3–4
Expiratory reserve volume (ERV), 64
Extracellular fluid gain, total, 78

Fasting growth hormone (hGH), 86
Fat
  storage, 83
  synthesis during pregnancy, 88
Fatty acids (*see also* Free fatty acids)
  conversion to glucose, 84–85
Femoral head, avascular necrosis of, *219*
Fetal asphyxia (see Asphyxia, fetal)
Fetal heart rate (FHR)
  baseline rate, 183
  measurement technique in animals, 43
  patterns, 195, 226
    following maternal exercise, 122
  responses to maternal exercise, 35, 36*t*
    bradycardia, 198, *199–201*
    related to exercise intensity, 196, *197*, 198
    summary of published literature, 196*t*
  variability, 183–184
    effects of atropine and propranolol, 185
Fetus(al)
  activity and maternal exercise, 198
  adaptations to asphyxial stress, 189
  blood
    hemoglobin, 157
    oxygen affinity, 157–158
    oxygen capacity, 158
  blood pressure, 183
  breathing movements and maternal exericse, 198, *202*
  circulation, 181, *182*
    baroreceptors, 186
    chemoreceptors, 185–186
    during asphyxial stress, 188–192
    hormonal, 186
    parasympathetic nervous system, 184–185
    regulation, 181, 185–186

Fetus(al) (*continued*)
  cotyledonary blood flow
    fetal cotyledonary venous PO$_2$ and placental O$_2$ exchange rate and, 169f–170
  distress, 35
  energy requirements, 92
  glucose utilization, 92
  metabolism and endocrinology, 32–33
  movements in relation to maternal exercise, *202*
  osmoregulation, 74
  outcome, 38–39
  oxygen consumption, 92
  oxygen supply, 155
  oxygenation, 175
    maternal exercise and, 122
  physiologic responses to maternal exercise, 36t
  placental blood flow
    "sluice flow relation", 170
  responses
    oxygen consumption, 31–32
    reasons for limited data, 31
  responses to maternal exercise
    circulation and, 35–36
    respiration and blood gases, 34–35
  temperature changes in response to exercise, 23–24
Fick equation, 9
Fluid balance, during exercise, 7
Folic acid, requirements, 104
Follicle stimulating hormone (FSH)
  changes during pregnancy, 74
  in relation to symptom-limited incremental exercise, 53, 54
Food restriction, effect on fetal growth, 99
Frank-Starling mechanism, 187
Free fatty acids (FFA)
  as energy substrate, 141
  concentrations, exercise effects on, 23
  concentrations during exercise, 139, *142*
  fasting blood levels, 88, *90*
  in gestational diabetes, 93
Fuel(s) (*see also* specific fuels)
  components and storage, 83–84
  interconversion of, 84–85
  metabolic, effect of pregnancy on, *93*
  metabolism in pregnancy, 83–95
    relationship to respiratory exchange ratio, 17, 18t
  supply, hormonal effects on, 86–88, *89*

Gastrointestinal system, adjustments to pregnancy, 62–63
Getting Ready to Be a Mother, 3
Gilbert v. General Electric Corporation, 5
Girls, pre-and postpubescent, mechanical efficiency, 13
Glomerular filtration rate (GFR), 69
Glucagon
  concentrations during exercise, 139, *142*
  functions, 140
  levels prior to and after exercise, *140*
  role in fuel metabolism, 86
Glucocorticoid(s), role in exercise, 144
Gluconeogenesis, 86

Glucose
  concentrations during exercise, 139, *142*
  conversion to fat, 84–85
  diffusion across placenta, 37
  fasting blood levels, 88, *90*
  fetal, 32, 39
  fluctuations in pregnancy, 93
  insulin closed delivery system and, *94*
  intolerance, 90
    maternal obesity and, 100
  levels prior to and after exercise, *140*
  maternal concentrations, 32
  metabolic fate, 91–92
  metabolism
    anaerobic vs aerobic, 190
    maternal responses in animals, 22
  plasma levels related to exercise intensity, 140, *143*
  tubular reabsorbtion, 69
  utilization, fetal, 92
  utilization during pregnancy, 139
Glucose tolerance, 87, 88
Glycogen
  storage in liver, 83, 84
Gonadotropin-releasing hormone (GnRH), 52
Growth retardation, fetal
  and maternal diet, 99
Growth retardation, intrauterine, 38

Haldane effect, 159
Heart
  capillary density and fiber-to-capillary ratio, 39
  disease, in pregnancy, 148
  size
    cardiac output and, 113, 116
    stroke volume and, 115
Heart rate (*see also* Fetal heart rate)
  cardiac output and, 114
  changes throughout pregnancy, 67
  during exercise related to work intensity, 130
  during maternal exercise, *118*
  effects on pregnancy, 130, *131*
  in excercise prescription, 228
  intrinsic, 114
  relationship to uterine blood flow, 28, *29*
  response to exercise, pregnancy and training, 31t
  target
    drawbacks to usage, 18
    use in prescribing exercise, 18
Heat
  dissipation, mechanism in pregnancy, 68
  excessive, as harmful to fetus, 123
Hematocrit
  during pregnancy, 68
  exercise effects on, 26
Hemodynamics, maternal
  at rest, 113–114
  changes during exercise, 129
  changes during pregnancy, 113–123
  pulmonary, 152, 154
Hemoglobin, 147

Bart's, 172
fetal, 157
   effects on placental oxygen transfer, 170, 171
   oxygen affinity, variations, 171–172
maternal, 155
concentration, 157
during exercise, 172
effects on placental oxygen transfer, 170–171
oxygen affinity, variations, 171
variants compatible with intrauterine development, 172
Hip pain, *219*
Historical perspectives, 1–6
Hormone(s) (*see also* specific hormones)
   affecting fuel supply in pregnancy, 86–88*f*
   changes during exercise, 144
   regulation of fetal circulation, 186
   responses to mild exercise
     in healthy, pregnant and diabetic patients, 139, *142*
   steroid, 86*t*
Horseback riding during pregnancy, 211
Human chorionic gonadotropin (hCG)
   changes during pregnancy, 74
   functions and regulation, 71
Human placental lactogen (hPL)
   effects on fuel metabolism, 86–87
   inhibition of human chorionic gonadotropin, 74
   related structure and function to pituitary hormones, 71
Human studies, on uterine blood flow during exercise, 121–122
Hydrogen ion concentration, arterial fetal, 36*t*
Hydrops fetalis syndrome, 172
5-Hydroxyindoleacetic acid, urinary, 30
20-α-Hydroxyprogesterone, 71
20-β-Hydroxyprogesterone, 71
17-Hydroxyprogesterone
   cortisone antagonism, 86
   mean plasma levels during pregnancy, 73*f*
17-α-Hydroxyprogesterone, mean plasma values, *70*
Hypercapnia, selective in fetus, 185
Hypertension
   edema and, 215
   maternal obesity and, 100
   pregnancy-induced, 136
   transient during weightlifting, 211
Hyperthermia
   exercise-induced
     effects on uterus and fetus, 32
   maternal, 203
Hypertrophy, 115, 116
Hyperventilation
   exercise-induced, 172, 206
   maternal-fetal respiratory relationships, 152, *153*
   respiratory consequences, 24–25
Hypoglycemia, exercise-related, 141
Hypothalamic control, progesterone and, 73–74
Hypothalamus, 186
Hypoxia
   fetal, 186
     cardiac output and, 35

selective in fetus, 185
metabolic consequences, 190–191
and reduction of fetal breathing movements, 198
maternal, 188

Inspiratory capacity, in pregnancy, 147
Insulin
   adjustments in diabetes, 93–95
   closed loop delivery system
     glucose levels with, *94*
   concentrations during exercise, 139
   counteraction of epinephrine, 85*t*
   effects of progesterone on, 87
   fetal, 39
   glucose utilization and, 92
   insensitivity, 90–91
   levels during pregnancy, 139
   levels prior to and after exercise, *140*
   prolactin effects on, 88
   pumps, 93–94
Insurance programs, pregnancy disability, 5
Intrauterine growth retardation, 203
Intrauterine transfusion, 171–172
Iron
   density of common foods, 102*t*–103*t*
   requirements
     in active nonpregnant women, 106–107
     for active pregnant woman, 109
     of pregnant sedentary women, 103
   supplementation, effects on active women, 107

Jogging (*see* Running)
Joint(s)
   flexibility, prenatal exercise for, 3
   increased mobility, 60

Kegel exercise, 205
Ketone(s)
   fasting blood levels, 88, 90*f*
   in gestational diabetes, 93
Ketosis, gestational, 91
Kidney(s)
   adjustments to pregnancy, 69
   blood flow to, 127
   regulation of phosphorus, 76
Knee pain, *218–219*

Labor, duration of, 136
Lactate
   blood concentrations, exercise and, 22–23
   compensatory blood flow redistribution and, 189
   diffusion across placenta, 38
   fetal concentrations, 32–33
   levels related to physical fitness, 134
   produced by anaerobic metabolism, 190
   ratio to pyruvate, 23
Lactic acid, production, 8
Left ventricular work, calculation during exercise, 130
Ligaments, relaxation of, 60
Limitations on physical activity, 123

Lipid metabolism, altered fetal, 39
Lipolytic center, progesterone and, 74
Locomotive system, physiological adjustments, 59–61
Long-term variability (LTV), of fetal heart rate, 184
Lordosis, 59, 60
Lung
   disease in pregnancy, 148
   responses to exercise during pregnancy, 148–152
   total capacity, 147
   volumes during pregnancy, 64–65
Lupus erythematosus, systemic, 220–221
Luteinizing hormone (LH)
   changes during pregnancy, 74
   in relation to symptom-limited incremental exercise, 53, *54*

Magnesium
   calcium metabolism and, 76
   levels during pregnancy, *75*
   requirements in pregnancy, 104
Manual for the Conduct of Classes for Expectant Parents, 3
Marie-Strumpell arthritis, 223
Maternal responses
   in animals
      blood gases, 24–25
      body temperature, 23–24
      cardiac output distribution, 26–30
      circulation, 25–26
      metabolism and, 22–23
      to physical working capacity, 22
      respiration, 24–25
      uterine oxygen consumption, 30–31
   oxygen consumption, 21–22
   to pregnancy and/or exercise, 31*t*
Maternal-fetal vascular interaction, 170
Mean arterial pressure (MAP), changes during pregnancy, 67, *68*
Mechanical efficiency, 12–14*t*
Median nerve compromise, 215–216
Medical screening, 225–226
Medroxyprogesterone acetate (Provera), 56
Medulla oblongata, 186
Melatonin, 53
Menarche delay, and vigorous physical activity, 51
Menstrual cycle (*see also* specific abnormalities)
   dysfunction and abnormalities
      exercise and, 7–8, 52
      management of, 56
   relationship to weight/height ratio, 51
MET activity, 11–12*t*
Metabolic acidosis, in fetal asphyxia, 188
Metabolic adaptation to pregnancy, 88–91
Mineralocorticoids, water metabolism and, 77–78
Moderation
   concept of, 1–2
   in physical activity, 3–4
Modern Motherhood, 2
Morning sickness, 71
Motor fitness, elements of, 59

Muscle relaxation, progesterone and, 73
Muscular strength activities, during pregnancy, 210–212
Musculoskeletal system, adjustments to pregnancy, 59–*61*
Myoendometrium, nutrient consumption, 36

Naloxone, 192
National Institute of Neurological and Communicative Disorders and Stroke, collaborative perinatal project, 91
Nerve compression syndrome(s)
   carpal tunnel, 215–*216*
   physiologic edema and, 215
   posterior tibial, 217–*218*
   ulnar, 216–*217*
Neurologic system, adjustments in pregnancy, 61
Neurotransmitter-hypothalamic function, effect of exercise on, 51–53
Nitrogen balance, 84
Nonaerobic activities, 212–213
Non-weight bearing exercise (*see also* Bicycling; Swimming)
   oxygen consumption and, 206
Norepinephrine
   changes related to exercise intensity, 141, *143*
   concentrations during exercise, 139, *142*
   effect
      on fetal heart rate, 185
      on fetal oxygen consumption, 31
      on uterine blood flow, 121
   increase with mild work loads, 141
   levels in pregnancy, 76
   production in response to stress, 186
   responses to exercise, *140*
   stimulation of uterus, 142
Nutrient(s) (*see also* specific nutrients)
   recommendations for active pregnant woman, 109–110
   requirements
      of active nonpregnant woman, 105–108*t*
      of pregnant sedentery women, 100–104
Nutritional advice, for pregnant women, 105
Nutritional needs, of physically active pregnant woman, 99–111
Nutritional risks during pregnancy, 104–105*t*

Obesity, maternal
   birth weight and, 100
   postpartum, 101
Obstetrical screening, 225–226
Oligomenorrhea, 56
Opioids, endogenous and modulation of hypoxic response, 192
Orthopaedic nerve compression syndrome(s) (*see* Nerve compression syndrome(s))
Osteitis condensans ilii, 221, *223*
Osteitis pubis, 221, *222*
Osteoporosis, 56
Outcome of pregnancy, related to physical fitness, 131, 134

Oxygen
  arterial content
    fetal, 36t
  arterial PO$_2$, 147
  arteriovenous differences, 154
  capacity
    of maternal blood, 157
    of fetal blood, 158
  carrying capacity, 147
  content as function of oxygen tension for maternal and fetal blood, 159
  cost of exercise, 14
    in pregnancy, 128–129
    of weight-bearing exercise, 12
  debt, 128
  deficit/debt, 15–16
  diffusion resistance, 164–165
  dissociation curves
    interrelations of maternal and fetal, 158–159f
    placental exchange, 37, 159–160
    major factors affecting, 155, 156t
  pulse, 16–17
  supply during pregnancy, 64–65
  ventilatory equivalent (VE/VO$_2$), 17
Oxygen affinity
  fetal, 157–158
  maternal, 155–157
    vs fetal, 158
Oxygen consumption (VO$_2$)
  during mild, moderate and VO$_2$ max exercise, 150f
  during pregnancy, 65, 66f, 147
  extra components during pregnancy, 61, 62t
  fetal, 36t, 92
    and umbilical blood flow, 168
  longitudinal studies, 206
  maternal
    effect of maternal exercise on, 39
    exercise and, 30
    responses, 31t
    responses in animal studies, 21–22
  measurement
    energy expenditure and, 10–11
    in animals, 40
  maximal, 8, 9–10
    defined, 9
    factors influencing, 13
    symptom limited testing, 10t
  organ, 189–190
    relationship to organ blood flow in asphyxia, 190
  placental, 161
  steady-level response, 15
  total peripheral resistance and, 25
  uterine, 30–31
Oxygen exchange
  mathematical model, 172, 173t
  mathematical model for prediction, 174
  reduction during exercise, 174
Oxygen partial pressure (PO$_2$)
  hemoglobin oxygen affinity and, 155
  umbilical, 166
  maternal
    effect on umbilical venous O$_2$ tension and exchange rate, 164
Oxygen saturation
  maternal vs fetal, 158–159
  curve
    fetal, 156
    maternal, 156
Oxygen tension
  decreased, 195
  gradient between umbilical and uterine venous blood placental oxygen consumption and, 161
  fetal, 34, 36t
  maternal
    decrease, as cause of fetal aphyxia, 188
    effect on oxygen placental transfer, 165–166
  maternal and fetal, 159–160f
Oxygen transfer, varying individual factors and, 165–172
Oxygen uptake
  importance of uterine blood flow, 166–167
  weight-dependent exercise and, 134
Oxygen-pulse ventilatory equivalents, 8
Oxyhemoglobin
  dissociation curve, 156
  maternal and fetal interrelationships, 158–159
  physiologic changes during pregnancy and, 155, 157
  saturation curve, 34

Pancreas, "artificial", 94–95
Paraesthesias, in hands, 61
Parasympathetic nervous system
  activity during fetal asphyxia, 191
  regulation of fetal circulation, 184–185
Parathyroid gland, calcium metabolism and, 74–76
Parathyroid hormone (PTH), 74, 75
Pelvic floor exercises, 205
Perfusion-perfusion inequalities, 162
Peripheral vascular resistance, estrogens and, 120
pH, arterial maternal
  during exercise, 172
  during pregnancy, 147
Phalen's test, 216
Phenoxybenzamine, 191
Phentolamine, 191
Phosphorus, 75
Physical fitness, maternal
  Apgar scores and, 136
  duration of labor and, 136
Physical training (see Training effect of exercise)
Physical work capacity (PWC)
  longitudinal studies, 206
  maternal response in animals, 22
Pituitary gland
  adjustments during pregnancy, 74
  function, effect of exercise on, 53, 54, 55
Pituitary-adreno-gonadal system, exercise and, 55–56
Placenta
  diffusing capacity
    carbon monoxide, 42–43, 162–163t
    effect on oxygen transfer, 165

238 Index

Placenta (*continued*)
   glucose, 32
      measurement technique in animals, 42–43
      oxygen, 163–164f
   exchange of carbon dioxide, 159
   heat transfer, 33–34
   hydrostatic pressure gradients, 187
   osmotic pressure gradients, 187
   oxygen consumption, 161
   oxygen flux, prediction of, 174
   oxygen transfer
      dependence on uteroplacental oxygen flow, 168
      geometry of vessels and, 160–161
      mathematical prediction model, 172, 174–175
   physiologic responses to maternal exercise, 36–38
   reserve capacity testing, 226
   shunts, 161–162
   site of diffusion resistance, 164–165
   transplacental diffusion
      maternal and fetal oxygen tensions, 159–160
   transport mechanisms, 37
   transport of amino acids, 33
   weight during pregnancy, 72
Placental lactogen (hPL) (*see* Human placental lactogen (hPL))
Placental protein 5 (PP5), 71
Plasma volume
   fetal, 36t
   maternal, 31t
      change during pregnancy, 66–67
      measurement technique in animals, 42
      changes in animals, 26, *27*
Postpartum exercise, instructions, 227–228
Postural exercises, for back pain, 219, *220*
Posture
   effects on cardiac output, 113–114
   effects on uterine blood flow, 120
Potassium
   deficiency, 108
   requirements, 108
Preeclampsia, excessive weight gain and, 101
Pregnancy associated plasma protein A (PAPP-A), 71
Pregnancy associated plasma protein B (PAPP-B), 71
Pregnancy Disability Amendment to Title VII, 5
Preload, 115
Preterm delivery, physical activity and, 207
Progestagens, placental, 71–74
Progesterone
   antagonism of cortisone, 86
   challenge testing, 56
   concentrations toward term, 23
   effects
      on uterine blood flow, 121
      on fuel metabolism, 87
      on uterus, 71–73
   increase during strenous exercise, 145
   inhibition of PTH, 75
   mean plasma levels during pregnancy, 73f
   mean plasma values, *70*
   production in placenta, 71
   replacement therapy for amenorrhea, 56
   respiratory alkalosis and, 147
   respiratory system changes and, 64
   role in fuel metabolism, 86
   secretion by corpus luteum, 69
Prolactin
   effects on fuel metabolism, 87
   evaluation in amenorrhea management, 56
   functions of, 74
   increase of gluconeogenesis, 88
   in relation to symptom-incremental exercise, 53, *55*
   levels, effect of running and amenorrhea, 53
   role in fuel metabolism, 86
   submaximal exercise in pregnancy and, *145*
Propranolol
   effect on fetal heart rate and variability, 185
   hypoxia-induced change and, 191
Prostaglandin(s), uterine blood flow and, 27, 121
Protein(s)
   catabolism to meet inadequate caloric intake, 61–62
   degradation, 83, 86
   major body, 83
   metabolism, exercise effects on, 23
   requirements
      of active nonpregnant woman, 106
      for active pregnant woman, 109
      of pregnant sedentary women, 101
   synthesis during pregnancy, 88
   total body, changes in pregnancy, 84
Proteinuria, edema and, 215
Psychoprophylaxis method of childbirth, 3
Pubarche, onset and vigorous physical activity, 51
Pulmonary diffusing capacity, 147
Pulmonary function testing
   in exercise laboratory, *149*
   pregnancy vs controls, 149t
   pregnancy vs postpartum, 148t
Pulmonary hemodynamics, 152, 154
Pulmonary responses, to exercise during pregnancy, 148–152
Pyruvate, 23, 189

Racket sports during pregnancy, 211
Radiosodium studies, of uterine blood flow, 121–122
Raynaud's syndrome, 122
Recommended Daily Dietery Allowance (RDA), for pregnancy, 63t, 75
Red cell volume
   changes in animals, 26, *27*
   during pregnancy, 67
Relaxin
   functions, 60, 69
   production of, 69
Renin
   aldosterone and, 77
   effect on uterine blood flow, 121
   production, 78
Renin-angiotensin system, 192
Residual volume (RV), 64
Respiration, fetal, 34–35

Respiratory acidosis, 188, 195
Respiratory alkalosis, 147, 152
Respiratory exchange ratio (R), 8, 17, 18t
   pregnant vs nonpregnant subjects during exercise, 139, 141
   during mild, moderate and VO$_2$ max exercise, 152, 153
Respiratory frequency
   during mild, moderate and VO$_2$ max exercise, 150
   maternal, 31t
   weight vs non-weight bearing exercises, 148
Respiratory gas transport, temperature changes and, 34
Respiratory minute volume, maternal responses, 31t
Respiratory system, adjustments to pregnancy, 64–65, 147
Rheumatoid arthritis, 219–220
Rib cage, adaption to pregnancy, 147
Riboflavin, requirements, 108
Running (jogging)
   during pregnancy, 208–209
   mechanical efficiency, 13
   number of women involved in, 5
   prescription guidelines, 18t
   relationship of distance/week and amenorrhea, 51

Saltatory pattern, 184
Schwangerschaftsprotein I (SP1), 71
Scuba diving during pregnancy, 211
Sex binding globulins, 70
Short-term variability, of fetal heart rate, 184
Shunts, placental, 161–162
Sinus node, vagal suppression of, 114
Sit-up exercises, 213
Skiing during pregnancy, 212
Skin, increased blood flow to, 68
Social class, birth weight and, 2
Sodium
   requirements
      in active nonpregnant women, 107–108
      for active pregnant women, 110
      for pregnant sedentary women, 104
   retention, 78
Speed, energy expenditure and, 12
Sports
   benefits of, 206
   during pregnancy, 211–212, 227
   related emergencies, 207, 208t
Sprains, sports related, 207, 208t, 207, 208t
Squat exercise, 205
Starvation
   during gestation and exercise, 88
   hormonal effects on fuel supply, 89
Steady-level exercise, 15
Step test, 14t
Steroid horomone(s) (see also specific hormones)
   effects on blood chemistry, 86t
   metobolism, effects of, 86t
Steroid(s)
   placental, 71–74
   production by corpus luteum, 69–70
Stress (see also Exercise, prenatal)
   adjustment to, 7
   diabetes and, 92
   hormones, 52
      interplay with anabolic insulin, 85–86
Stroke volume
   afterload and, 115–116
   cardiac output and, 67, 115
   contractility and, 116
   during maternal exercise, 118
   effects of pregnancy on, 130, 131
   estrogen effect on, 120
   heart size and, 116
   maternal, 31t
   preload and, 115
   related to trimester, 114
   variables affecting, 115
Submaximal exercise, 15
Surgery, in animal experimentation, 40, 41
Sweat
   electrolyte composition, 107t
   potassium losses in, 108
   production, exercise and, 23
   sodium loss by, 107–108
Swelling, during pregnancy, 215
Swimming
   during pregnancy, 210
   freestyle, efficiencies for, 13
Sympathetic nervous system
   activation during exercise, 142
   activity during fetal asphyxia, 191
   role in fetal circulation regulation, 185–188
Sympathoadrenal responses, to exercise, 140
Systole, left ventricular, 115

Tachycardia, fetal
   carbon dioxide content and, 185
   defined, 183
   fetal distress and, 35
   as protective mechanism, 195
   following maternal exercise, 122
   vagal suppression of sinus node and, 114
Tailor-sitting position(s), 3
Tea, iron absorption and, 103
Temperature
   body core and possible teratogenic effects, 203, 208
   correction for blood gas analysis, 24
   effects on fetal metabolism during exercise, 174–175
   fetal, 33–34, 38
      oxygen consumption and, 31–32
   maternal and fetal
      measurement techniques in animals, 42
Tennis during pregnancy, 211
Teratogenicity, of hyperthermia, 34, 203, 208
Testosterone
   anabolic changes in pregnancy, 70
   concentration in pregnancy, 76
   in relation to symptom-limited incremental exercise, 53, 54
Thelache delay, and vigorous physical activity, 51
Thermoregulatory control center, progesterone and, 74

Third trimester, physiological changes, 60–61
Thyroid gland, adjustments to pregnancy, 74
Thyroid-stimulating hormone (TSH), exercise and, 53, 55
Thyrotropin (TSH), 74
Thyroxin-binding globulin (TBG), 74
Tibial nerve compression, posterior, 217–218
Tidal volume
   during mild, moderate and VO$_2$ max exercise, 31t, 151, 152
   during pregnancy, 31t, 64
   increased, 206
Tinel's sign, 218
Total lung capacity (TLC), 64
Total peripheral resistance, exercise effects on, 25
Toxemia, sodium restriction and, 104
Training effect of exercise
   bicycling, 210
   effect on catecholamine response, 144
   for pregnant women, 207
   maternal physiologic variables, 31t
Treadmill testing
   in animals, 40
      uterine blood flow and, 28, 29
      uterine oxygen consumption and, 30
   β-endorphin release and, 52
   blood pressure response during, 25–26
   evaluation of exercise on pregnant women, 14t
   fetal blood glucose concentrations and, 32
   hyperventilation and, 206
   release of met-enkephalin and, 52
   with bicycle, 14t
   work efficiency during, 13
Treatise of Midwifery, 1
Triiodothyronine, effect on fetal oxygen consumption, 31

Ulnar nerve compression, 216–217
Umbilical cord
   arterial PO$_2$, 174
      placental oxygen transfer and, 166, 167
      venous oxygen tension and O$_2$ exchange rate and, 167
   blood flow, 36t
      catecholamine effect on, 195
      in control of fetal blood volume, 187–188
      insufficient, as cause of fetal aphyxia, 188
      importance on fetal oxygen delivery and placental oxygen transfer, 169
   venous oxygen tension, 160, 161
Unemployment compensation funds, 5
United States Childrens' Bureau, recommendations for moderation in physical activity, 3
Urinary system, adjustments to pregnancy, 69
Uterine blood flow
   cardiovascular changes and, 116–117
   catecholamines and, 121
   controlling mechanisms, 120
   estrogen effects on, 120–121
   exercise effects on, 28–29
      animal studies, 121
      human studies, 121–122
   factors affecting, 26–28
   insufficient, as cause of fetal aphyxia, 188
   magnitude, time course and effects of posture, 120
   measurement technique in animals, 40–42
   progesterone effects on, 121
   reduction, 195
      in fetal asphyxia, 190
   relationship to placental oxygen transfer, 167
   renin, angiotensin and prostaglandins and, 121
   response to pregnancy, exercise and training, 31t
   resting values, 120
Uteroplacental circulatory deficiencies, 208
Uterus (*see also* Uterine blood flow)
   alteration of size and progesterone, 71–73
   dimension increase during pregnancy, 59–60
   estrogen effects on, 73
   stimulation by norepinephrine, 142
   vascular resistance and exercise, 28–29

Vagus nerve, regulation of fetal circulation, 184–185
Valsalva maneuver, avoidance, 211
van't Hoff-Arrhenius law, 32, 174
Variability of fetal heart rate
   defined, 183–184
   long-term (LTV), 184
   short-term (STV), 184
   vagus nerve and, 185
   variability of oscillating frequency, 184
Vascular resistance, measurement in animals, 40–42
Vasopressin
   blood flow and, 186
   response to hypoxia, 186, 191–192
Vegetarian diets, 101, 103
Venous return, impaired during maternal exercise, 117–120
Ventilatory equivalent(s)
   during mild, moderate and VO$_2$ max exericse, 151
   elevation of, 206
   for oxygen (V$_E$/VO$_2$), 17
Ventricular function, ejection-phase indices, 116
Ventricular percent fractional shortening, 119f
Vital capacity, 147
Vitamin B6, 104
Vitamin C, requirements, 108
Vitamin D, requirements, 103
Vitamin E, requirements, 104, 108
Vitamin(s)
   requirements in pregnancy, 104, 108
   water-soluble, tubular reabsorbtion, 69
VO$_2$ max exercise
   pulmonary function testing and, 148–152

Walking, mechanical efficiency, 13
Water
   excretion, increase dietary protein and, 106
   loss, electrolytes associated with, 107t
   metabolism
      adrenal gland and, 76–77
      mineralocorticoids and, 77–78
   requirements

    of active nonpregnant women, 107
    for active pregnant women, 110
    retention, 61
Weight (*see* Birth weight; Body weight)
Weight lifting, during pregnancy, 210–211
Weight-bearing exercises (*see also* specific exercises)
    oxygen consumption and, 206
    pulmonary function results and, 148
Weight-dependent exercise (*see also* specific exercises)
    oxygen uptake and, 134
Work (*see also* Physical working capacity)
    efficiency during treadmill testing, 13
    relative vs. absolute, aerobic exercise and, 10, *11*
    vs exercise, psychological implications, 122–123

Work capacity, maternal maximal
    related to maternal and fetal pH and lactate, 134
Work load
    oxygen cost and, 13
    oxygen uptake vs., 9–10
Working mothers
    birthweight and, 2, 203
    number of, 5
Wrist extension splint, neutral, 216, *217*

Yoga, 212

Zinc, 104